MW01258982

Authoritative Communities

The Search Institute Series on Developmentally Attentive Community and Society

Series Editor
Peter L. Benson, Search Institute, Minneapolis, Minnesota

Series Mission
To advance interdisciplinary inquiry into the individual, system, community, and societal dynamics that promote developmental strengths; and the processes for mobilizing these dynamics on behalf of children and adolescents.

DEVELOPMENTAL ASSETS AND ASSET-BUILDING COMMUNITIES:
Implications for Research, Policy, and Practice
Edited by Richard M. Lerner and Peter L. Benson

OTHER PEOPLE'S KIDS:
Social Expectations and American Adults' Involvement with Children
Peter C. Scales with Peter L. Benson, Marc Mannes, Nicole R. Hintz, Eugene C. Roehlkepartain, and Theresa K. Sullivan

WHAT DO CHILDREN NEED TO FLOURISH?
Conceptualizing and Measuring Indicators of Positive Development
Edited by Kristin Anderson Moore and Laura H. Lippman

MOBILIZING ADULTS FOR POSITIVE YOUTH DEVELOPMENT:
Strategies for Closing the Gap between Beliefs and Behaviors
Edited by E. Gil Clary and Jean E. Rhodes

AUTHORITATIVE COMMUNITIES:
The Scientific Case for Nurturing the Whole Child
Edited by Kathleen Kovner Kline

A Continuation Order Plan is available for this series. A continuation order will bring delivery of each new volume immediately upon publication. Volumes are billed only upon actual shipment. For further information please contact the publisher.

Kathleen Kovner Kline
Editor

Authoritative Communities

The Scientific Case for Nurturing the Whole Child

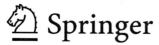 Springer

Kathleen Kovner Kline, M.D.
Dartmouth Medical School
Hanover, NH 03755
Kline.Kathleen@tchden.org

ISBN 978-0-387-72720-2   e-ISBN 978-0-387-72721-9

Library of Congress Control Number: 2007933182

Series Preface

As a society, we have lost our focus when it comes to nurturing our youngest generations. We either neglect the young altogether, attending only to more powerful voting blocs or larger demographic groups, or we wring hands over one crisis or another. Rarely do we invest enough time or resources to turn the tide on any of the challenges before us.

This book series seeks to offer an alternate, more hopeful focus. Instead of just investing in individual problems (often with little success), this series focuses on the nature of and strategies to build "developmentally attentive communities." Such communities attend to providing the foundation of experiences, boundaries, guidance, support, and opportunities that help young people begin life on a positive trajectory. Our thesis—supported by a growing body of evidence—is that young people who grow up in such communities are better equipped for life and more likely to avoid or overcome the challenges they face in contemporary life.

Authoritative Communities: The Scientific Case for Nurturing the Whole Child adds important and compelling evidence to this case while also crystallizing and expanding the vision in powerful ways. By gathering these essays by preeminent scholars into an accessible volume, Kathleen Kovner Kline offers an invaluable scientific foundation to support an inclusive and holistic vision of communities that love, support, and encourage young people while also setting firm boundaries and high expectations—the kind of "authoritative" approach that we know from parenting literature is key to young people's healthy development.

The volume makes several important and unique contributions to the literature on community youth development. First, it builds on a widely acclaimed report, *Hardwired to Connect*, which represented the wisdom of 33 national youth development leaders in seeking to frame a new agenda for youth in the United States. That report (the summary of which is included in this volume) stimulated a broad dialogue about society's responsibility to its young people among policy makers, practitioners, and researchers. This volume will, we believe, sustain this conversation into the future.

The second unique contribution is that it draws extensively on neurobiology and related fields, introducing insights from brain research and genetics into the dialogue about positive youth development, which has been primarily the domain of the social sciences. The thoughtful examinations of nature and nurture, adolescent brain development, and related issues add important new dimensions to our understanding of young people's developmental pathways through childhood and adolescence.

Perhaps most significant, however, is that this volume (and the report that stimulated it) emphasizes the scientific case for attending much more intentionally to the moral, religious, and spiritual development of young people. Though positive youth development has often paid lip service to the importance of spirituality in youth development, rarely has the field been as explicit and as expansive in examining this dimension of life as part of community building. My sense is that this theme will become more and more visible in research, policy, and practice, and I commend Kline and her colleagues for being at the forefront of this trend.

The challenges we face in moving toward a more developmentally attentive society are sometimes daunting. However, one can take courage in knowing that leaders in the field are building a compelling case and broad consensus about what's needed and what it will take to bring about positive change. The framework, research, and recommendations presented in this book have much to offer as we engage in this important and compelling agenda.

Peter L. Benson, Ph.D.
Search Institute
Series Editor

Preface

The scholarly papers and commentaries in this book provided the intellectual foundation for the report titled *Hardwired to Connect*, which was issued by the Commission on Children at Risk in Washington, D.C., on September 9, 2003. These papers were presented at a multidisciplinary conference at Dartmouth Medical School for the purpose of investigating the social, moral, and spiritual foundations of child well-being. The first chapter here consists of the summary report from that conference, "Hardwired to Connect: The New Scientific Case for Authoritative Communities." This report is the synthesis and multidisciplinary statement of the 33 members of the Commission on Children at Risk, in their effort to forge a new framework for addressing the needs of youth in the United States.

The organization of this book largely reflects the conference's explorations of our "hardwired connections" in light of cutting-edge work from the brain and behavioral sciences. We first examine neurobiology, as it shapes our earliest development and some of our most basic drives, learning from studies of animals as well as of humans. Following the developmental process itself, we then look at the emergence of conscience and morality, and the "prosocial self." Next, the role of religion and spirituality is explored from the vantage point of new material available to us from technologies of neuroimaging, as well as voluminous evidence from the social sciences. We also choose to pay particular attention to adolescence, as it is a time of onset of many emotional and behavioral problems for young people. As the child's world expands, we focus on the influence of increasing connections in the broader community, including the media. Finally, the commentaries provide insights from leaders on the front lines of children's mental health.

In Part II, "Primal Connections," Larry J. Young and Darlene D. Francis in Chapter 2 introduce us to the biochemistry of connection; that is, the neurotransmitters and receptors that are activated when we fall in love with our mates and our children. We learn that the bonds we feel, and the drives to protect and care for our families, are rooted in chemical interactions deep within the brain. In mammals, the experience of being intensely cared for brings with it many forms of physical and emotional resilience. By looking closely at several generations of rat mothers and pups, we also see that the propensity to care for one's offspring can be passed on both through inherited traits and by the experience of having been intensely nurtured. Whether the parental drive to nurture arises from temperament or social learning, offspring reap the benefits of increased emotional and physical health through several generations.

In Chapter 3, Stephen J. Suomi invites us to learn about the connection between nature and nurture by introducing us to a troop of rhesus monkeys. In a subgroup of these monkeys, we see the relationship between heritable traits that appear to be genetically linked and risk factors for emotional and behavioral disturbances. Suomi's studies demonstrate that these behavioral patterns are not determined by genes alone but rather by the interactions between genes and environment. By enriching the nurturing environment of vulnerable individuals, inherited tendencies toward apparent anxiety, depression, and alcohol abuse can be ameliorated.

Turning specifically to human infants, Robert Karen offers in Chapter 4 a compelling lesson in the history of our knowledge of the importance of mother–infant attachment. He begins in the 1940s with the observations of child psychoanalyst John Bowlby regarding the impact of early separations from the mother on a child's behavior and character. Karen documents the elaboration of this insight by many other researchers, particularly Mary Ainsworth. Whereas the importance of secure early childhood attachment has become a basic tenet of child psychology and the foundation of effective treatment interventions, Karen explores why it has been difficult to implement these insights in the policy arena.

In Part III, we look to the child's development of "higher" functions such as a sense of meaning and morality. In Chapter 5, Barbara M. Stilwell describes the conscience as "a dynamic entity within the self continuously prompting responses to moral issues." Stilwell describes her empirically derived domains for understanding the development of conscience. She goes on to explore the characteristic features of conscience through early, middle, and late adolescence, as well as the formative influences that shape its development.

As an expert in pediatric prevention research and health promotion, Michael D. Resnick discusses prosocial development in Chapter 6. He reviews the evolution of the current adolescent public health emphasis toward a dual strategy of enhancing protective factors and reducing risk factors. Drawing from studies of resilience in the face of adversity, as well as characteristics of high-functioning children, Resnick elaborates on a number of protective factors that appear to enhance prosocial development, including a strong sense of connectedness to family and other adults and institutions in the community, as well as opportunities to develop academic and social competence.

From the vantage point of modern psychology and psychiatry, Paul C. Vitz presents us in Chapter 7 with a history of our understanding of the moral and spiritual dimensions of the human person. Beginning with Freud, Vitz chronicles the theoretical frameworks promoted by leaders of various psychological movements such as psychoanalysis, attachment theory, object relations theory, and humanist, existential, transpersonal, cognitive behavioral, and positive psychologies.

Given that the human experience of religion and spirituality is mediated by the activity of the brain, we begin Part IV, "Connecting to the Transcendent," with perspectives from neuroimaging and developmental psychology. Andrew B. Newberg and Stephanie K. Newberg offer intriguing data regarding the impact of specific religious practices on brain function. With evidence from brain imaging and knowledge of brain function, Newberg and Newberg describe the relationship between certain spiritual experiences described by practitioners and specific changes in brain function. In addition, they attempt to link what is now known regarding physiologic brain development over the course of childhood with what others have delineated as stages of spiritual development in youth.

In Chapter 9, Byron R. Johnson uses the term *organic religion* to represent the effect of religious activities, practices, and beliefs over time. Johnson has reviewed more than 600 studies examining the relationship between religion and a variety of health outcomes for children, youth, and families. He presents the empirical facts regarding the prosocial and protective effects of religion, and notes that religion appears to have its positive effect on mental and physical health outcomes, based not only on the behaviors and attitudes that it prohibits but also on the behaviors and attitudes that it promotes.

Whereas previous chapters have examined the potent impact that intense parental nurture has upon the psychological well-being of children, W. Bradford Wilcox examines in Chapter 10 the effect of religious affiliation and practice upon parenting styles and behavior. Using data from two separate national surveys, Wilcox is able to describe in some detail the similarities and differences among parents of different religious groups. In addition, he examines the teaching of certain religious leaders regarding parenting and reflects upon the rationale for faith communities' concerns with parental guidance and support.

Julie E. Thomas and Lisa A. Wuyek continue our examination of the role of faith traditions in promoting child well-being by introducing us to a Buddhist perspective on parenting. Focusing on the concept of bodhichitta, similar to compassionate love, Thomas and Wuyeck explore a number of Buddhist concepts and practices useful in confronting the challenges and enhancing the joys of parenthood. They also review the literature regarding the use of Buddhist practices in the context of therapeutic intervention.

Because the teen years are a time when new interests, abilities, and desires bring with them increased risks for many emotional and behavioral problems, we take a special look in Part V at the changing biological, social, and spiritual connections of adolescence. Developmental psychobiologist Linda Patia Spear demonstrates that many of the aspects of teenage behavior that are most challenging to adults are rooted in developmental changes in the structure and capacity of the teenage brain. Not only have these adolescent proclivities been noted by concerned adults throughout history, but the same, quintessential adolescent drives toward risk taking, novelty seeking, and peer affiliation have been seen in other mammalian species as well. Understanding the biologically driven changes underpinning adolescent behavior is crucial lest we mistake immaturity for pathology or fail to provide the structure and opportunities that allow teens to grow safely into adults.

From the purview of psychological anthropology, David Gutmann looks cross-culturally in Chapter 13 at the role of fathers, grandfathers, and other

senior men in the socializing of young males. He introduces us to the features
of certain traditional rites of passage that have been used to mark a young
man's transition into manhood. Administered by male elders, these rites
often emphasize virtues such as strength, bravery, and perseverance while
connecting the young man to the spiritual traditions of his community.

Psychologist Lisa Miller reviews several aspects of the development of
spirituality and religiousness among adolescent girls and boys. She identifies
personal devotion as the most highly protective dimension of religiousness.
That protective effect of personal spirituality appears most strongly associated
with emotional resilience for teenage girls. Miller suggests that traditions that
acknowledge the confluence of physical maturation and spiritual maturity may
do much to support the emotional well-being of adolescent girls.

Leading Part VI, "Connecting to Community," psychiatrist James P.
Comer uses his childhood experience of growing up in the African American
community to analyze the factors that promote success for children. Noting that
many of the critical factors have deteriorated in our poorest neighborhoods,
Comer recounts the way in which the School Development Program, begun in
New Haven, Connecticut, and replicated elsewhere, has organized schools to
strengthen connections between families, teachers, and cultural institutions. He
also describes a special social skills training program, which provides inner-
city children with experiences in mainstream community institutions that are
requisite to achievement.

Competing with the human connections in a child's life are the ever more
ubiquitous involvements with various electronic media through the Internet,
television, movies, and video games. Leonard A. Jason and Kerri L. Kim
relate recent findings regarding both the positive and negative aspects of
children's media use. They pay particular attention to the effects of children's
exposure to violent and sexual content, as well as effects on academic and
social functioning. Jason and Kim conclude with strategies to help parents
structure and supervise their children's media use.

Bill Stanczykiewicz weaves together the intellectual theory behind the civil
society movement with the sociological data that support the role of vibrant
community life and positive youth outcomes. Drawing from many years of
experience in youth policy, Stanczykiewicz richly portrays the power of local
community leaders to transform their neighborhoods for the well-being of
their young people.

In our final section, we have invited leaders in the thick of promoting
healthy child development to give us their viewpoints. With the astute eye of
a seasoned child psychiatrist, Elizabeth Berger walks us through the developmental progression of child character development. She gives us an insider's
view of the growing child's perspective, demonstrating the cumulative effect
of everyday firm and loving interactions at home and, as the child matures, at
school. Locating the critical generation of good citizenship in healthy families
and well-functioning schools, Dr. Berger makes a passionate plea for us to
mobilize the will and resources to assist families in need and renew our educational system.

   As leaders in the motherhood movement, Enola Aird and the Mothers' Council laud the work of the Commission on Children at Risk but also challenge it. They praise its validation of the importance of nurturing, especially mothering, as foundational to the well-being of children and the vitality of communities. They claim "bonding" as a feminist issue and a human rights issue. They argue, however, that the commission does not go far enough to specifically examine the primacy of parents and the real supports that mothers and fathers need to do their essential work well. They also critique its timidity in confronting social and institutional values that undermine healthy childhood ecology.

   Since the release of the *Hardwired to Connect* report, members of the Commission on Children at Risk have been invited to speak across the nation in a variety of venues. They have addressed academics and leaders in the health care professions, public policy, education, psychology, theology, social work, youth services, and many parent and community coalitions. The listeners have been intrigued by our organizing motif ("Hardwired to Connect") as an analogy about the human person with great explanatory power on multiple levels. They have also embraced the framework of authoritative communities as a most useful way to organize and enhance their personal and institutional engagements with young people. We commend this volume to you in the same spirit and hope that it will serve as a valuable tool for all those committed to the biological, social, moral, and spiritual health of the next generation.

2007

Kathleen Kovner Kline, M.D.

Dartmouth University

Hanover, New Hampshire

USA

Foreword: The Crisis in American Childhood

Authoritative Communities: The Scientific Case for Nurturing the Whole Child is a response to the crisis in the ecology of childhood. It addresses fundamental issues underlying the rising rates of mental problems and emotional distress among U.S. children and adolescents. With contributions from children's doctors, research scientists, and mental health and youth service professionals, this book does several things: It identifies the crisis; it presents what these experts believe to be a main cause of the crisis; it looks to the fundamental social, moral, and spiritual foundations of child well-being for solutions to the crisis; and, most important, it introduces a new concept, *authoritative communities*, intended to help youth service professionals, policy makers, and the entire society do a better job of addressing the crisis.

The crisis in contemporary childhood comes in two parts.

The first part is the deteriorating mental and behavioral health of U.S. children. We are witnessing high and rising rates of depression, anxiety, attention deficit, conduct disorders, thoughts of suicide, and other serious mental, emotional, and behavioral problems among children and adolescents.

The second part is how we as a society are thinking about this deterioration. We are using medications and psychotherapies. We are designing more and more special programs for "at risk" children. These approaches are necessary. But they are not enough. Why? Because programs of individual risk assessment and treatment seldom encourage us as a society to recognize, and can even prevent us from recognizing, the broad *environmental* conditions that are contributing to growing numbers of suffering children.

In large measure, what is causing this crisis of American childhood is a lack of connectedness, by which we mean two kinds of connectedness: close connections to other people and deep connections to moral and spiritual meaning.

Where does this connectedness come from? It comes from groups of people organized around certain purposes—what scholars call social institutions. In recent decades, the U.S. social institutions that foster these two forms of connectedness for children have gotten significantly weaker. That weakening, these authors argue, is a major cause of the current mental and behavioral health crisis among U.S. children.

Much of this book is a presentation of scientific evidence—largely from the field of neuroscience, which concerns our basic biology and how our brains develop—showing that the human child is "hardwired to connect." We are hardwired for other people and for moral meaning and openness to the transcendent. Meeting these basic needs for connection is essential to health and to human flourishing.

Because in recent decades we as a society have not been doing a good job of meeting these essential needs, large and growing numbers of our children are failing to flourish. The chapters in this volume will deepen your understanding of children's essential needs.

Authoritative communities will solve the crisis in American childhood. Such communities are groups that live out the types of connectedness that our children increasingly lack. They are groups of people who are committed to one another over time and who model and pass on at least part of what it means to be a good person and live a good life. Renewing and building them is the key to improving the lives of U.S. children and adolescents.

Authoritative community is a new public policy and social science term, developed for the first time in the *Hardwired to Connect* report, which serves as the first chapter in this book. In the report is a definition of authoritative communities, an analysis of their role in society, and proposals for strengthening them. This concept is intended to help all those in our society working to understand and improve the lives of children.

Among scholarly projects on children at risk, this book is distinctive in several ways. For what may be the first time, this project on children's mental and emotional health brings together prominent neuroscientists and children's doctors with social scientists who study civil society. As a result, this book represents an early serious effort to integrate the "hard science" of infant attachment and child and adolescent brain development with sociological evidence of how civil society shapes outcomes for children. Call it a new—watch out, big word coming—bio-psycho-social-cultural model of child development. This new model is intended both to deepen our understanding of today's crisis of childhood and to provide practical help to youth professionals, policy makers, and others working to improve the lives of our children.

For what may be the first time, a diverse group of scientists and other experts on children's heath is publicly recommending that our society pay considerably more attention to young people's moral, spiritual, and religious needs.

It is not unheard of, but it is not common either, for doctors and other professionals involved in the delivery of social and medical services to recommend a fundamental social change model, as opposed to an improved service delivery model, as a key to improving the mental and emotional lives of children.

In their common concern for the crisis in childhood, the contributors to this book have come together from across the philosophical and political spectrum.

This book introduces the concept and argues for the importance of *authoritative communities*. This concept is the project's major innovation and, potentially, its most important contribution. What's new is not just the term itself but, more important, what it seeks to designate. For what may be the first time, a concept has been developed to help policy makers, youth service professionals, scholars, journalists, philanthropists, and others to identify the specific traits across social institutions that are most likely to produce good outcomes for children. A healthy society for children will consist of a great variety of overlapping authoritative communities. But right now, there are just not enough of them.

How can we join together to renew and build authoritative communities? Achieving this goal asks something of all of us: youth service organizations and youth service professionals; all levels of government; employers; philanthropists and foundations; religious and civic leaders; scholars; educators; and families and individuals.

A common commitment to authoritative communities as the means to solve the crisis in American childhood would constitute fundamental social change in our society. Nothing less will do.

David Blankenhorn
President
Institute for American Values

Acknowledgments

The Commission on Children at Risk is an independent, jointly sponsored initiative of the YMCA of the USA, Dartmouth Medical School, and the Institute for American Values. The commission is composed of 33 children's doctors, research scientists, and mental health and youth service professionals. Its mission has been to investigate the social, moral, and spiritual foundations of child well-being, evaluate the degree to which current practices and policies in the United States recognize those foundations, and make recommendations for the future. The concept of *authoritative communities* was introduced in the commission's report to the nation, *Hardwired to Connect*, which was the product of interdisciplinary deliberation, a comprehensive literature review, and the evaluation of commissioned papers.

I have served as the commission's principal investigator and would like to express my appreciation to the commission members for their scholarly contributions, their sharp and probing observations, dynamic exchanges, and their commitment to young people in both their personal and their professional lives.

The commission, and what has become the Hardwired to Connect Project, owe a debt of gratitude to many individuals and institutions. The project would not have been possible without the generous support of its sponsors, the YMCA of the USA, Dartmouth Medical School, and the Institute for American Values. I am particularly grateful for the leadership and foresight of David Blankenhorn of the Institute for American Values and Ken Gladish of the YMCA. I am deeply thankful to Chuck Stetson for helping to conceive this project and for his generous financial support. I am also grateful to the Bodman Foundation for its financial support of the planning phase of the project and to the John Templeton Foundation for its financial support, particularly in the dissemination phase. The research, editorial, administrative, and other contributions of Josephine Abbatiello, David Blankenhorn, Robert Boisture, Eden Fisher Durbin, Maggie Gallagher, Ken Gladish, Norval Glenn, Ann Hartshorn, Audrey Hayes, Mia Hockett, Brian Hershisnik, Andrew Kline, Art Maelender, Kate Marlborough, Charity Navarette, Bonnie Robbins, Alex Roberts, Mary Schwarz, Tammy Smith, Erin Streeter, Richard Wilkins, and the administrators of Dartmouth Medical School have been invaluable and are deeply appreciated.

I have been privileged to work with Gene Roehlkepartain, Kay Hong, and Mary Byers of Search Institute, who have performed yeomen's work in shaping this edited volume and graciously included it in the Search Institute Series on

Developmentally Attentive Community and Society. Finally, I am grateful to Springer for making this scientific research and practical reflection available to all those engaged in building and renewing "authoritative communities" for our children.

Contents

Part I   A Report to the Nation   1

1. Hardwired to Connect: The New Scientific Case
    for Authoritative Communities   3
    The Commission on Children at Risk

Part II   Primal Connections   69

2. The Biochemistry of Family Commitment and Youth
    Competence: Lessons from Animal Models   71
    Larry J. Young and Darlene D. Francis

3. How Mother Nurture Helps Mother Nature: Scientific Evidence
    for the Protective Effect of Good Nurturing on Genetic
    Propensity Toward Anxiety and Alcohol Abuse   87
    Stephen J. Suomi

4. Investing in Children and Society: What We Have Learned
    from Seven Decades of Attachment Research   103
    Robert Karen

Part III   Meaning and Morality   121

5. The Consolidation of Conscience in Adolescence   123
    Barbara M. Stilwell

6. Best Bets for Improving the Odds for Optimum Youth
    Development   137
    Michael D. Resnick

7. Moral and Spiritual Dimensions of the Healthy Person: Notes
    from the Founders of Modern Psychology and Psychiatry   151
    Paul C. Vitz

Part IV   Connecting to the Transcendent   163

8. Hardwired for God: A Neuropsychological Model
    for Developmental Spirituality   165
    Andrew B. Newberg and Stephanie K. Newberg

9. A Tale of Two Religious Effects: Evidence for the Protective
    and Prosocial Impact of Organic Religion   187
    Byron R. Johnson

10. Focused on Their Families: Religion, Parenting,
    and Child Well-Being   227
    W. Bradford Wilcox

11. Minding the Children with Mindfulness: A Buddhist
    Approach to Promoting Well-Being in Children   245
    Julie E. Thomas and Lisa A. Wuyek

Part V   The Changing Connections of Adolescence   261

12. The Psychobiology of Adolescence   263
    Linda Patia Spear

13. Elders and Sons   281
    David Gutmann

14. Spirituality and Resilience in Adolescent Girls   295
    Lisa Miller

Part VI   Connecting to Community   303

15. Promoting Well-Being Among At-Risk Children: Restoring
    a Sense of Community and Support for Development   305
    James P. Comer

16. Sex, Guns, and Rock 'n' Roll: The Influence of Media
    in Children's Lives   323
    Leonard A. Jason and Kerri L. Kim

17. The Civil Society Model: The Organic Approach to Building
    Character, Competence, and Conscience in Our Young People   339
    Bill Stanczykiewicz

Part VII   Commentaries   353

18. Caring and Character: How Close Parental Bonds
    Foster Character Development in Children   355
    Elizabeth Berger

19. Gather Around the Children   369
    Enola Aird

Index   375

Contributors

Elizabeth Berger is a board-certified child and adolescent psychiatrist with 30 years' experience treating children and families. She has been on the faculty of the Columbia University College of Physicians and Surgeons and of the Northwestern University Medical School and is a spokesperson for the American Academy of Child and Adolescent Psychiatry. Dr. Berger has appeared in numerous panels and public forums as well as on radio and television addressing social policy issues and parents' concerns about their children. She is the author of the parenting book *Raising Kids with Character: Developing Trust and Personal Integrity in Children.*

James P. Comer is the Maurice Falk Professor of Child Psychiatry at the Yale University School of Medicine's Child Study Center. He has concentrated his career on promoting a focus on child development as a way of improving schools. His efforts in support of healthy development of young people are known internationally. Among numerous other publications, Dr. Comer is the author, coauthor, or coeditor of *Waiting for a Miracle: Why Schools Can't Solve Our Problems, and How We Can* and *Leave No Child Behind: Preparing Today's Youth for Tomorrow's World.* Dr. Comer is perhaps best known for the founding of the Comer School Development Program in 1968, which promotes the collaboration of parents, educators, and community to improve social, emotional, and academic outcomes for children that, in turn, helps them achieve greater school success. His concept of teamwork has improved the educational environment in more than 500 schools throughout America.

Darlene D. Francis is an assistant professor of psychology and public health in the School of Public Health at the University of California, Berkeley.

David Gutmann is a professor of psychiatry and education at Northwestern University. He is the author of *Reclaimed Powers: Men and Women in Later Life.*

Leonard A. Jason is a professor of psychology at DePaul University and the director of the Center for Community Research. He is a former president of the Division of Community Psychology of the American Psychological Association, from which division he received the 1997 Distinguished Contributions to Theory and Research Award.

Byron R. Johnson is professor of sociology and director of the Center for Religious Inquiry Across the Disciplines (CRIAD) at Baylor University. He is also a fellow at the Witherspoon Institute in Princeton, New Jersey. He formerly directed the Center for Research on Religion and Urban Civil Society at the University of Pennsylvania and most recently was a lecturer in the Politics Department at Princeton University. Professor Johnson's research focuses on quantifying the effectiveness of faith-based organizations to confront various social problems. His recent publications have examined the efficacy of the "faith factor" in reducing crime and delinquency among at-risk youth in urban communities, and he has conducted several studies examining the impact of faith-based programs on recidivism reduction and prisoner reentry.

Robert Karen is a clinical psychologist in private practice and an award-winning author. His four books include *The Forgiving Self: The Road from Resentment to Connection* and *Becoming Attached: First Relationships and How They Shape Our Capacity to Love.* He has written for the *Atlantic Monthly, New York, O (The Oprah Magazine),* the *Nation,* the *Yale Review,* the *Psychoanalytic Review,* and *Contemporary Psychoanalysis,* among other publications.

Kerri L. Kim is a contributor to *Creating Communities for Addiction: The Oxford House Model.*

Kathleen Kovner Kline, M.D., is an assistant professor of psychiatry at the University of Colorado Health Sciences Center and an adjunct faculty member at Dartmouth Medical School. She serves on the Medical Staff of Children's Hospital in Denver. At the University of Colorado and at Dartmouth, she has taught child and adolescent development and psychopathology to medical students, pediatricians, family practitioners, psychiatrists, child and adolescent psychiatry fellows, and trainees in psychology and social work. Her clinical practice has included treating child and adult patients in acute hospital and outpatient settings, directing diagnostic and psychopharmacology clinics, and consultation to treatment centers for delinquent and severely emotionally impaired youth. She has a history of involvement with grass-roots, community service, and religious institutions and a particular interest in the role of character-shaping institutions in the prevention of psychosocial maladjustment.

Lisa Miller is an associate professor in the Clinical Psychology Program, Teachers College, Columbia University, and president-elect of the Division of Religion and Psychology, American Psychological Association.

Andrew B. Newberg, M.D., is assistant professor in radiology and psychiatry at the University of Pennsylvania Health System. He is the coauthor of *Why God Won't Go Away: Brain Science and the Biology of Belief* and *The Mystical Mind: Probing the Biology of Religious Experience.*

Stephanie K. Newberg is assistant director, Center City and Wynnewood Offices, Council for Relationships, Philadelphia.

Michael D. Resnick is professor of pediatrics and public health and director of research in the Division of General Pediatrics and Adolescent Health at the University of Minnesota. He has been principal or co-investigator on numerous federal and foundation research projects focusing on health and risk behaviors, resiliency and protective factors in the lives of young people, with a particular emphasis on issues related to adolescent sexual behaviors and violence. Dr. Resnick is currently director of the Healthy Youth Development Prevention Research Center, funded by the CDC, conducting research and evaluation studies on best practices in pregnancy prevention and promotion of healthy youth development, as well as providing leadership training to postgraduate health professionals specializing in community-based prevention research.

Linda Patia Spear is Distinguished Professor of Psychology at the State University of New York at Binghamton. Her area of research is behavioral neuroscience, with a focus on how prenatal drugs such as cocaine and ethanol, along with environmental factors, can influence subsequent behavior. Her work has provided a critical data resource for policy decisions by the Food and Drug Administration and the Environmental Protection Agency. Her other interests include developmental psychobiology, psychopharmacology, and neurobehavioral teratology.

Bill Stanczykiewicz is president and CEO of the Indiana Youth Institute in Indianapolis. He is a frequent speaker on the value of nonprofit youth development services and a community approach to addressing the problems of children, and he has been featured at such national events as the National League of Cities conference, Search Institute's national Healthy Communities Healthy Youth conference, Harvard University's seminar on community renewal and civic engagement, and on ABC's *Good Morning America*. He also works closely with Indiana's state and national legislators, providing them with data and information that aid in the formulation of public policy on children's issues.

Barbara M. Stilwell is professor emeritus of child and adolescent psychiatry at Indiana University School of Medicine in Indianapolis. Her research interests have been in the development and functioning of the conscience in normal and psychiatrically impaired development. She is coauthor, with Matthew R. Galvin, M.D., and S. Mark Kopta, M.D., of the book *Right vs. Wrong: Raising a Child with a Conscience*, published by Indiana University Press in 2000.

Stephen J. Suomi is chief of the Laboratory of Comparative Ethology at the National Institute of Child Health and Human Development (NICHD), National Institutes of Health (NIH), in Bethesda, Maryland. Dr. Suomi has received international recognition for his extensive research on biobehavioral development in rhesus monkeys, beginning with research in which he successfully reversed the adverse effects of early social isolation previously thought to be permanent. His latest research focuses on (1) the interaction between genetic and environmental factors in shaping individual developmental trajectories; (2) continuity versus change and the relative stability of individual differences throughout development; and (3) the degree to which findings from monkeys studied in captivity generalize to monkeys living in the wild and to humans living in different cultures.

Julie E. Thomas is an associate professor in the Department of Psychology at Youngstown State University in Ohio. She has consulted as a Faculty in Residence as part of the Tri County Partnership for Excellence in Teaching (Title II grant) since fall 2001, serving as a clinical psychologist consultant to pertinent schools in the area and to the undergraduate students in the Preservice Teacher Education Program at YSU. To address the emotional needs of middle school children and those of the teachers and parent/family members, she helped create the Emotional Resource Network (ERN) at Western Reserve Middle School. ERN consists of staff members within the school system and representatives from the community agencies.

Paul C. Vitz is professor of psychology, emeritus, New York University. Besides his interest in how things religious relate to psychology, he is also involved in the general topic of psychology and art. His work focuses on the relationship between psychology and Christianity. He has published more than 100 articles and essays. His books include *Psychology as Religion: The Cult of Self-Worship* and *Defending the Family: A Sourcebook.*

W. Bradford Wilcox is assistant professor of sociology at the University of Virginia. He is the author of *Soft Patriarchs, New Men: How Christianity Shapes Fathers and Husbands,* as well as numerous scholarly articles and book chapters. He is an expert on religion and family life and is regularly featured in media outlets such as the *New York Times,* the *Washington Post,* and *USA Today.*

Lisa A. Wuyek's clinical and research interests are focused on the anxiety disorders and exposure therapy. Her current research is investigating the importance of attention and context in exposure, psychometric properties of anxiety measures, and the implementation of treatment manuals.

Larry J. Young is an associate professor of psychiatry and behavioral sciences at Emory University. His work explores the molecular-, cellular-, and system-level mechanisms that are involved in innate behaviors. Currently studying oxytocin and vasopressin receptor sites in the brains of two vole species, Young is attempting to identify their involvement (if possible) for monogamous/promiscuous behavioral patterns in each vole species. His research focuses on the social attachment and general social behavior and how specific genes may regulate the expression of these behaviors.

I
A Report to the Nation

1 Hardwired to Connect: The New Scientific Case for Authoritative Communities

The Commission on Children at Risk

The Two-Part Crisis

In the midst of unprecedented material affluence, large and growing numbers of U.S. children and adolescents are failing to flourish. In particular, more and more young people are suffering from mental illness, emotional distress, and behavioral problems. Let's call this first aspect of the crisis *epidemiological*.

The second part of the crisis is *intellectual*. It concerns failures of understanding. The result is our inability as a society to respond effectively to these deteriorations in child and adolescent well-being. Let us look briefly at both parts of the crisis.

1. Our Waiting Lists Are Too Long

Many of us on the Commission on Children at Risk are children's doctors and mental health professionals. Every day we see children and adolescents who are suffering. We are seeing far too many of them. One of the main reasons we formed this commission is that our waiting lists are too long.

Scholars at the National Research Council estimated in 2002 that at least one of every four adolescents in the United States is currently at serious risk of not achieving productive adulthood.[1] According to another recent study, about 21% of U.S. children ages 9 to 17 have a diagnosable mental or addictive disorder associated with at least minimum impairment.[2] These high numbers appear to reflect actual increases in these problems, not changes in methods or rates of treatment.[3]

Despite increased ability to treat depression, the current generation of young people is more likely to be depressed and anxious than was its parents' generation.[4] According to one study, by the 1980s, U.S. children as a group were reporting more anxiety than did children who were psychiatric patients in the 1950s.[5] High levels of anxiety, or neuroticism, are not only problems in themselves but are also associated with major depression,[6] suicide attempts,[7] alcohol abuse,[8] marital problems,[9] and a wide variety of physical ailments, including asthma, heart disease, irritable bowel syndrome, and ulcers.[10]

Several studies have found than an estimated 8% of U.S. high school students suffer from clinical depression. Other studies, including World Health Organization surveys and a study showing possible errors in school-based depression screening, suggest that the total number of U.S. children suffering from serious depression (clinical or otherwise) may be higher than 8%.[11]

About 20% of students report having seriously considered suicide in the past year.[12] A recent study of mental health problems among college students at a large midwestern university finds that, over the past 13 years, the number of students being seen for depression doubled; the number of suicidal students tripled; and the number of students seen after a sexual assault quadrupled.[13] A growing body of research also finds that children entering out-of-home care for mental and developmental problems are more disturbed than in the past.[14]

Beyond the specific areas of mental illness and emotional and behavioral disorders, recent additional indicators of U.S. child and adolescent well-being are mixed at best. A recent report from the Annie E. Casey Foundation, *Children at Risk: State Trends 1990–2000*, finds that 8 of 11 indicators of child well-being— all material and demographic indicators, such as living in poverty, living with a household head who is a high school dropout, and living in a single-parent family—improved at least slightly between 1990 and 2000.[15] A similar study from 2001, using an index of child and youth well-being consisting of 28 mostly material and demographic indicators, reports that overall U.S. child well-being, after dropping sharply from 1975 to the early 1990s, rose during the middle and late 1990s, while still remaining, as of 1998, lower than it was in 1975.[16]

It is important to note that most of this good news is linked to broad recent improvements in our *material* well-being, which in turn are closely connected to the astonishing economic growth that characterized most of the 1990s, as well as to impressive recent drops in U.S. crime rates. We are heartened by these changes. But *despite them*, U.S. young people not only appear to be experiencing sharp increases in mental illness and stress and emotional problems but also continue to suffer from high—we as a commission believe unacceptably high—rates of related behavioral problems such as substance abuse, school dropout, interpersonal violence, premature sexual intercourse, and teenage pregnancy.

For example, there has been a recent, and welcome, downward trend in recent years in U.S. births to teenagers.[17] At the same time, according to the Centers for Disease Control and Prevention, the United States is still the world leader among developed countries in the proportion of births occurring to teenagers.[18] Similarly, the number of high school students who say that they have never had sexual intercourse rose by almost 10% between 1991 and 2001.[19] Yet about one of every three U.S. teenagers is sexually active.[20] One consequence is high levels of sexually transmitted diseases, particularly among adolescent girls and young women, who are biologically more susceptible to chlamydia, gonorrhea, and HIV.[21]

Almost half of U.S. teenagers report having used marijuana. The use of other illegal drugs by teenagers appears to be increasing. As many as one in three teenagers report having engaged in binge drinking. In spite of an aggressive antismoking campaign, frequent cigarette use among teenagers has risen slightly during the past decade.[22] About 11% of U.S. teenagers drop out of high school.[23] More than one of three U.S. adolescents report having been involved in a physical fight at school in the past year, and about 9% report having been threatened or injured with a weapon while on school property.[24]

Overall, the nature of childhood suffering and death in the United States has changed dramatically in recent decades. For example, since the 1950s, death rates among U.S. young people due to unintentional injuries, cancer, and heart disease have all fallen by about 50%. Death rates overall have dropped by about 53%.

But during this same period, homicide death rates among U.S. youth rose by more than 130%. Suicide rates—the third leading cause of death among U.S. young people, and famously recognized more than a century ago by Emile Durkheim, one of the fathers of modern sociology, as a key indicator of social connectedness—rose by nearly 140%.[25] More and more, what is harming and killing our children today is mental illness, emotional distress, and behavioral problems.[26]

The Curious Case of the Children of Immigrants

Consider this disturbing paradox. Low birth weight and infant mortality are actually higher among babies of U.S.-born women than among babies of immigrant mothers—despite the immigrant mothers' generally lower socioeconomic status, and despite the fact that immigrant mothers typically receive less prenatal care.[27] Similarly, adolescents from immigrant families are less likely than U.S.-born adolescents to experience school absences due to health or emotional problems and are also *less* likely to report engaging in risky behaviors, from early sex to substance use, delinquency, and violence.

Even more unsettling is the fact that, as one recent study points out, whereas children in immigrant families "are healthier than U.S.-born children in U.S.-born families," this "relative advantage tends to decline with length of time in the United States and from one generation to the next." Thus, as the children of immigrants live in the United States for longer periods of times, they "tend to be less healthy and to report increases in risk behaviors. By the third and later generations, rates of most of these behaviors approach or exceed those of U.S.-born white adolescents."[28]

The implication of these findings is unmistakable. For the children of immigrants, and for U.S. children overall, some of the basic foundations of childhood appear currently to be at best anemic, in the sense of weak and inadequate to foster full human flourishing, and at worst toxic, inadvertently depressing health and engendering emotional distress and mental illness.

Our waiting lists are too long.

2. Our Intellectual Models Are Inadequate

The Pharmacological Model

The psychopharmacological revolution of recent years has yielded enormous benefits for millions of suffering patients. Moreover, mental illness is still undertreated in the United States, not overtreated, among children and adolescents, and especially among those living in less affluent communities. Indeed, we as a commission believe that the current lack of resources to treat children with major mental illness is a serious problem that must be addressed.[29]

But as mental health professionals, and as a society, we must also probe deeper. Why are apparently growing numbers of our children suffering from depression, anxiety, attention deficit, conduct disorders, thoughts of suicide, and other serious mental and emotional problems? In the field of medicine, any steady increase in an illness prompts doctors not only to treat (more and more) individual patients but also to examine the larger environments that would appear to be contributing to the spread of disease and poor health. We should do the same today in the field of mental health. Even though psychotropic drugs and related psychotherapies and treatments permit us as professionals to pull many drowning children out of the river, surely we must still ask: Why are so many of today's children in the river?

The tension is between a few of us taking action to treat individual victims of a calamity and all of us, or at least many of us, taking action to eliminate or reduce the calamity. To use a bit of jargon, the tension is between a treatment (or deficit) model and a prevention (or ecological) model.

Obviously, we need both. But we as a commission are saddened and disturbed to conclude that, today in the United States, just as we are making significant progress in many areas of individual treatment, especially those using psychotropic drugs and specific psychotherapies, we are collectively *regressing* in the area of prevention. We as a society seem to be inattentive, and at times even indifferent, to some of the basic foundations of overall child and adolescent well-being. *We are steadily losing ground when it comes to keeping our children out of the river in the first place.*

Consider this analogy. What if environmental experts today focused almost exclusively on remediating some of the worst consequences of pollution—perhaps by encouraging people to wear masks or to stay inside on certain days—while acting as if nothing can or should be done about the pollution in the environment?

Thankfully, a focus on prevention now permeates much of the medical field and much of our approach to public (physical) health. Yet we mental health workers, more than almost any other group of related professionals, have been comparatively slow to make this crucial transition from private to public, from treatment alone to treatment plus prevention. We today urgently challenge ourselves and our mental health colleagues—as we urgently challenge all of our fellow citizens—to become much better at thinking ecologically, and to do much more, in the area of child and adolescent mental health, to become environmental advocates of childhood.

Moreover, we have already learned from the medical field that preventive public health seldom consists only of targeted treatments and services delivered by trained professionals. Instead, much broader approaches and partnerships, deeply rooted in the institutions of civil society, must be mobilized to attack foundational problems that contribute to disease. The same is almost certain to be true of preventive mental health.

The At-Risk Model

We call our group the Commission on Children at Risk for two reasons. One is that we recognize both the usefulness and prevalence of the term *at risk*. The second is that we wish publicly and respectfully to insist on the term's important limitations.

Certainly, when it comes to helping children in need, no term is more widely used or more conceptually influential among scholars, philanthropists, youth service workers, policy makers, journalists, and other opinion leaders. In particular, the language and categories of *at risk* strongly guide most current scholarly and public policy discussions of youth problems and programs.

The term seems partly to have originated in the insurance industry, which has long used the concept of "risk" as a way of developing mathematical models aimed at predicting future insurer liability under various circumstances and therefore determining the costs of providing insurance to various groups of individuals. As we commonly use it today, however, the term *at risk* comes to us primarily from the field of epidemiology, a branch of medical science that deals with the incidence, distribution, and control of disease in a population.

Specifically, the term refers to a methodology for identifying individuals or groups within a population that are vulnerable to disease. The term carries with it the implication that what is necessary are specific treatments or interventions aimed at reducing the incidence or severity of the disease. Thus the *at-risk* model, as we use it today, is essentially a disease-based model of understanding.

From these quite specific roots, the term has grown to its current influence and ubiquity in the fields of youth studies and youth programming. The at-risk model of thinking about youth problems has some important uses. At times, this model gestures toward the goal of prevention. But as a way of thinking, today's at-risk model does not take us nearly far enough.

First, the model tends to focus on individual pathology and dysfunction. It typically locates the problem as "inside" the person, rather than as stemming at least partly from the environment. Consider, say, a student who drops out of high school. The at-risk model would lead us to ask: What is wrong with this student? (What's the "disease"?) Does he need special instruction? Medication? Counseling? Does she need to attend a special class? Find a mentor? Should the school hire credentialed specialists to try to help her and other students who appear to be "at risk" of dropping out?

These are important questions. But are they the only questions? Are they even the most important ones? We believe that the answer is no. Regarding school dropouts, for example, it seems clear that much of this problem in the United States today is traceable to deficits that are not just personal and individual, calling for treatment by professionals in clinical and quasi-clinical settings, but also social and communal. For example, what if the poor quality of the school itself is a problem, not just for the minority of students who drop out or contemplate doing so, but also for the majority of the students? From another angle, what if one important factor associated with dropping out is living in a father-absent home? (In fact, research tells us that it is.)[30] Yet the bias of the at-risk model is consistently *against* recognizing and confronting those dimensions of a problem that are structural, systemic, and social, and *in favor* of interventions that are clinical, highly targeted, and oriented to individual pathology.

Second, a frequent corollary of the bias toward individual pathology is the notion that meeting the needs of at-risk youth is largely a task for professionals. For this reason, the at-risk model sometimes recognizes,[31] but seldom places primary emphasis on, issues such as family structure or the role of local, voluntary civic and religious institutions in improving children's lives.

Third, the at-risk model typically encourages us to focus on the most extreme and advanced manifestations of problems. In that respect, the at-risk model closely resembles what doctors serving soldiers in combat call a "triage" approach. Based on the presumptions of a short time frame and scarce resources, the triage model seeks to determine which wounded soldiers to help, and in what order, in order to maximize the number of survivors.

But when the population in question is an entire generation of a society's children and youth, rather than a small number of wounded soldiers on a battlefield, the ideas contained in the triage approach are largely inappropriate. For example, when it comes to improving life for our children, short-term thinking is important, but longer-term thinking is equally important. Also, we are by far the materially richest society in the world. That fact does not mean that our resources for helping children are limitless, but neither does it mean that we can afford to do nothing other than try to prevent the most seriously wounded among us from dying.

For these and other reasons, as Bill Stanczykiewicz of the Indiana Youth Institute has stressed, it is seldom a good idea to focus only on the most troubled children exhibiting the worst extremes of the problem. Of course, pathology must be treated. But treating pathology is not the same as positive youth development. The at-risk model focuses on illness. The ecological model focuses on health. The former emphasizes the need to direct help to a few of us. The latter emphasizes the need to shift probabilities for most of us. As a result, the former seeks to solve a problem when it is big. The latter recognizes that arguably the wisest way to solve a big problem is to solve it when it is small. *Both approaches are necessary.* But today, in our view, we as a society do not have the balance right. As a result, our currently dominant ways of thinking about the crisis are inadequate. Our deepest challenge today is to think and act much more ecologically—to broaden our attention to the environmental conditions creating growing numbers of suffering children.

The New Scientific Case

If too many of our children are in the river, and if our current approaches to helping them are insufficient, what is to be done? That is the central question with which this commission has struggled.

To try to find answers, we have looked carefully at recent scientific findings in our respective fields. We are heartened by them. We believe that these findings fit together into a discernible whole. Taken together, they tell us a story. Moreover, we believe that this scientific story can help to guide us as a society toward a better, truer understanding of the crisis of American childhood.

Essentially, science is increasingly demonstrating that the human person is hardwired to connect.[32]

First, a great deal of evidence shows that we are hardwired for close attachments to other people, beginning with our mothers, fathers, and extended family, and then moving out to the broader community.

Second, a less definitive but still significant body of evidence suggests that we are hardwired for meaning, born with a built-in capacity and drive to search for purpose and reflect on life's ultimate ends.

Meeting the human child's deep need for these related aspects of connectedness—to other people and to meaning—is essential to the child's health and development.

Meeting this need for connectedness is primarily the task of what we are calling authoritative communities—groups of people who are committed to one another over time and who model and pass on at least part of what it means to be a good person and live a good life.

The weakening of authoritative communities in the United States is a principal reason—arguably *the* principal reason—why large and growing numbers of U.S. children are failing to flourish. As a result, strengthening these communities is likely to be our best strategy for improving the lives of our children, including those most at risk.

The 10 Main Planks

Here are the 10 main planks of the new scientific case for authoritative communities:

1. The mechanisms by which we become and stay attached to others are biologically primed and increasingly discernible in the basic structure of the brain.
2. Nurturing environments, or the lack of them, affect gene transcription and the development of brain circuitry.
3. The old "nature versus nurture" debate—focusing on whether heredity or environment is the main determinant of human conduct—is no longer relevant to serious discussions of child well-being and youth programming.
4. Adolescent risk taking and novelty seeking are connected to changes in brain structure and function.
5. Assigning meaning to gender in childhood and adolescence is a human universal that deeply influences well-being.
6. The beginning of morality is the biologically primed moralization of attachment.
7. The ongoing development of morality in later childhood and adolescence involves the human capacity to idealize individuals and ideas.
8. Primary nurturing relationships influence early spiritual development—call it the spiritualization of attachment—and spiritual development can influence us biologically in the same ways that primary nurturing relationships do.
9. Religiosity and spirituality significantly influence well-being.
10. The human brain appears to be organized to ask ultimate questions and seek ultimate answers.

Let us look at each of these propositions in greater depth.

1. *The mechanisms by which we become and stay attached to others are biologically primed and increasingly discernible in the basic structure of the brain.*

Let's start with the human infant. Here is how Allan N. Schore of the UCLA School of Medicine puts it: "The idea is that we are born to form attachments, that our brains are physically wired to develop in tandem with another's, through emotional communication, beginning before words are spoken."[33]

Let him say it a bit more formally. Schore has done extensive research on affect regulation—how we regulate our emotions and behaviors—among young children. He presents a large body of interdisciplinary data underscoring the importance of infant attachment and suggesting that "the self-organization of the developing brain occurs in the context of a relationship with another self, another brain. This relational context can be growth-facilitating or growth-inhibiting, and so it imprints into the developing right brain either a resilience against or a vulnerability to later forming psychiatric disorders."[34]

Let's look at other ways in which this proposition appears to hold true. Recent animal studies have helped to clarify the role of the neuropeptides, oxytocin, and vasopressin in male–female bonding.[35] In females, the presence of large numbers of oxytocin receptors in the reward circuitry located deep in the cortex of the brain suggests that social bonding manifests itself biochemically. In males, the presence of large numbers of vasopressin receptors in the brain suggests the same phenomenon. In a sense, then, these pair-bonded couples can be described as being "addicted" to one another.

In the area of parental care, in several animal species it has been shown that attachment hormones help trigger parental care, which in turn helps trigger the release of more attachment hormones. For example, as male marmosets begin to care for their offspring, their levels of prolactin increase, which likely reinforces the bonding process. Thus, we see social behavior and biology involved in an intricate dance of mutual reinforcement, in which caretaking, among other things, boosts some of the very neurotransmitters that appear to facilitate caregiving.[36]

Other studies implicate numerous other neurotransmitters and hormones in the human bonding process. These hormones include dopamine, prolactin, endogenous opioid peptides, and steroid hormones such as estrogen, testosterone, and progesterone.[37]

In a preliminary study, Rebecca Turner and her colleagues at the University of California show that the hormone oxytocin enters a female's bloodstream during sexual intercourse, affecting the brain and limbic system in ways that appear to promote emotional intimacy and bonding (also sometimes known as "love").[38] Oxytocin is also released during birth and lactation and appears to strengthen the mother's attachment to the baby.[39]

Similarly, in males, the steroid hormone testosterone is associated with both sexual desire and aggression. Researchers have found that for men, getting married—becoming sexually and intimately bonded with a spouse—seems to lower testosterone levels. The result is a diminished biological basis for violent male behavior and male sexual promiscuity and infidelity. Researchers also report, not surprisingly, that drops in testosterone seem also to be connected to better fathering. Call it a "neuroendocrine basis" for recognizing that male connectedness resulting from marriage tends to guide men away from bars, brawling, and tomcatting around and toward washing the dishes and making sure the kids do their homework.[40]

To take another example, at the Ohio State University Medical Center, Janice K. Kiecolt-Glaser and her colleagues have conducted a series of studies examining the connections between close sexual relationships, especially those of married couples, and physiologic processes such as immune, endocrine, and cardiovascular functioning. These researchers report growing evidence linking relationship intimacy to better health, including stronger immune systems and physical wounds taking less time to heal. Conversely, high-conflict (anti-intimate) marital relationships appear to weaken the immune system and increase vulnerability to disease, especially among women, including worsening the body's response to proven vaccines and lengthening the amount of time required for physical wounds to heal.[41]

In short, brain researchers and other scientists are now clearly mapping out what might be called the biochemistry of connection.

2. *Nurturing environments, or the lack of them, affect gene transcription and the development of brain circuitry.*

Let's start by looking at rats.[42] Specifically, let's look at how the parenting of rat pups influences their basic health, including their capacity to respond successfully to stress, and how such environmentally engineered traits, in part because they also become expressed genetically, can then be passed from generation to generation.

The neuroscientist Larry Young of Emory University finds that, for rats, early nurturing experiences "have a powerful effect on emotional reactivity of the offspring" and also produce "permanent changes in behavioral responses to stressful situations." Specifically, "rats that received more maternal stimulation as pups have altered levels of stress hormone receptors (glucocorticoid receptor) in the hippocampus, a brain region that plays a central role in the regulation of the stress response."[43]

That's good. These well-cared-for rats are healthier and more capable. But there is more. In fact, something quite extraordinary has apparently happened. Abundant maternal attention—good mothering—not only measurably enhances a pup's emotional and physiologic resilience but can also be passed on by that pup to future generations. As Young describes it: "Not only do these differences in maternal attention predict emotionality of the offspring, they also predict how the offspring will mother their own pups. That is, the offspring of high-licking [high-nurturing] mothers also showed high levels of licking [nurturing] towards their own pups in adulthood."[44]

And how, exactly, does this intergenerational transmission occur?

On the one hand, cross-fostering experiments—in which some of the young are transferred at birth to genetically unrelated mothers—show that some of this positive transmission can occur nongenetically, simply through the pup's own social experience of having been so intensively licked and groomed as a baby. At the same time, however, Young reports that "the underlying neural systems believed to mediate these behaviors are also changed."

As a result, these positive traits have effectively become *biologically patterned* in the pup. They even influence genetic transcription! That is, the well-mothered pup will be predisposed, *at the cellular level*, to pass on this same confluence of good nurturing and physiologic resilience to the next generation. Call it passing on the neurobiological ties that bind.[45]

These are rats. What about humans? In fact, the presence in humans of many of these same hormones connected to sexual bonding, birth, and lactation suggests that they may also be relevant to human behavior and relationships. Available human data,[46] as well as these and other similar findings from animal studies,[47] suggest that our deep need for attachment and connectedness to others can be traced back to the brain's deepest centers of reward and gratification.

Even as children grow into adolescence, parental presence can have an impact on their biology. Several recent studies have explored the connections between adult male pheromones and the age at which adolescent girls reach sexual puberty.

Pheromones are chemical substances secreted by the body that, when inhaled through the nose by others, can help to stimulate one or more behavioral responses. Researchers have found that, for an adolescent girl, living in close proximity to her biological father tends to slow down the onset of puberty. Conversely, living with a biologically unrelated adult male—for example, a stepfather or mother's boyfriend—seems to speed up the onset of puberty. Why? In part, the researchers suggest that exposure to an unrelated male's pheromones accelerates a girl's physical sexual development, whereas exposure to her father's pheromones has exactly the opposite effect.[48]

> 3. *The old "nature versus nurture" debate—focusing on whether heredity or environment is the main determinant of human conduct—is no longer relevant to serious discussions of child well-being and youth programming.*

Social contexts can alter genetic expression. That extraordinary fact is why the traditional "nature versus nurture" debate is obsolete.

A social environment can change the relationship between a specific gene and the behavior associated with that gene. Changes in social environment can thus change the transcription of our genetic material at the most basic cellular level.

This fact turns the entire "nature versus nurture" debate inside out. For it turns out that there is no "versus" in it at all. It is futile to ask which one is dominant. Instead, new scientific findings are teaching us to marvel at how wonderfully the two interact—not like boxers, with each one trying to knock the other out, but more like dancers, with each subtle move producing a reciprocating move.[49]

For parents, community leaders, and youth service providers, this is important news. It is also sobering news. The various social environments that we create or fail to create for our children matter a great deal, for both good and ill. They matter not only because of all the soft reasons with which we are familiar, such as the desire to "help" a child or be a "good influence" on a child, but also because of the hardest facts now flowing from our microscopes and laboratories. These hard facts tell us that the environments we create influence our children's genetic expression.

To see more clearly how this phenomenon works, let's first turn to some research with monkeys. Stephen Suomi of the National Institute of Child Health and Human Development has done extensive research on rhesus monkeys. In particular, Suomi has studied how genes and social contexts interact to influence behavioral outcomes. Here is one of the main questions he has sought to answer. In one social context, a gene clearly seems to put an individual monkey "at risk"; that is, the gene seems to predispose that monkey toward negative outcomes. In a different social context, however, the very same gene appears to have either no effect on behavior or, amazingly, even the opposite effect on behavior. (That is, in some environments the supposedly "risky" gene actually served to reduce the likelihood of bad behavioral outcomes.) Why?

About 15% to 20% of rhesus monkeys appear to carry a heritable trait associated with anxiety. In situations that most young monkeys would experience as novel and interesting, these anxious monkeys typically withdraw and become quite timid and nervous. To an outside human observer, they clearly resemble a human child lingering on the edge of the playground, fretfully looking down, afraid to join the other children.

Compared with other monkeys in similar situations of potential stress, these anxious monkeys generate significantly more "stress hormones," such as cortisol. Also, when given unlimited access to a sweetened alcohol solution, these anxious monkeys participate much more readily and heavily in this "monkey happy hour" than do their less-stressed-out peers—an alcohol consumption pattern closely resembling what many alcohol counselors and medical professionals among us humans would call "self-medication," in which anxious or depressed patients seek to relieve their suffering by abusing alcohol.

Yet when members of this same minority of supposedly genetically "at risk" infant monkeys are cross-fostered at birth, and placed under the care of particular female rhesus monkeys that have been identified as being especially capable and nurturing—what might be called "supermom" monkeys—an extraordinary change takes place in these young rhesus monkeys. The tendency toward anxiety and timidity disappears. So does the tendency to abuse alcohol. What has happened? An *improved social environment has modulated a heritable vulnerability*.[50]

Suomi has also wrestled with the genetic and social influences on aggression and impulsivity. In some rhesus monkeys, a variation in one of the genes associated with the neurotransmitter serotonin seems to predispose the monkeys not toward anxiety but instead toward aggression and poor impulse control. These aggressive monkeys also drink a lot of alcohol at monkey happy hour, and they are more likely than either anxious monkeys or the other monkeys to engage in "binge drinking." Typically, these overly aggressive young monkeys are not well-liked or accepted by the other monkeys, for obvious reasons. As a result, they fare quite poorly in monkey society, with high rates of mortality.

Yet when these same genetically "at risk" monkeys are raised in supportive environments, the harmfully aggressive behavior disappears, as does the excessive and binge drinking. But there is more. These potentially "at risk" monkeys not only survive, they flourish. They do very well. They appear to be especially successful in making their way to or near the top of the rhesus monkey social hierarchy! What has happened? *An improved social environment has changed a heritable vulnerability into a positive behavioral asset.*

Recall again the old "nature versus nurture" paradigm. According to that framework, what is going on with these aggression-prone rhesus monkeys? Are they genetically vulnerable or environmentally vulnerable? Is it nature or nurture? The answer, we now know, *is both and neither.*

Whether a particular gene or combination of genes ends up helping or hurting these monkeys depends largely on the social context![51]

Among humans, research to date points to a similar phenomenon. Human gene expression, as well as brain growth and structure at the neuronal level, can apparently be altered as a function of experience.[52]

For example, the same physiologic trait—such as cardiovascular reactivity, measured by an unusual spike in blood pressure in response to stress—can be linked to either positive or negative behavioral outcomes, depending on social context. As the researcher W. T. Boyce puts it, "Both extreme vulnerability and uncommon resilience can be found in the same highly reactive children depending on the basic stressfulness or supportiveness of the surrounding social context."[53]

In the past decade, prompted largely by the 1994 publication of Charles Murray and Richard Herrnstein's *The Bell Curve: Intelligence and Class Structure in American Life,* there has been much public discussion of the meaning and role of general intelligence, as measured by IQ tests, in U.S. society. Some of this discussion has been based on the premise, which is present in *The Bell Curve,* that the genetic, or heritable, component of IQ is quite high. One implication of such a premise, also repeatedly suggested in *The Bell Curve,* is that social environments, including the interventions of public policy, can have little impact on intelligence and are therefore largely futile.[54]

However, the more recent research findings summarized in this report— as well as some specific scholarly analyses of *The Bell Curve*[55]—support a quite different presumption. Social environments matter. They can affect us at the cellular level to reduce genetically based risks and even help to transform such risks into behavioral assets. They can also help substantially to raise intelligence and measures of intelligence. The old "nature versus nurture" debate is obsolete. The two interact in complex ways that add up to good news—a reason for optimism—for those who seek to improve the social environments for U.S. children and adolescents.

4. *Adolescent risk taking and novelty seeking are connected to changes in brain structure and function.*

In recent years, considerable academic and public attention has focused on brain development during the first 3 years of life.[56] This focus has been important, but incomplete. For example, recent advances in neuroimaging demonstrate that the period of significant brain growth, maturation, and remodeling extends into the third decade of human life.[57]

In particular, recent research is producing important insights into adolescent brain development. More important, today's increases in mental health and emotional problems among U.S. young people suggest that we as a society should do more to recognize adolescence as an especially critical period of life.

Adolescence is partly a social and cultural construction. At the same time, there is also something nearly universal about it: Adolescence emerges as a key period of change and transition in the life cycle of many mammalian species and in most known human societies.[58]

In general, the journey away from the protection of the family, and toward the wider social world, is a time of peril. Characterized by increased risk taking and peer affiliation in many species, this period of transition also often sees high rates of certain forms of adolescent mortality. For example, homicides, suicides, and accidents account for about 85% of all deaths among early to late U.S. adolescents.[59]

Why are teenagers the way they are? There are many valid answers to this question, but here is one of the best: Current research suggests that alterations in brain structure and function may best account for some of the most distinctive behavioral and psychological changes that typically accompany adolescence.

Specifically, recent neuroscientific evidence demonstrates that considerable maturational changes are seen through adolescence in the prefrontal cortex and related brain regions—regions of the brain that are critical for cognitive functions such as judgment and insight.[60]

Some of these brain transformations are quite dramatic. Adolescents can experience a decline of nearly 50% of the connections to some regions of the brain.

Consider an example. It appears that alterations in levels of activity of the neurotransmitter dopamine in parts of the adolescent brain can produce in these young people, in comparison to adults, a relative "reward deficiency."[61] Translation: For the adolescent, *any* pleasurable stimulus, from music to drugs, may need to be especially powerful and intense in order to pass the adolescent brain's recently altered ("reward deficient") threshold of interest, pleasure, or excitement. Thus, many teens' quest for adventure, novelty, and risk may simply reflect their efforts to feel good.

Teenagers may also suffer the consequences of risk taking more intensely than do adults. For example, young people who abuse alcohol and drugs may be biologically primed to suffer more harm than adults who do the same thing. Why? Here's a clue: "[T]he brain of the adolescent differs considerably from the adult in a number of neural systems prominent in the action of these drugs."[62]

In general, adolescents do not appear inherently to suffer from higher rates of mental illness than do adults. But they do seem to suffer disproportionately from moodiness and unhappiness. For example, one study finds that between childhood and early adolescence—from about the 5th to the 7th grade—the proportion of young people who say that they feel "very happy" drops by about 50%.[63] The developmental psychobiologist Linda Spear suggests that this (relatively mild and transient) anhedonia may be directly linked to changes in the dopamine function of the adolescent brain.

In short, scientific research is increasingly demonstrating that adolescence is a biological as well as a social phenomenon. The teenage propensity for risk taking, novelty seeking, excitement, and peer affiliation is partly biologically based. This conclusion highlights the importance of the social environments that we create, or fail to create, for our adolescents. As stressed throughout this report, the interplay between environment and biology is profound, and its consequences run deep. *Social context can alter genetic expression and impact neurocircuitry itself.*

We as a society are doing a remarkably poor job of addressing our adolescents' partly hardwired needs for risk, novelty, excitement, and peer affiliation. Wishing that teenagers were different won't make them so. Treating immaturity as pathology will cure very little. Pressuring young people to focus on other priorities will only go so far. Worst of all, leaving them largely to their own devices, with one another as their main sources of wisdom regarding how to take risks and pursue novelty, has shortcomings those of us in the mental health field see every day.

Meeting the challenge of this special period of life requires a society-wide mobilization of a particular kind—one that understands and embraces, rather than denies or walks away from, what is distinctive about adolescence, and one that carefully guides the adolescent need for risk, novelty, excitement, and peer approval toward authentic fulfillment, leading toward maturity.

5. *Assigning meaning to gender in childhood and adolescence is a human universal that deeply influences well-being.*

In recent years, dozens of studies of the behavior of young children show that boys and girls differ significantly in a number of areas, including who they want to play with, the toys they prefer, fantasy play, rough-and-tumble play, activity level, and aggression.[64]

Some portion of these differences is likely attributable to (just as the differences are also reinforced by) environmental factors, including boys and girls being treated differently by parents and other caregivers. But a number of basic differences in gender role behavior are also biologically primed and even established prenatally. In particular, male and female brains appear to develop differently *in utero*, each responding to gonadal hormones released by the ovaries (in females) and the testes (in males). During this period of fetal development, for example, the male brain appears to develop in ways that heighten its sensitivity to testosterone, which in turn is linked (among humans and in a diversity of other animal species) to aggression.[65]

At the same time, as we have stressed often in this report, social contexts can affect biological systems.[66] In the area of gender identity, when the young child (typically at about 18 to 24 months of age) begins to show a deep need to understand and make sense of her or his sexual embodiment, the child's relationships with mother and father become centrally important. For the child searching for the meaning of his embodiment, both the same-sex-as-me parent and the opposite-sex-from-me parent play vital roles. So the process of early gender identity is not only physiologic but also familial and psychosocial.[67] The resulting gender identity continues to develop and is deeply influential throughout the life cycle.

Moreover, puberty and adolescence—a time of rapid physical, sexual, and reproductive maturing, guided in part by increases in estrogenic hormones in females and in testosterone in males[68]—is a time in which human communities across time and cultures typically mobilize themselves quite purposely to define and enforce the social meaning of sexual embodiment and thereby seek to guide burgeoning adolescent strength, energy, aggression, and sexuality in prosocial directions. These mobilizations are commonly expressed through sex-specific rituals, tests, and rites of passage.

For young women, many world rituals suggest that with menarche come heightened introspective powers, greater spiritual access, and an enriched inner life.[69] For boys, such rituals tend to involve tests of endurance, stamina, bravery, and physical capacity.[70]

For these and other reasons, the need to attach social significance and meaning to gender appears to be a human universal.

In much of today's social science writing, and also more generally within elite culture, gender tends to be viewed primarily as a set of traits and as a tendency to engage in certain roles. Yet the current weight of evidence suggests that this understanding, although accurate, is seriously incomplete. Gender also runs deeper, near to the core of human identity and social meaning—in part because it is biologically primed and connected to differences in brain structure and function, and in part because it is so deeply implicated in the transition to adulthood.

In recent decades, many adults have tended to withdraw from the task of assigning prosocial meaning to gender, especially in the case of boys. For some people, actual and desired changes in sex roles, including a desire for greater androgyny, make some of our culture's traditional gender formulations appear anachronistic and even potentially harmful. We recognize the important issues at stake here.

But neglecting the gendered needs of adolescents can be dangerous. Boys and girls differ with respect to risk factors for social pathology. For example, adolescent girls' capacity for pregnancy places them at special risk for lower educational achievement and future poverty related to teenage childbearing. Boys' aggressive tendencies put them at increased risk for being perpetrators and victims of homicide, suicide, or injuries. Similarly, what works best in efforts at prevention and intervention often varies significantly according to gender.[71] We recognize the perils of oversimplifying or exaggerating gender differences. But as the medical world has discovered, the risk of not attending to real differences that exist between males and females can have dangerous consequences.

Ignoring or denying this challenge will not make it go away. Indeed, when adults choose largely to neglect the critical task of sexually enculturating the young, they are left essentially on their own—perhaps with some help from Hollywood and Madison Avenue—to discover the social meaning of their sexuality. The resulting, largely adolescent-created rituals of transition are far less likely to be prosocial in their meaning and outcomes.

Young people have an inherent need to experience the advent of fertility, physical prowess, and sexual maturing within an affirming system of meaning.

6. *The beginning of morality is the biologically primed moralization of attachment.*

Recall a point stressed earlier in this report: The human infant, as the anthropologist Sarah Blaffer Hrdy puts it, is "born to attach."[72] Now we want to relate that finding to the issue of morality. Why? Because for the child, this born-to-attachedness is the essential foundation for the emergence of conscience and of moral meaning.

In this sense, if the fundamental idea of morality is love of neighbor, we can therefore say, speaking scientifically as well as poetically, that the human child is talked into talking and loved into loving.[73]

In her empirical study of the development of conscience, Barbara Stilwell of the Indiana University School of Medicine describes the child's quest for parental approval as the foundation for the emergence of conscience: "Moralization is a process whereby a value-driven sense of *oughtness* emerges within specific human behavioral systems, namely, the systems governing attachment, emotional regulation, cognitive processing, and volition."

Moreover, this "moralization of attachment" is partly hardwired: "Biological substrates prepare us to moralize experience under the tutelage of available morally tuned support systems." The process begins as early as infancy:

> Very early in development, infant attachment and parent bonding interact to form a *security-empathy-oughtness* representation within the child's mind.... Physiological feelings associated with security and insecurity combine with intuitively perceived, emotionally toned messages that certain behaviors are parent-pleasing or nonpleasing; prohibited, permitted, or encouraged; while other behaviors gain no attention at all. A bedrock value for human connectedness guides the child's readiness to behave in response to parent wishes and attentiveness.[74]

What happens when this "bedrock value for human connectedness" is ignored or denied? Evaluating seven decades of attachment research, Robert Karen writes, "[A]ll of the [early] researchers, though unaware of one another's work, had unanimously found the same symptoms in children who'd been deprived of their mothers—the superficial relationships, the poverty of feeling for others, the inaccessibility, the lack of emotional response, the often pointless deceitfulness and theft, and the inability to concentrate in school."[75]

In sum, our sense of right and wrong originates largely from our biologically primed need to connect with others. In this sense, moral behavior—good actions—stems at least as much from relationships as from rules. Thwarting the child's need for close attachments to others also thwarts basic moral development, the social consequences of which can be stark and tragic.

This finding also suggests that our moral sense is an integral part of our personhood. An important implication is that the moral needs of children are not merely personal and private. They are also social and shared. They are needs that, in a good society, will command the attention and resources of the community as a whole.

Conversely, ignoring the moral needs of children can be a form of child neglect.

7. *The ongoing development of morality in later childhood and adolescence involves the human capacity to idealize individuals and ideas.*

The moralization of attachment that begins with the infant–parent bond later extends outward, to the larger community, as growing cognitive capacity and widening networks of relationships lead young people to identify new and additional sources of moral meaning. For the developing child and adolescent, then, forming a moral identity is an ongoing and increasingly complex process. In a society that cares about moral conduct, it cannot be left on autopilot.

What may be particularly important in this process is what the psychiatrically trained anthropologist David Gutmann calls "the human capacity for awe, worship, and idealization." Summarizing cross-national research on the development of adolescent moral and social identity, Gutmann describes how the adolescent in human societies "discovers the ideal self outside of the self," typically by recognizing "an equivalence between his own, usually inchoate, origin myth and the founding legacy of some worthy group, vocation, profession, religion, or nation."[76] Acquiring a mature moral identity, he writes, is largely

> based on a profound redirection of the idealizing tendency, from being introversive and reflexive (that is, fixed on the self) to being focused on some worthy version of otherness. We can say that adulthood has been achieved when narcissism is transmuted, and thereby detoxified, into strong, lasting idealizations and into healthy narcissism.... Instead of himself, the true adult venerates ideal versions of his community, his vocation and his family.[77]

This process can happen in a good or bad way, but either way, it happens. Several years ago in a television commercial for Nike, Charles Barkley, the basketball star, famously declared, "I am not a role model." He was wrong. Because of the "idealizations" to which we humans are perhaps distinctively prone, we clearly tend to imitate—in moral terms, we tend to become—those whom we admire, whether those persons wish it or not. Accordingly, the challenge for civil society is to expose young people to morally admirable persons. As Barbara Stilwell puts it:

> What really holds potential for making a moral impact on a midadolescent is a powerful connection with individual adults whom he comes to admire or even idealize. It is that teacher, coach, counselor, religious youth worker, Big Brother, neighbor, stepparent, grandparent, police officer, or other individual in the community who can inspire him to make moral sense of the social confusion of his surroundings.[78]

We can put this another way. In the sometimes dense language of the social sciences, "moral" often appears as "prosocial," and what promotes prosocial conduct is described as "protective." Fair enough. So listen to Michael Resnick of the University of Minnesota:

> Numerous researchers ...have demonstrated the protective impact of extrafamilial adult relationships for young people, including other adult relatives, friends' parents, teachers, or adults in health and social service settings. This sense of connectedness

to adults is salient as a protective factor against an array of health-jeopardizing behaviors of adolescents ...and has protective effects for both girls and boys across various ethnic, racial, and social class groups.[79]

8. *Primary nurturing relationships influence early spiritual development—call it the spiritualization of attachment—and spiritual development can influence us biologically in the same ways that primary nurturing relationships do.*

The famous Swiss psychologist Jean Piaget once observed that "the child spontaneously attributes to his parents the perfections and abilities which he will later transfer to God if his religious education gives him the possibility."[80]

At least regarding monotheistic religion, ample research now suggests that children's conceptions of God—who God is and how God acts—initially stem partly from their actual day-to-day experiences with their parents, and partly from their magnified, idealized conceptions of who their parents are.[81] The first tendency, attributing to God traits that come from experiences with parents, is an example of what might be called the *spiritualization of attachment*. The latter tendency, attributing to God those larger-than-life traits that the child had first attributed to one or both of the parents, is an example of the drive to idealize. In addition, many religious traditions reinforce these related phenomena when they teach children that God is like a father or mother.

Children often associate both maternal and paternal qualities with God, and their early positive or negative experiences with their parents can predispose or hinder their development of religious faith later in life. In some cases, the image of God is more strongly influenced by the child's experience with the parent of the opposite sex, or with the preferred parent.[82]

At the same time, some religions and spiritual traditions are nontheistic, and not all conceptions of God are personal. Some children may describe God as being "like the sun" or "like a cool breeze." In these cases as well, many of the descriptions of God, and the qualities that children are likely to associate with the divine, relate to trust and a sense of security and peace—descriptions and attributes that are quite similar to those associated with the experience of healthy parental nurture.

As the child matures in religious faith, her or his images of God become more complex and developed, fed by a diversity of ideas and experiences other than those linked to parents. For this reason, among others, religious and spiritual commitments can never be crudely reduced to mere surrogates for early parental attachments.[83] At the same time, the child's earliest experiences of parental attachment and idealization, and the happiness or disappointment that comes with them, can lay an important foundation for the beginnings of religious comprehension and may set a course in spiritual and religious development that will influence the rest of the child's life.

But there's more. We have seen that, along with the drive to idealize, attachment helps to shape early religious experience. But influence also goes in the other direction. Religious experience also appears at times to do some of what attachment does. For example, in her work with HIV-infected men and women, Gail Ironson of the University of Miami discovered that, among these patients, spirituality is positively associated with long-term survival. The benefits of spirituality and religiosity associated with increased survival included lower levels of stress hormones (cortisol), more optimism, and commitment to helping others.[84]

Thus we discover an amazing fact: The physiologic and emotional resilience that Ironson finds associated with spirituality is the same kind of resilience that, as the report has shown, is associated with effective early parental nurture.[85] In short, the two kinds of connectedness analyzed in this report—connection to others and connection to the transcendent—seem to influence the same biological systems in quite similar ways. This phenomenon may help explain why some people find, in their religious faith and spiritual practice, some of the very sources of security and well-being that were not available to them from their parents.

9. *Religiosity and spirituality significantly influence well-being.*

Paul C. Vitz of New York University puts it this way: "Emerging in contemporary psychology is a general belief that the good life involves a significant spiritual component."[86] Regarding our children, what are the implications of this general belief? Religion is a truth claim, not a therapy or a youth policy or a way to network more effectively or improve one's health. Going to a house of worship or embracing a religious creed because "it's good for you" may make practical sense for some,[87] but ultimately such a strategy assumes that some of the possible consequences of the thing are the same as the thing itself. They are not.

At the same time, one way of assessing a phenomenon is to examine some of its consequences. And when the phenomenon itself tends to center on "things unseen"[88] and the most vexing and enduring philosophical problems known to human beings, a strategy of selectively isolating a few of the more likely by-products, while obviously insufficient, may at least be one valid way to approach the subject. For this reason, we as a commission report that seeking connectedness to the transcendent through religious and spiritual belief and practice appears frequently to yield psychological benefits and reduce the risk of certain pathologies.[89] This generalization is as true for children as it is for adults.

By almost any measure, U.S. young people are quite religious.[90] About 96% of U.S. teenagers say that they believe in God.[91] More than 40% report that they pray frequently. About 36% are members of a church or religious youth group.[92] Notwithstanding these robust social facts, however, Byron Johnson of Baylor University reports that, to date, the influence of religion on U.S. young people has been "grossly understudied."[93] At the same time, existing research is highly suggestive. For adults, religious faith and practice appear to have a sizable and consistent relationship with improved health and longevity, including less hypertension and depression, a lower risk of suicide, less criminal activity, and less use and abuse of drugs and alcohol.[94]

Religious practice also correlates with higher levels of reported personal happiness, higher levels of hope and optimism, and a stronger sense that one's life has purpose and meaning. Part—but almost certainly not all— of the explanation for these findings is that people who are religiously active appear to benefit from larger social networks and more social contacts and support. Byron Johnson stresses: "The beneficial relationship between religion and health behaviors and outcomes is not simply a function of religion's constraining function or what it discourages—opposing drug use, suicide, or delinquent behavior—but also through what it encourages—promoting behaviors that can enhance hope, well-being, or educational attainment."[95]

For adolescents, religiosity is significantly associated with a reduced likelihood of both unintentional and intentional injury (both of which are leading causes of death for teenagers).[96] Compared with their less religious peers, religious teenagers are safer drivers and are more likely to wear seatbelts. They are less likely to become either juvenile delinquents or adult criminals.[97] They are less prone to substance abuse.[98] In general, these young people are less likely to endorse engaging in high-risk conduct or to endorse the idea of enjoying danger.[99]

Looking at the other side of the developmental coin, religiously committed teenagers are more likely to volunteer in the community. They are more likely to participate in sports and in student government.[100] More generally, these young people appear to have higher self-esteem and more positive attitudes about life.[101] Much of this research is based on large national studies.[102] Whereas these and similar findings demonstrate clear correlations between religiosity and good outcomes for young people, they do not prove a causal connection.[103] (Definitive proof regarding causation is all but impossible in social science research.) Yet there are good reasons to suspect that causal factors may be involved.

First, religious involvement appears to increase social connectedness. It also commonly exposes young people to messages about good behavior and connects them to other young people who are presumably sympathetic to those messages.

Second, positive religious coping mechanisms—including a framework of meaning as well as specific religious practices, such as the cultivation of gratitude[104]—may help children and others deal with stressful situations and orient them toward specific goals.[105]

Third, it can be helpful to compare the influences of what the sociologist James Coleman calls *purposive* institutions, such as corporations, state welfare agencies, or even clubs or athletic leagues, to the influences of *primordial* institutions, such as religious groups and (even more primordial) the family. One major distinction is that primordial institutions are more likely to treat children as ends in themselves rather than largely as means to one or more particular ends, such as buying a product or winning a game. For example, because religious institutions are inherently oriented to passing on a body of belief and practice from one generation to the next, they tend to demonstrate what Coleman calls "an intrinsic interest" in "the kind of person the child is and will become."[106] Consequently, religious institutions are more likely than many others to offer a shared vision of the good life, communal support for good behavior, a long-term rather than short-term outlook, and thick networks of relationships that are multigenerational rather than unigenerational.

Fourth, some research indicates correlations between religiosity and several aspects of good parenting, including expressions of affection, monitoring, effectively establishing discipline, and parental involvement in children's schools. One recent study finds that these correlations are stronger for poor and working-class families than they are for middle- and upper-class families.[107] The domains of religiosity, parenting style, and child outcomes appear to affect one another in complex ways. For example, one study focusing on adolescent alcohol abuse points to the value of those families that provide "an important social context for the development of adolescent religiosity," partly due to the fact that "religious commitment, in turn, reduces the risk for alcohol use among teens."[108] In general, according to W. Bradford Wilcox of the University of Virginia, religious commitment on the part of parents appears to be associated with "significantly higher investments in parenting and better parenting environments."[109]

Finally, for adolescents, one religious quality that appears to be especially beneficial, in terms of the range of mental health and lifestyle consequences that we are describing is what some scholars call personal devotion, or the young person's sense of participating in a "direct personal relationship with the Divine."[110] Personal devotion among adolescents is associated with reduced risk-taking behavior. It is also associated with more effectively resolving feelings of loneliness,[111] greater regard for the self and for others,[112] and a stronger sense that life has meaning and purpose.[113]

These protective effects of personal devotion are twice as great for adolescents as they are for adults.[114] This particular finding clearly reinforces the idea, found in many cross-national studies, of adolescence as a time of particularly intense searching for, and openness to, the transcendent.[115] For this reason, we believe that our society as a whole, and youth advocates and youth service professionals in particular, should pay greater attention to this aspect of youth development. This task will not be easy. Because we are a philosophically diverse and religiously plural society, many of our youth-serving programs and social environments for young people will need to find ways respectfully to reflect that diversity and pluralism.

But that is a challenge to be embraced, not avoided. Denying or ignoring the spiritual needs of adolescents may end up creating a void in their lives that either devolves into depression or is filled by other forms of questing and challenge, such as drinking, unbridled consumerism, petty crime, sexual precocity, or flirtations with violence. Here is how Lisa Miller of Columbia University puts it: "A search for spiritual relationship with the Creator may be an inherent developmental process in adolescence."[116]

10. *The human brain appears to be organized to ask ultimate questions and seek ultimate answers.*

Human beings have a basic tendency to question in order to know. Why am I here? What is the purpose of my life? How should I live? What will happen when I die? Exploring these questions of ultimate concern, and making choices and judgments about what we value and love, are characteristic human activities. They reflect the deep human drive to order and draw meaning from experience and are part of what distinguishes us as a species.[117]

Calling these activities "religious" partly misses the point, as they are more an aspect of personhood than a result of institutionalized religion. Better, perhaps, simply to call them human. At the same time, across time and cultures, this distinctively human pursuit has been closely connected to spiritual seeking and experience and to religious belief, ritual, and practice.

Recent advances in neurobiology also suggest that these spiritual and religious experiences stem partly from processes and structures that are deeply embedded in the human brain.

For example, the neuroscientists Eugene d'Aquili and Andrew B. Newberg have used brain imaging to study individuals involved in spiritual practices such as contemplative prayer and meditation. During such states, they have found an increase in activity in a number of frontal brain regions, including the prefrontal cortex.[118] They report that these "experiences are based in observable functions of the brain. The neurological roots of these experiences would render them as convincingly real as any other of the brain's perceptions. In this sense ...they are reporting genuine, neurobiological events."[119]

This research suggests that the human need to know what is true about life's purpose and ultimate ends is connected to brain functions underlying many spiritual and religious experiences. These findings are one reason why these researchers suggest that human beings appear to have "no choice but to construct myths to explain their world."[120]

These findings may also help to explain why modern psychiatry in recent years has appropriated some spiritual practices, such as mindfulness, in an effort to alleviate patients' suffering and enhance their functioning.[121]

Studies also reveal that children whose parents have low levels of religiosity report levels of personal religiosity quite similar to those of other children—additional evidence to support the thesis that the need in young people to connect to ultimate meaning and to the transcendent is not merely the result of social conditioning but is instead an intrinsic aspect of the human experience.[122]

Even the intensified search for meaning commonly seen during adolescence may be in part biologically determined, given that the brain regions that are activated during religious experiences, such as the prefrontal cortex, are also among the regions undergoing considerable developmental change during adolescence.

Authoritative Communities

Recall the twin dimensions of the crisis of American childhood: first, disturbingly high and apparently rising rates of depression, anxiety, attention deficit, conduct disorders, thoughts of suicide, and other forms of mental and emotional stress among U.S. children and adolescents; second, influential intellectual models of individual risk assessment and treatment that, while valuable, seldom encourage us to recognize, and often prevent us from recognizing, the broad environmental conditions that are contributing to growing numbers of suffering children.

In search of solutions, we have considered the weight of scholarly evidence in our respective fields. As part of our literature review, we have also paid special attention to recent research findings from the field of neuroscience and in the behavioral sciences. We are impressed by mounting scientific evidence suggesting that, in two basic ways, the human child is hardwired to connect.

First, we are hardwired to connect to other people.

Second, we are hardwired to connect to moral meaning and to the possibility of the transcendent.

Meeting these basic needs for connectedness is essential to health and to human flourishing.

These data, and our reflections on them, lead us in turn to a fundamental conclusion and recommendation: We believe that building and strengthening authoritative communities is likely to be our society's best strategy for ameliorating the current crisis of childhood and improving the lives of U.S. children and adolescents.

Here's the core proposition: *Authoritative communities are groups that live out the types of connectedness that our children increasingly lack.*

Here's the core rationale: *If children are hardwired to connect, and if the current ecology of childhood is leading to a weakening of connectedness and therefore to growing numbers of suffering children, building and renewing authoritative communities is arguably the greatest imperative that we face as a society.*

The 10 Main Characteristics of an Authoritative Community

Here's the definition: As an ideal type,[123] an authoritative community (or authoritative social institution) has 10 main characteristics:

1. It is a social institution that includes children and youth.
2. It treats children as ends in themselves.
3. It is warm and nurturing.
4. It establishes clear limits and expectations.
5. The core of its work is performed largely by nonspecialists.
6. It is multigenerational.
7. It has a long-term focus.
8. It reflects and transmits a shared understanding of what it means to be a good person.
9. It encourages spiritual and religious development.
10. It is philosophically oriented to the equal dignity of all persons and to the principle of love of neighbor.

This definition owes much to the work of others. It is largely consistent with a number of previous attempts to think environmentally and institutionally about problems facing U.S. children and youth. Several decades ago, Diana Baumrind coined the term *authoritative parenting*, distinguishing it as superior to permissive, authoritarian, and neglectful parenting.[124] Since then, numerous studies have shown that authoritative parenting—warm and involved, but also firm in establishing guidelines, limits, and expectations—tends to correlate with the best psychological and behavioral outcomes for children.[125] Indeed, for this reason, one of the chief missions of what we are calling authoritative communities is to help parents be authoritative parents.

James P. Comer of Yale University, in his work with the New Haven, Connecticut, public schools, has done much to show how schools can improve children's education, and their lives, by becoming authoritative communities.[126] Martin Seligman and the positive psychology movement have attempted to identify those individual, family, and communal characteristics that promote psychological heartiness, resilience, and character strengths.[127]

Search Institute of Minneapolis has proposed 40 "assets" that contribute to optimal child and youth development. These include external or community assets, such as "family support" and the availability of "youth programs," as well as internal or characterological assets, such as high "achievement motivation" and a "sense of purpose" in life.[128]

In recent years, scholars such as Robert N. Bellah,[129] Peter L. Berger,[130] Don Eberly,[131] Amitai Etzioni,[132] Francis Fukuyama,[133] Robert D. Putnam,[134] and others[135] have helped to launch an important national discussion of the importance of "mediating structures" and "civil society" in addressing both youth problems and overall societal vitality.

We are grateful for, and depend on, these and other contributions. The primary value of *authoritative community* as an analytic and diagnostic tool is that it seeks to spell out those basic group traits or qualities that, across a wide diversity of social institutions, appear to be most likely to improve probabilities for U.S. children and youth.

What exactly do authoritative communities look like? How does being in one feel? Looking from the outside, how can we tell more precisely whether a particular group is or is not one? Let's go through the 10 major characteristics, examining each one in a bit more detail.

1. *It is a social institution that includes children and youth.*

Whatever their other virtues, neither the U.S. Army nor AARP (formerly the American Association of Retired Persons) meets this criterion. Families with children, including extended families, do. So do all civic, educational, recreational, community service, business, cultural, and religious groups that serve or include persons under age 18. There are a lot of them. They come in all shapes and sizes. The diversity is astonishing. One of them that almost everyone has heard of is the YMCA—the organization that is helping to sponsor this report.

Even relatively informal institutions can meet the standard. The weekly Father–Daughter Saturday morning pancake breakfast at the downtown

Kiwanis Club, and the without-an-office, volunteer-run "Mommy and Me" group that involves 10 neighborhood families and gets together when it can, would be two examples.

2. *It treats children as ends in themselves.*

The rule is not that children can never be treated instrumentally, as a means to an end, such as winning a trophy at the debate tournament, or the basketball championship, or having the largest school band in the district, or selling lots of cookies. The rule is that children can never be treated merely as means to an end and that they must always, at the same time, be treated as ends in themselves. Authoritative communities, according to this criterion, relate to the whole person of the child and care about the child for his or her own sake.

3. *It is warm and nurturing.*

Rules matter, but so do close relationships. The central importance for the child of attachment and connectedness to others is a central theme of this report.[136] To frame the issue negatively, a style that combines firm rules for the child with cold, distant relationships with adult caregivers is not authoritative. It is authoritarian, and its consequences for children are usually less than optimal.[137] To frame the issue positively, children typically learn to be what they admire, and having warm, nurturing relationships with admirable adults is arguably the single finest way to help children learn.

4. *It establishes clear limits and expectations.*

Close relationships matter, but so do clear rules and expectations. Children need adults to set clear standards and a positive vision of the goals they are to achieve and the people they are to become. Again, to frame the issue negatively, a style that combines warmth and affection for the child with no, or few, or unclear, limits and boundaries—and therefore few if any clear adult expectations regarding the child's conduct and character—is not authoritative. It is what Diana Baumrind and others call permissive, and its consequences are also less than optimal.[138]

5. *The core of its work is performed largely by nonspecialists.*

Specialists and experts have their place. Some leaders may even have professional degrees. But in authoritative communities, the main action is largely in other hands. Accordingly, while many (though by no means all) authoritative communities pay some individuals to do work, and while many may rely, at least in part, on various types of professionals and various forms of expertise, the basic ethos and mode of operation of an authoritative community differ from those of fully "professionalized" and expert-led organizations. Authoritative communities are more likely to be largely defined and guided by family members, volunteers, and citizen-leaders.[139]

Further, although many authoritative communities may value and seek to make use of technocratic efficiency—arguably the hallmark theme of modern professionalism—technocratic efficiency is seldom their basic purpose or style. In this regard, language is often revealing. Authoritative communities are less likely to use words such as *client* or *services*, for example, and more likely to use words such as *neighbor*, *friend*, and *family*. They are also more likely to employ moral reasoning and offer moral judgments.

6. *It is multigenerational.*

An authoritative community ideally brings together people of all ages: the young, the middle-aged, and the old. A sizable body of scholarship confirms what most people sense intuitively: Children benefit enormously from being around caring people in all stages of the life cycle. They benefit in special ways from being around old people, including, of course, their grandparents.[140]

In addition, a community that is multigenerational is significantly more likely to reflect, as a core part of its identity, the quality of *shared memory*, a key dimension of human connectedness and a vital component of civil society. Shared memory says: This is where we came from. This is what happened. This helps explain why we are who we are. We heard the stories; we tell the children; we remember.

Shared memory can help to deepen identity and define character, largely by giving the child clear access to lessons and admirable persons from the past. In this way, shared memory can deepen our connectedness not just to other persons currently living but also to persons who have died, and also, in some respects, to persons not yet born.

7. *It has a long-term focus.*

Me first. Instant gratification. What have you done for me lately? These are some of the slogans of a social environment in which all connections to others, even including marriages, are increasingly viewed as contingent, nonpermanent, and prospectively short-term. Perhaps the most celebrated observer of American democracy, Alexis de Tocqueville, called this set of values "individualism" and warned at length of its capacity eventually to separate the American from ancestors, descendants, and contemporaries, throwing him "back forever upon himself alone" and threatening in the end "to confine him entirely within the solitude of his own heart."[141]

An authoritative community cuts the other way. It connects us to others and to posterity in ways that extend our time horizon.[142] An authoritative community cares about today and tomorrow, but it also recognizes and takes into account the immediate and distant future—often including, especially in the case of religious organizations, the perspective of eternity. An authoritative community cares about the children of its children. For this reason, authoritative communities are more likely to generate two social realities that, especially from the perspective of child well-being, are vital to human flourishing: first, enduring and frequently permanent relationships with others; and, second, trust.[143]

8. *It reflects and transmits a shared understanding of what it means to be a good person.*

The psychologist Jerome Kagan of Harvard University says, "After hunger, a human's most important need is to know what's virtuous."[144] More than anyone or anything else, authoritative communities must and can meet this basic human need.

For this reason, an authoritative community stands for certain principles and, in its treatment of children, seeks to shape and launch a certain type of person. Put a bit more formally, an authoritative community clearly embodies a substantive conception of the good and includes effective communal support for ethical behavior.

A multigenerational Fencers' Club displays its "Code of Honor" on its wall—members will "graciously extend themselves" to welcome newcomers and will "treat themselves, each other, and our facility with the highest degree of respect"—and requires its members to follow it. A YMCA summer camp teaches children the motto "Better Faithful Than Famous." And the children know and appreciate what it means. A high school teaches the value of respect for others by requiring it, and teaches the meaning of charity in part by encouraging students to do charitable things. A mother tells her teenage son, "That's not what we do in this family." And the son knows and appreciates what she means. These are examples of authoritative communities demonstrating and teaching conceptions of what it means to be a good person and lead an ethical life.

Because of our society's philosophical and religious pluralism, and because of the remarkable complexity and variety of our civil society, these institutionally embodied conceptions of the good will be richly diverse and anything but uniform, even as there is some area of common moral ground. In a pluralistic society, there is great diversity among authoritative communities.

9. *It encourages spiritual and religious development.*

An authoritative community recognizes that religious and spiritual expression is a natural part of personhood.

Pretending that children's religious and spiritual needs do not exist, or arguing that it is too hard to address them in ways that respect individual conscience and pluralism, is for an authoritative community a form of denial and even self-defeat.[145]

10. *It is philosophically oriented to the equal dignity of all persons and to the principle of love of neighbor.*

Sometimes also described as either the principle of "equal moral regard" or as the "golden rule" ethic, this credo is also evident in characteristic no. 2 (above) and constitutes what almost all moral philosophers view as the necessary minimum foundation of any philosophical stance consistent with basic human and moral values.

The principle that one should love one's neighbor as oneself is found in many religions.[146] For believers, the call to neighbor love commonly flows from the belief that all persons are created in the image of God. But the "golden rule" ethic is not restricted to religion, nor does it require or presuppose religious reasoning for its validity. In the late 18th century, the German philosopher Immanuel Kant, in the second formulation of his so-called categorical imperative, famously insisted that "all rational beings stand under the law that each of them should treat himself and all others never merely as means but always at the same time as an end in himself."[147]

Today, that basic principle, which can also be summarized as the principle of equal human dignity, is the starting point for almost all liberal moral thought. It has become the essential universal moral law. In our own country, the signers of the U.S. Declaration of Independence in 1776 affirmed as a "self-evident" truth—made clear by both "Nature and Nature's God"—the idea that all persons possess equal dignity ("all men are created equal"). In 1863, President Abraham Lincoln echoed the Declaration in his Gettysburg Address when he insisted that, at its core, the United States is "dedicated to the proposition" of equal human dignity. Internationally, the United Nations Universal Declaration of Human Rights of 1948 states in Article 1, "All human beings are born free and equal in dignity and rights."

Including this philosophical orientation as a basic trait of authoritative communities is important because, as many analysts of civil society point out, there are examples of immoral, and therefore harmful, civil society. (An example would be the Ku Klux Klan.) Therefore, any formal institutional definition, or ideal type, must necessarily address the issue of morality.

At the same time, it is important to stress that the call to neighbor love and the principle of equal human dignity constitute a floor, not a ceiling. They are necessary philosophical starting points, but they are only starting points. Many—probably most—real-life authoritative communities will clearly embody and seek to pass on to children numerous other moral norms and specific spiritual and religious values that richly add to, without negating, the foundational moral principle.

What Happens When Authoritative Communities Get Weaker?

In recent years, social institutions reflecting these 10 characteristics appear to have gotten significantly weaker in the United States.

For starters, consider the family, arguably the first and most basic association of civil society, and a central example of what should be an authoritative community. The family is usually the source of the most enduring and formative relationships in a child's life. As 24 civil society scholars and leaders put it in 1998: "As an institution, the family's distinguishing trait is its powerful combination of love, discipline, and permanence. Accordingly, families can teach standards of personal conduct that cannot be enforced by law, but which are indispensable traits for democratic civil society."[148] These traits include honesty, trust, loyalty, cooperation, self-restraint, civility, compassion, personal responsibility, and respect for others.[149]

Over the course of three decades, from the mid-1960s through at least the mid-1990s, U.S. families overall got steadily weaker. For example, during these years, U.S. adults became significantly less likely to get and be married.[150] Marriage is important in part because it is one of society's principal ways of supporting and sustaining the consistent, enduring, nurturing relationships that children require of parents and kin.[151]

Structurally, very high rates of divorce[152] and increasing rates of unwed childbearing[153] have led in recent decades to a significant disintegration of the two-parent family. One result of this trend is that, virtually with each passing year, a smaller and smaller proportion of U.S. children are living with their own biological, married parents.[154] One particularly harmful aspect of this trend is the widespread absence of fathers in children's lives.[155] Another related aspect is the effective disconnection in our society of so many adult males from what the psychiatrist Erik Erikson called generativity, or the concern for establishing and guiding the next generation.[156]

Finally, this particular community's loss of authority has been not only structural but also broadly cultural. As a social value, familism has lost much ground in recent decades to other and in some cases competing values, such as individualism and consumerism.

Since about 1995, a number of these family-weakening demographic trends appear to have either slowed down considerably or come to a halt. Some evidence suggests the proportion of U.S. children living in homes headed by married couples (now about 73%) may even have increased slightly since the late 1990s. Similarly, the number of U.S. children residing with two biological parents may also have increased in recent years.[157] Among African Americans, for example, there has been a clear increase since 1995 in the proportion of children living in two-parent, married-couple homes.[158] Some recent research also suggests that U.S. rates of divorce are modestly decreasing[159] and that levels of reported marital happiness, which declined steadily from the early 1970s through the early 1990s, have stabilized and may be slightly increasing.[160]

This is good news. But these recent changes, though suggestive, are not large or definitive, and it remains to be seen whether the decades-old trend toward family fragmentation in the United States is about to be replaced by a trend toward reintegration. Much of the answer, of course, will depend on what U.S. leaders and citizens in the near future choose to value and decide to do.

For children, the family is the first and probably most important authoritative community. But what are the trends regarding the vitality of the many other relationships-rich, values-shaping institutions of U.S. civil society?[161] There has been much recent scholarly research in this area, much of it prompted by and centered on Robert D. Putnam's now famous 1995 essay, "Bowling Alone," and his book, *Bowling Alone: The Collapse and Revival of American Community*, published in 2000.[162]

Putnam presents evidence suggesting that the great majority of U.S. social institutions focusing on what he terms civic engagement—political clubs and parties, civic and community groups based on face-to-face relation-ships and activities, houses of worship and other religious organizations, unions and other workplace associations, philanthropic organizations, and a vast array of informal social networks and institutions, from card-playing groups to family meals—have declined significantly in recent decades. In the late 1990s, Putnam's thesis was widely debated by scholars. This scholarly attention has been fruitful and has led to some valuable findings and important qualifications.[163] But today there is also a rough scholarly consensus: Putnam was right. Those U.S. social institutions that most directly build and sustain our connectedness to one another and to shared meaning have deteriorated significantly in recent decades.

So here is the story thus far: on the one hand, a large body of evidence, including recent findings from the field of neuroscience, suggesting that the human person is hardwired to connect to other people and to moral and spiritual meaning; and on the other hand, a long-term weakening of precisely those social groups that connect us to one another and to shared meaning. Is it logical to conclude that the diminishment of these authoritative communities is at least partly responsible for the steady rise in the proportion of U.S. children suffering from mental, emotional, and behavioral problems? We believe that the answer is yes.

Other scholars seem to agree with us. A recent analysis of 269 studies, dating back to the 1950s, links steady increases in self-reported anxiety and depression among U.S. young people primarily to the decline of "social connectedness."[164] A major population-based study from Sweden—that is, a study focusing on *all* Swedish children—concludes that children living in one-parent homes have more than double the risk of psychiatric disease, suicide or attempted suicide, and alcohol-related disease, and more than three times the risk of drug-related disease, compared with Swedish children living in two-parent homes. These findings remained after the scholars controlled for a wide range of demographic and socioeconomic variables.[165]

To us, the Swedish study is important not only because of its large scale and rigorous controls[166] but also because Sweden has long been a world leader in developing social policies that ameliorate the economic and material consequences of growing up in one-parent homes. As a result, the higher rates of mental and emotional problems experienced by Swedish children in one-parent homes would appear to be less likely to stem solely or even primarily from economic circumstances. Obviously, the lack of money can be a critical problem. But another obviously important—and partially independent—problem is the fracturing of the child's primary authoritative community.[167]

Looking more broadly at organizations and institutions that help to build what some scholars call social capital[168] by fostering face-to-face civic engagement, Robert Putnam carried out a small but fascinating experiment in *Bowling Alone* to test the hypothesis that higher levels of social connect-edness correlate with significantly better outcomes for children and youth. On the one hand, he highlighted the Annie E. Casey Foundation's 10 leading indicators of child well-being for 1999 and the foundation's research based on those indicators, which was carried out on a state-by-state basis. Putnam and his colleagues then developed their own list of 14 leading indictors of social connectedness, which they called the Social Capital Index, and similarly carried out their research related to these indicators on a state-by-state basis. Putnam then compared the state rankings on child well-being to the state rankings on social connectedness and social capital. Here is what he found: "Statistically, the correlation between high social capital and positive child development is as close to perfect as social scientists ever find in data analyses of this sort." This robust correlation held true even after Putnam controlled for a range of socioeconomic and demographic characteristics.[169]

Numerous other studies similarly support the proposition that the thinning out of social connectedness is contributing significantly to a range of childhood problems, including child abuse and adolescent depression, and conversely, that thickening the networks of meaningful relationships contributes significantly to better outcomes for children and youth.[170] Combined with the mounting evidence about the harmful consequences of the weakening of marriage and of the two-parent home,[171] these findings lead us to conclude that strengthening authoritative communities is an urgent national priority for all of us who are seeking to understand and confront the crisis of childhood in the United States.

Renewing Authoritative Communities

Of course, as with any set of problems this large and multifaceted, there can be no such thing as the one ideal solution. Many proposals, many solutions, are necessary. We have noted, for example, the great importance of pharmacological and therapeutic interventions and of programs based on the at-risk model of youth services, even as we have insisted on the important limitations of those approaches.

More broadly, our commission, focusing as we have on the spread of mental, emotional, and behavioral problems among U.S. young people, has largely neglected many other issues relevant to children and youth. For example, in this report we touch only briefly upon issues of material insecurity and economic status and well-being. Nor does this report focus directly on issues of physical health.[172] Yet these are obviously important issues, requiring their own careful analyses and recommendations.

At the same time, as a social change goal, and in light of the scientific evidence summarized in this report, we believe that strengthening authoritative communities constitutes a logical and necessary response to the "deconnection" that appears to be contributing to the suffering of so many of our children. For this reason, we recommend and hope to participate in a serious national conversation, leading to sustained national action and directed toward achieving the goal of strengthening authoritative communities.

A brief word about strategy. Building authoritative communities is more an "us" strategy than a "them" strategy. We think that's fitting. "Them" strategies can be valuable and certainly have their place. The main idea linking such strategies is that some other person or group should do something. The experts should focus on it. The professionals should fix it. The media should highlight it. The government should get busy. Parents should wise up. Teenagers should have to. There ought to be money for it; there ought to be a program.

All of us at times have supported "them" strategies, often for very good reasons. But an "us" strategy is quite different. It is much broader and more radical. Its focus is cultural, not merely political or programmatic. It aims less at a specific intervention than a fundamental social shift—a change that involves the society as a whole. A "them" strategy is about getting a specific thing done. An "us" strategy includes getting specific things done, but it is more fundamentally about guiding an entire society in a certain direction.

For obvious reasons, an "us" strategy is much harder to carry out, and in almost every sense is more costly, than a "them" strategy. An "us" strategy is most appropriate for those fundamental societal problems that simply cannot be delegated to specialists or solved by "them." Today's crisis of childhood in the United States is one of those problems—arguably our single most important one.

Most successful movements for social change employ both "them" and "us" strategies. But the deepest and most lasting social changes—think of the impact of the civil rights, women's, and environmental movements—ultimately require something from almost all of us. Regarding the current suffering of our children, we as a commission believe that nothing less than an "us" strategy is adequate to the challenge we face.

Building Authoritative Communities in Low-Income Neighborhoods

What is the relevance of this report's findings for our neediest children living in our poorest, most troubled neighborhoods? Put a bit more sharply, is the basic challenge of revitalizing authoritative communities the same for all of us everywhere, regardless of economic context and neighborhood conditions?

To us, the answer to this last question is both yes and no. The answer is yes, insofar as the basic needs of children, and the importance of authoritative communities, do not vary significantly according to skin color, economic circumstance, or place of residence. Moreover, many youth problems—from early sex to drug use to delinquency to involvement in violence—that some in the past may have tended to view largely as inner-city or poor people's problems are in fact present and spreading today in many middle-class and affluent neighborhoods.[173] In general, "them" problems in our society are getting rarer with each passing year, while "us" problems are becoming more common.

But the answer is also no, insofar as what will be required to renew authoritative communities in tough, low-income neighborhoods is different from, and in many ways more than and harder than, what will be required in our nation's safer, more affluent communities. Building those authoritative communities that can improve the lives of our neediest children will require special, intensive attention and investment—not only from the leaders and residents of these low-income neighborhoods but also from the nation as a whole. This special challenge, as much as any discussed in this report, is an urgent "us" challenge, an important national priority.

What is distinctive—and harder—about this task in low-income neighborhoods? Listen to Ernie Cortés. Besides the civil rights movement, the community organizing movement has emerged as one of the most serious and promising efforts in recent generations for positive social change in low-income neighborhoods. One of the leading organizations in this movement is the Industrial Areas Foundation, and one of the IAF's most prominent organizers is Ernesto Cortés Jr. of San Antonio, Texas.[174] According to Cortés, the processes and methods of effective community organizing are quite different today compared with those used by earlier generations of organizers.

What is the essential difference? In earlier generations, organizers in low-income neighborhoods sought to mobilize a vibrant civil society—families, churches, civic and educational groups, all kinds of neighborhood associations—for social and political change. Today, these forms of civil society frequently cannot be mobilized, because they are too weak and depleted. Too often, they are nonexistent. As a result, the first task of today's community organizer is less to mobilize civil society than to renew and even re-create it. Posing the challenge to today's organizers, Cortés asks: "It's been said *ad nauseam* that it takes a village to raise a child. Well, do we know what it means to build a village?"[175]

We are convinced that building the village—in short, building authoritative communities, in some cases from the ground up—must become a primary goal for all those who are committed to reducing poverty and inequality in the United States and to improving the life prospects of our neediest children.

This challenge must involve the society as a whole, not just government. But to be successful, this work of renewal will also require greater attention and investment from all levels of government. First, the crisis-level weakening and disappearance of authoritative communities in these neighborhoods demand this level of intervention. In addition, a range of other problems in these neighborhoods—joblessness, poverty, crime, lack of medical and mental health care, and others—is making everything harder, including the critical task of revitalizing authoritative communities. Addressing these problems in part through improved public policies is therefore one necessary component of any serious strategy for revitalizing authoritative communities in these neighborhoods.

There are grounds for optimism. Some (though not enough) inspiring work is being done in this area. James P. Comer's work with public schools in New Haven,

Connecticut, has convincingly demonstrated the capacity of public schools in low-income neighborhoods to become genuine authoritative communities.[176]

Recognizing the positive family and civic effects of religious involvement, and also that religious institutions are frequently among the strongest civic institutions in low-income neighborhoods,[177] scholar-leaders such as Robert Michael Franklin, the former president of the Interdenominational Theological Seminary, are examining ways in which urban churches can provide more and better leadership in efforts to rebuild marriage, strengthen fatherhood, and revitalize family and civic life in low-income neighborhoods.[178]

The Annie E. Casey Foundation's "Making Connections" program, launched in 1999, is a major, 10-year investment by the foundation to bring together diverse leadership and organizing coalitions in a number of low-income neighborhoods around the country. A major premise of this initiative is that family strengthening and neighborhood strengthening go together, each enhancing the other.[179]

This insight is important. The community shapes families. A number of scholars have documented the strong community effects on child and family well-being.[180] But causation flows in the other direction as well: Families shape the community.

Consider, for example, the role of marriage. Married couples tend to be more civically engaged.[181] Research also indicates that married-couples families are significantly less likely to experience poverty than other family types, including those with at least two potential earners. Even after controlling for other relevant variables, current research suggests that marriage in low-income neighborhoods can play an independent role in reducing the likelihood of poverty and improving economic well-being.[182]

Some research also suggests that well-functioning marriages in poor communities do more than other close relationships to reduce the likelihood that economic pressure will in turn either cause emotional distress or cause parents to lose confidence in their efficacy as parents.[183]

Linda M. Burton and Anne C. Crouter of Pennsylvania State University, as well as other scholars, have done a series of studies investigating the complex interactions between family structure and process on the one hand, and neighborhood life and development on the other, especially when viewed from the perspective of child and adolescent well-being.[184]

This research, as well as the important community-level work being done by James P. Comer, the Annie E. Casey Foundation, the Industrial Areas Foundation, and numerous others, points toward what we believe can and should be a new model for leaders and organizations working to reduce poverty and inequality in the United States.

This new model seeks to combine the (usually more top-down) professional delivery of social services with a strong focus on bottom-up, citizen-led community organizing. It also seeks to combine the techniques and insights of family therapy and family and marriage education with the techniques and insights of neighborhood empowerment and development.

Social Change

Will we as a society find the will, identify the material and moral resources, and engage in the hard thinking necessary to improve the lives of our children by building and renewing authoritative communities? We do not know. But we do know that the answer to that question is not hardwired, either biologically or historically.

At this time in our society, in this vital area of our communal and civic life, what happens to us will depend mostly on us. Our future in this respect is less an externally structured or preordained process than an event in freedom and an act of choice. In that spirit, and with hope and solidarity, we offer the following goals and recommendations.

Goals

1. To deepen our society's commitment to those values that build and sustain authoritative communities and to reconsider our commitment to those values that often replace or undermine them. The former include enduring marital relationships and family connectedness, community action and civic engagement, and concern for the moral and spiritual well-being of all children. The latter include "me first" and consumerism as ways of living, materialism, and the notion of the individual person as self-made and owing little to others or to society.

2. To increase measurably in the next decade the proportion of U.S. children who are members of authoritative communities and whose lives are improved through their participation in them.

3. To win support for a major shift in public policy, in which policy makers at all levels seek to meet youth needs by utilizing and empowering authoritative communities.

   The old model is essentially mechanistic and problem oriented. It focuses on specific youth deficits and responds to those deficits with direct government regulations and government-initiated programs, often including an emphasis on "new" programs. This directly governmental approach tends to be top-down, bureaucratic, centralized, rigidly secular, ethically bland, and expert driven.

   The new model is essentially ecological. It focuses on what children need to thrive and responds to those needs by building and empowering nearby authoritative communities that can most effectively meet them. The new model therefore tends to favor decentralization, a rich diversity of approaches, moral and spiritual robustness, and community-based leaders. The basic aim of the new model is to improve child well-being by creatively using the tools and resources of public policy to strengthen authoritative communities.

Recommendations

Concerning All Community Members

1. We recommend that all adults examine the degree to which they are positively influencing the lives of children through participating in authoritative communities and try where possible to do a better job.
2. We recommend that all families with children and youth-included organizations and initiatives examine the degree to which they meet the 10 basic criteria for authoritative communities and try where possible to strengthen themselves in accordance with those criteria.[185]

Concerning Families, Neighborhoods, and Workplaces

3. A child's first and typically most important authoritative community is her or his family. We recommend that we reevaluate our behavior and our dominant cultural values, and consider a range of changes in our laws and public policies, in order to increase substantially the proportion of U.S. children growing up with their two married parents who are actively and supportively involved in their lives.
4. We recommend that some U.S. "work-family" advocates change their priorities, putting less emphasis on policies that free up parents to be better workers and more emphasis on policies that free up workers to be better parents and better guides for the next generation. Examples of the latter include flexible and reduced work hours, teleworking, job sharing, part-time work, compressed work weeks, career breaks, job protection and other benefits for short-term (up to 6 months) parental leave, and job preferences and other benefits, such as graduated reentry and educational and training benefits, for long-term (up to 5 years) parental leave. We suspect that, if more leading advocates and analysts were to reconsider their priorities, at least some corporate decision makers might follow suit. Perhaps the new emphasis could be conveyed by a new label, "family-work." This shift would benefit not only families but also neighborhoods and civic life generally.
5. We recommend that large employers reduce the practice of continually uprooting and relocating married couples with children.

Concerning Adolescents

6. We recommend a creative society-wide effort to respond more effectively to adolescents' needs for risk taking, novelty seeking, and peer affiliation. The goal is to provide healthy opportunities for young people to meet these needs in the context of significantly greater adult support, participation, and supervision. "Integral to these efforts," as

Michael Resnick of the University of Minnesota reiterates, "is a philosophical commitment that young people are resources to be developed, not problems to be solved."[186]

7. We recommend that authoritative communities attend more purposively to the gendered needs of adolescents. Equal opportunity and equal rights do not mean that boys and girls have identical patterns of development. The goal is to address their needs for meaning and sexual identity in prosocial ways, including mentoring, rites of passage, opportunities for adventure, exploration and service, discussions about the meaning of fertility, and guidance regarding the appropriate means of managing sexual and aggressive energies. Much more than it is today, adolescence should become a time for adult engagement with, not retreat from, young people.

Concerning Moral and Spiritual Development

8. We recommend that youth-serving organizations purposively seek to promote the moral and spiritual development of children, recognizing that children's moral and spiritual needs are as genuine, and as integral to their personhood, as their physical and intellectual needs. For organizations that include children from diverse religious backgrounds or no religious background, this task admittedly will be difficult. But it need not be impossible and should not be neglected. In a society in which pluralism is a fact and freedom a birthright, finding new ways to strengthen, and not ignore or stunt, children's moral and spiritual selves may be the single most important challenge facing youth service professionals and youth-serving organizations in the United States today.

Concerning Private and Public Resources

9. We recommend that a major funding priority for philanthropists who want to help children at risk should be the goal of empowering and extending the influence of authoritative communities.

10. We recommend that corporate foundations and charitable giving programs reconsider the practice of refusing even to consider giving grants to faith-based organizations whose mission is to improve the lives of children.

There is nothing inherently improper about religiously informed efforts to help children, and these efforts, just like purely secular efforts, should be judged strictly by the (secular) results that they produce. The issue is understandably difficult and complex. In a pluralistic society such as ours, there are significant differences in viewpoints and values, and tolerance for these differences is essential. But religious and philosophical pluralism is a challenge to be embraced, not avoided by arbitrary exclusiveness.

11. We recommend that the U.S. Congress, as well as state legislators, shift their approach to providing social services for children, seeking wherever possible to use and empower authoritative communities to deliver services and meet human needs.

12. We recommend a special national commitment of both private and public energy and resources to rebuild authoritative communities in disadvantaged, low-income neighborhoods.

13. With Isabel V. Sawhill of the Brookings Institution and her colleagues,[187] we recommend that, in order to improve the life prospects of children in low-income families and neighborhoods, the United States in the near term allocate an additional 1% of its gross domestic product to children, and especially to the goal of strengthening those authoritative communities that affect the lives of children in low-income, troubled neighborhoods.

14. We recommend that the U.S. Congress create a new federal tax credit for individual contributions of up to $500 ($1,000 for married couples) to charitable organizations whose primary purpose is improving the lives of children and youth.

    The goals of this policy change are to increase charitable giving and volunteerism and to diversify and decentralize the financial supports for authoritative communities and other nonprofit youth-serving organizations.

Concerning Scholars

15. We recommend more and stronger partnerships between scholars and youth-serving organizations. Access to relevant research findings, scholarly analysis, and evaluation tools can help youth leaders do a better job. Connectedness to front-line leaders and local communities and organizations can help scholars do a better job, both professionally and as individuals.

16. Building in part on Robert Putnam's work showing correlations between high levels of social capital and good outcomes for children, we recommend that interested scholars develop scientific measures of the reach and effects of authoritative communities in the United States.

    Doing this work would permit scholars to examine correlations between authoritative communities and child outcomes. It would also permit scholars to develop data, including trend line data, on the vitality of U.S. authoritative communities and their precise effects on child well-being.

17. We recommend that scholars and others consider revising their methodology to include families in the definition of civil society.

    This issue might at first glance appear to be of purely academic interest, but it is not. Conceptually separating families from civil society has many practical consequences—most of which, in our view, tend to be unhelpful and even potentially harmful. For example, based in part on this conceptual exclusion of families from civil society, researchers and policy makers often simply assume that family structure is not a legitimate area for inclusion in policy recommendations.[188] It is. More generally, as this report has tried to demonstrate, it is important for policy makers and society as a whole (not just scholars) to view the environment of childhood holistically, transcending the largely arbitrary intellectual dichotomy between family life and civic and public life.[189]

Concerning Immediate Next Steps

18. We recommend that youth service and civic leaders across the country, drawing on this report as well as other resources, help to lead a new and sustained national conversation about the crisis of childhood in the United States and the most effective ways to meet that crisis.

Authoritative Communities: A Summary

The 10 Main Planks

1. The mechanisms by which we become and stay attached to others are biologically primed and increasingly discernible in the basic structure of the brain.
2. Nurturing environments, or the lack of them, affect gene transcription and the development of brain circuitry.
3. The old "nature versus nurture" debate—focusing on whether heredity or environment is the main determinant of human conduct—is no longer relevant to serious discussions of child well-being and youth programming.
4. Adolescent risk taking and novelty seeking are connected to changes in brain structure and function.
5. Assigning meaning to gender in childhood and adolescence is a human universal that deeply influences well-being.
6. The beginning of morality is the biologically primed moralization of attachment.
7. The ongoing development of morality in later childhood and adolescence involves the human capacity to idealize individuals and ideas.
8. Primary nurturing relationships influence early spiritual development—call it the spiritualization of attachment—and spiritual development can influence us biologically in the same ways that primary nurturing relationships do.
9. Religiosity and spirituality significantly influence well-being.
10. The human brain appears to be organized to ask ultimate questions and seek ultimate answers.

The 10 Main Characteristics of an Authoritative Community

1. It is a social institution that includes children and youth.
2. It treats children as ends in themselves.
3. It is warm and nurturing.
4. It establishes clear limits and expectations.
5. The core of its work is performed largely by nonspecialists.
6. It is multigenerational.
7. It has a long-term focus.
8. It reflects and transmits a shared understanding of what it means to be a good person.
9. It encourages spiritual and religious development.
10. It is philosophically oriented to the equal dignity of all persons and to the principle of love of neighbor.

The Commission on Children At Risk

Peter L. Benson, Search Institute; Elizabeth Berger, American Academy of Child and Adolescent Psychiatry; David Blankenhorn, Institute for American Values; T. Berry Brazelton, Harvard Medical School; Robert Coles, Harvard University; James P. Comer, Yale University; William J. Doherty, University of Minnesota; Kenneth L. Gladish, YMCA of the USA; David Gutmann, Northwestern University; Thomas R. Insel, Emory University; Leonard A. Jason, DePaul University; Byron R. Johnson, Baylor University; Robert Karen, Adelphi University; Kathleen Kovner Kline, Dartmouth Medical School; Susan Linn, Harvard Medical School; Arthur C. Maerlender Jr., Dartmouth Medical School; Lisa Miller, Columbia University; Andrew B. Newberg, University of Pennsylvania; Stephanie K. Newberg, Pennsylvania Council for Relationships; Stephen G. Post, Case Western Reserve University; Alvin F. Poussaint, Harvard Medical School; Michael D. Resnick, University of Minnesota; Allan N. Schore, UCLA School of Medicine; Christian Smith, University of North Carolina at Chapel Hill; Linda Patia Spear, Binghamton University; Bill Stanczykiewicz, Indiana Youth Institute; Barbara M. Stilwell, Indiana University School of Medicine; Stephen J. Suomi, National Institute of Child Health and Human Development; Paul C. Vitz, New York University, Emeritus; Judith Wallerstein, Center for the Family in Transition; W. Bradford Wilcox, University of Virginia; Larry J. Young, Emory University.

Notes

1. J. Eccles & J. Appleton Gootman (eds.), *Community programs to promote youth development* (Washington, DC: National Academies Press, 2002).
2. *Mental health: A report of the Surgeon General* (Rockville, MD: U.S. Department of Health and Human Services, Substance Abuse and

Mental Health Services Administration, Center for Mental Health Services, National Institutes of Health, National Institute of Mental Health, 1999): 123.

3. R. J. Haggerty, "Child health 2000: New pediatrics in the changing environment of children's needs in the 21st century," *Pediatrics*, 96 (1995): 807–808; "Mental illness: More children are on prescription drugs for psychiatric disorders," *Mental Health Weekly Digest*, January 27, 2003.

4. *Practice parameters for the assessment and treatment of children and adolescents with depressive disorders* (Washington, DC: American Academy of Child and Adolescent Psychiatry, 1998): 2.

5. J. M. Twenge, "The age of anxiety? Birth cohort change in anxiety and neuroticism, 1952–1993," *Journal of Personality and Social Psychology*, 79, no. 6 (2000): 1007–1021.

6. P. G. Surtees & N. W. Wainwright, "Fragile states of mind: Neuroticism, vulnerability and the long-term outcome of depression," *British Journal of Psychiatry*, 169, no. 3 (1996): 338–347; R. M. Bagby, R. T. Joffe, J. D. A. Parker, V. Kalemba, & K. L. Harkness, "Major depression and the five-factor model of personality," *Journal of Personality Disorders*, 9 (1995): 224–234.

7. W. H. Coryell, R. Noyes, & J. D. House, "Mortality among outpatients with anxiety disorders," *American Journal of Psychiatry*, 143, no. 4 (1986): 508–510. A recent British study reports that about 10% of U.K. teenagers ages 15 to 16 have committed acts of deliberate self-harm. See *Youth and self harm: Perspectives* (Oxford: University of Oxford, Centre for Suicide Research, 2003).

8. D. L. Chambless, J. Cherney, G. C. Caputo, & B. J. G. Rheinstein, "Anxiety disorders and alcoholism: A study with inpatient alcoholics," *Journal of Anxiety Disorders*, 1 (1987): 29–40.

9. K. D. O'Leary & D. A. Smith, "Marital interactions," *Journal Review of Psychology*, 42 (1991): 191–212.

10. R. J. Edelman, *Anxiety: Theory, research and intervention in clinical and health psychology* (New York: John Wiley, 1992).

11. World Health Organization, *Health behavior in school-aged children, 1996* [Electronic file] (Calverton, MD: Macro International, 2001); S. Matthey & P. Petrovski, "The Children's Depression Inventory: Error in cutoff scores for screening purposes," *Psychological Assessment*, 14, no. 2 (2002): 146–149.

12. "Youth risk behavior surveillance: United States, 2001," *Morbidity and Mortality Weekly Report*, 51 , no. SS-4 (Washington, DC: Centers for Disease Control and Prevention, 2002).

13. S. A. Benton, J. M. Robertson, W.-C. Tseng, F. B. Newton, & S. L. Benton, "Changes in counseling center client problems across 13 years," *Professional Psychology: Research and Practice*, 34 , no. 1 (2003): 66–72.

14. *National Conference on Research in Child Welfare*, June 21, 1999 [Electronic file] (St. Paul, MN: Amherst H. Wilder Foundation, 1999); B. D. Fabry, A. L. Reitz, & W. C. Luster, "Community treatment of extremely troublesome youth with dual health/mental retardation diagnoses: A data based case study," *Education and Treatment of Children*, 25, no. 3 (August 2002): 339.

15. *Children at risk: State trends 1990–2000* (Baltimore: Annie E. Casey Foundation, 2002).

16. P. Scommegna, "New index tracks children's well-being," *Population Today*, 29, no. 8 (2001): 1–3. See also Federal Interagency Forum on Child and Family Statistics, *America's children: Key national indicators of well-being, 2002* (Washington, DC: Government Printing Office, July 2002); *Trends in the well-being of America's children and youth, 2000* (Washington, DC: U.S. Department of Health and Human Services, 2000); and "A century of children's health and well-being" (Washington, DC: Child Trends, December 1999). See also *The Child Indicator*, especially vol. 3, no. 4 (Washington, DC: Child Trends, 2001). For international comparisons and perspectives, see J. Micklewright & K. Stewart, *The welfare of Europe's children* (Bristol, U.K.: Policy Press, 2000); Jonathan Bradshaw (ed.), *The well-being of children in the U.K.* (Plymouth, U.K.: Plymbridge, 2002).

17. The fertility rate of unmarried teenagers has fallen in recent years from its high point of 46.4 births per 1,000 unmarried women ages 15 to 19 in 1994 to 37.4 in 2001. See *Births to unmarried women—End of the increase?* (Washington, DC: AmeriStat, Population Reference Bureau, 2003).

18. *Teen pregnancy, 1999* (Washington, DC: Centers for Disease Control and Prevention, 2001).

19. "Youth risk behavior surveillance: United States, 2001," *Morbidity and Mortality Weekly Report, 51*, no. SS-4 (Washington, DC: Centers for Disease Control and Prevention, 2002).

20. Ibid.

21. *Tracking the hidden epidemics: Trends in STDs in the United States, 2000* (Washington, DC: Centers for Disease Control and Prevention, 2001).

22. "Youth risk behavior surveillance: United States, 2001," *Morbidity and Mortality Weekly Report, 51*, no. SS-4 (Washington, DC: Centers for Disease Control and Prevention, June 2002).

23. National Center for Education Statistics, *Digest of Education Statistics, 2000* (Washington, DC: U.S. Department of Education, 2001).

24. "Youth risk behavior surveillance: United States, 2001," *Morbidity and Mortality Weekly Report, 51*, no. SS-4 (Washington, DC: Centers for Disease Control and Prevention, 2002).

25. "Death rates for leading causes of death among persons 1-24 years of age: United States, 1950–1999" (Hyattsville, MD: National Center for Health Statistics, 2002). See also E. Durkheim, *Suicide: A study in sociology* (New York: Free Press, 1951).

26. For more information and analysis regarding mental health trends among U.S. children and youth, see Appendix A of the complete report (available at www.americanvalues.org).

27. R. A. Hummer et al., "Race/ethnicity, nativity, and infant mortality in the United States," *Social Forces*, 77, no. 3 (1999): 1083–1118.

28. D. J. Hernandez & E. Charney (eds.), *From generation to generation: The health and well-being of children in immigrant families* (Washington DC: National Academy Press, 1998): 5–6, 107.

29. One indicator (but by no means the only indicator) of this underinvestment is the shortage of child and adolescent psychiatrists in the United States. For example: "While the U.S. Bureau of Health Professions projects that the number of child and adolescent psychiatrists will increase by about thirty percent to 8,312 by 2020 if the funding and recruitment remain stable at the current level, this is far less than the estimated 12,624 needed to meet demand." See *Critical shortage of child and adolescent psychiatrists* (Washington, DC: American Academy of Child and Adolescent Psychiatry, Work Force Fact Sheet, November 28, 2001).

30. S. McLanahan & G. Sandefur, *Growing up with a single parent: What hurts, what helps* (Cambridge, MA: Harvard University Press, 1994): 40–43; S.-L. Pong & D.-B. Ju, "The effects of change in family structure and income on dropping out of middle or high school," *Journal of Family Issues*, 21 (March 2000): 147–169; R. B. McNeal Jr., "Extracurricular activities and high school dropouts," *Sociology of Education*, 68 (1995): 62–81.

31. *Mental health: A report of the Surgeon General* (Rockville, MD: U.S. Department of Health and Human Services, Substance Abuse and Mental Health Services Administration, Center for Mental Health Services, National Institutes of Health, National Institute of Mental Health, 1999): 63–64.

32. The word *hardwired*, which we use throughout this report and include in the report's title, is more a metaphor than a technical term. We use it here to mean biologically primed and discernible in the basic structure and systems of the brain.

33. Schore continues: "If these things go awry, you're going to have seeds of psychological problems, of difficulty coping, stress in human relations, substance abuse, those sorts of problems later on." Quoted in B. Carey, "Shaping the connection: Studies renew interest in effects of the parent-child bond," *Los Angeles Times*, March 31, 2003. See also J. Kendall, "Fierce attachments," *Boston Globe*, June 29, 2003.

34. A. N. Schore, *Affect dysregulation and disorders of the self* (New York: W.W. Norton, 2003): xv; see also Schore, *Affect regulation and the origin of the self: The neurobiology of emotional development* (Mahwah, NJ: Lawrence Erlbaum, 1994) and *Affect regulation and repair of the self* (New York: W.W. Norton, 2003).

35. L. J. Young, D. D. Francis, & T. R. Insel, "The Biochemistry of Family Commitment and Youth Competence: Lessons from Furry Mammals," Commission on Children at Risk, Working Paper 18 (New York: Institute for American Values, 2002) (chapter 2, this volume). See also T. R. Insel & L. J. Young, "The neurobiology of attachment," *Nature Reviews Neuroscience*, 2, no. 2 (2001): 129–136.

36. A. Dixson & L. George, "Prolactin and parental behaviour in a male New World primate," *Nature*, 299 (1982): 551–553.

37. S. Taylor, *The tending instinct: How nurturing is essential to who we are and how we live* (New York: Times Books, 2002).

38. R. A. Turner, M. Altemus, T. Enos, B. Cooper, & T. L. McGuinness, "Preliminary research on plasma oxytocin in normal cycling women: Investigating emotional and interpersonal distress," *Psychiatry: Interpersonal and Biological Processes*, 62, no. 2 (1999): 77–114.

39. C. Pedersen & A. Prange, "Induction of maternal behavior in virgin rats after intracerebroventricular administration of oxytocin," *Proceedings of the National Academy of Sciences of the United States of America*, 76, no. 12 (1979): 6661–6665.

40. P. B. Gray, S. M. Kahlenberg, E. S. Barrett, S. F. Lipson, & P. T. Ellison, "Marriage and fatherhood are associated with lower testosterone levels in males," *Evolution and Human Behavior*, 23 (2002): 193–201. See also A. Mazur & J. Michalek, "Marriage, divorce, and male testosterone," *Social Forces*, 77 (1998): 315–320; A. Booth & J. M. Dabbs Jr., "Testosterone and men's marriages," *Social Forces*, 72 (1993): 463–477.

41. J. K. Kiecolt-Glaser, L. McGuire, T. Robles, & R. Glaser, "Psychoneuroimmunology: Psychological influences on immune function and health," *Journal of Consulting and Clinical Psychology*, 70, no. 3 (2002): 537–547; J. K. Kiecolt-Glaser & T. L. Newton, "Marriage and health: His and hers," *Psychological Bulletin*, 127, no. 4 (2001): 472–503; Kiecolt-Glaser et al., "Marital conflict and endocrine function: Are men really more physiologically affected than women?" *Journal of Consulting and Clinical Psychology*, 64, no. 2 (1996): 324–332; W. B. Malarkey, J. K. Kiecolt-Glaser, D. Pearl, & R. Glaser, "Hostile behavior during marital conflict alters pituitary and adrenal hormones," *Psychosomatic Medicine*, 56 (1994): 41–51; Kiecolt-Glaser et al., "Negative behavior during marital conflict is associated with immunological down-regulation," *Psychosomatic Medicine*, 55 (1993): 395–409. In another study, these researchers found that changes in hormone levels are more accurate than what spouses say about the quality of the marriage as predictors of marital success and divorce. See Janice K. Kiecolt-Glaser, C. Bane, R. Glalser, & W. B. Malarkey, "Love, marriage, and divorce: Newlyweds' stress hormones foreshadow relationship changes," *Journal of Clinical and Consulting Psychology*, 71, no. 1 (2003): 176–188. Related findings on the connection between marriage and improved health for women and men are reported in David De Vaus, "Marriage and mental health," *Family Matters*, 62 (2002): 26–32.

42. A brief word about animal studies. We should never simply assume that findings from animal studies pertain directly, or even indirectly, to humans. But in some cases, findings from animal studies are at least suggestive. Moreover, in practical terms, studies involving animals are important and necessary for students of human society, because these studies have numerous advantages that could never, or almost never, be present in studies of humans. For example, in the case of studying humans, it is typically impossible to include control groups. To take another example, because the human life cycle is so much longer than that of most other animals, studies focusing on questions of intergenerational transmission over time must typically involve animal subjects.

43. L. J. Young et al., "The biochemistry of family commitment and youth competence: Lessons from furry mammals," Commission on Children at Risk, Working Paper 18 (New York: Institute for American Values, 2002): 13 (chapter 2, this volume).

44. Ibid., 14.

45. M. J. Meaney, "Maternal care, gene expression, and the transmission of individual differences in stress reactivity across generations," *Annual Review of Neuroscience, 24* (2001): 1161–1192. We are not stating that the genes themselves have changed. We are stating that social environment can affect genes at the level of transcription. To use an analogy, if we imagine genes as an alphabet, social environments can affect which letters of this alphabet are transcribed, how often they are transcribed, and in what order they are transcribed, which in turn will help to determine the makeup or content of the "words" that are the biochemical messengers in our nervous system. Thus, we can begin to glimpse the complexity and even beauty of this nature–nurture dance. Environment has influenced genetic transcription in the parental generation, which helps to shape parental behavior, which in turn influences genetic transcription in the offspring's generation, which helps to shape the offspring's parental behavior.

46. For example, studies of institutionalized children in Romania suggest that a severely degraded social environment can result in enduring biological as well as psychological dysfunction. See M. Carlson & F. Earls, "Social ecology and the development of stress regulation," in L. R. Bergman, R. B. Cairns, L.-G. Nilsson, & L. Nystedt (eds.), *Developmental science and the holistic approach* (Mahwah, NJ: Lawrence Erlbaum, 2000): 229–248.

47. See L. J. Martin, D. M. Spicer, M. H. Lewis, J. P. Gluck, & L. C. Cork, "Social deprivation of infant rhesus monkeys alters the chemoarchitecture of the brain: Subcortical regions," *Journal of Neuroscience, 11* (1991): 3347–3358.

48. B. J. Ellis, S. McFadyen-Ketchum, K. A. Dodge, G. A. Pettit, & J. E. Bates, "Quality of early family relationships and individual differences in the timing of pubertal maturation in girls: A longitudinal test of

an evolutionary model," *Journal of Personality and Social Psychology*, 77, no. 2 (1999): 387–401; B. J. Ellis & J. Garber, "Psychosocial antecedents of variation in girls' pubertal timing: Maternal depression, stepfather presence, and marital and family stress," *Child Development*, 71, no. 2 (2000): 485–501.

49. See also D. S. Moore, *The dependent gene: The fallacy of nature versus nurture* (New York: W. H. Freeman, 2002).

50. S. J. Suomi, "Developmental trajectories, early experiences, and community consequences," in D. P. Keating & C. Hertzman (eds.), *Developmental health and the wealth of nations: Social, biological, and educational dynamics* (New York: Guilford Press, 1999): 189–200.

51. S. J. Suomi, "How mother nurture helps mother nature: Scientific evidence for the protective effect of good nurturing on genetic propensity toward anxiety and alcohol abuse," Commission on Children at Risk, Working Paper 14 (New York: Institute for American Values, 2002): 18–19 (chapter 3, this volume); see also S. J. Suomi, "Attachment in rhesus monkeys," in J. Cassidy & P. R. Shaver (eds.), *Handbook of attachment: Theory, research, and clinical applications* (New York: Guilford Press, 1999): 181–197.

52. J. A. Kleim, E. Lussnig, E. R. Schwarz, T. A. Comery, & W. T. Greenough, "Synaptogenesis and FOS expression in the motor cortex of the adult rat after motor skill learning," *Journal of Neuroscience*, 16 (1996): 4529–4535. R. S. Dumas, "Genetics of childhood disorders: XXXIX. Stem cell research, part 3: Regulation of neurogenesis by stress and antidepressant treatment," *Journal of the American Academy of Child and Adolescent Psychiatry*, 41 , no. 6 (June 2002): 745–748.

53. W. T. Boyce, "Biobehavioral reactivity and injuries in children and adolescents," in M. H. Bornstein & J. L. Genevro (eds.), *Child development and behavioral pediatrics* (Mahwah, NJ: Lawrence Erlbaum, 1996): 35–58. Cited in Linda P. Spear, "The adolescent brain and age-related behavioral manifestations," *Neuroscience and Biobehavioral Reviews*, 24 (2000): 430.

54. C. Murray & R. Herrnstein, *The bell curve: Intelligence and class structure in American life* (New York: Free Press, 1994). For a more recent iteration and defense of this thesis, see Murray, "IQ and income inequality in a sampling of sibling pairs from advantaged family backgrounds," *American Economic Review*, 92, no. 2 (2002): 339–343.

55. See M. Daniels, B. Devlin, & K. Roeder, "Of genes and IQ," in B. Devlin, S. E. Fienberg, D. P. Resnick, & K. Roeder (eds.), *Intelligence, genes, and success: Scientists respond to* The Bell Curve (New York: Springer-Verlag, 1997): 45–70. For a more general and speculative critique of physiological or genetic reductionism, see O. James, "They muck you up," *Psychologist*, 16, no. 6 (2003): 294–295.

56. See L. Eliot, *What's going on in there? How the brain and mind develop in the first five years of life* (New York: Bantam, 1999); and R. Shore, *Rethinking the brain: New insights into early development* (New York: Families and

Work Institute, 1997). See also the journal *Zero to Three*, published by the National Center for Clinical Infant Programs, Arlington, VA.

57. J. N. Geidd et al., "Brain development during childhood and adolescence: A longitudinal MRI study," *Nature Neuroscience, 2* , no. 10 (1999): 861–863. See also M. D. De Bellis et al., "Sex differences in brain maturation during childhood and adolescence," *Cerebral Cortex, 11*, no. 6 (2001): 552-557.

58. L. P. Spear, "The adolescent brain and age-related behavioral manifestations," *Neuroscience and Biobehavioral Reviews, 24* (2000): 418.

59. C. E. Irwin Jr., "Risk taking behaviors in the adolescent patient: Are they impulsive?" *Pediatric Annals, 18* (1989): 122–133.

60. E. R. Sowell, P. M. Thompson, C. J. Holmes, T. L. Jernigan, & A. W. Toga, "In vivo evidence for post-adolescent brain maturation in frontal and striatal regions," *Nature Neuroscience* 2, no. 10 (1999): 859-861; L. P. Spear, "The adolescent brain and age-related behavioral manifestations," *Neuroscience and Biobehavioral Reviews, 24* (2000): 424–425.

61. L. P. Spear, ibid.

62. M.D. De Bellis et al., "Hippocampal volume in adolescent-onset alcohol use disorders," *American Journal of Psychiatry, 157* (2000): 737–744; L. P. Spear, "The adolescent brain and age-related behavioral manifestations," *Neuroscience and Biobehavioral Reviews, 24* (2000): 426.

63. R. Larson & M. H. Richards, *Divergent realities: The emotional lives of mothers, fathers, and adolescents* (New York: Basic Books, 1994); see also R. Larson & L. Asmussen, "Anger, worry, and hurt in early adolescence: An enlarging world of negative emotions," in M. E. Colten & S. Gore (eds.), *Adolescent stress: Causes and consequences* (New York: Aldine de Gruyter, 1991): 21–41.

64. K. J. Zucker & R. Green, "Gender identity and psychosexual disorders," in J. M. Weiner (ed.), *Textbook of child and adolescent psychiatry* (Washington, DC: American Psychiatric Press, 1997).

65. See, e.g., J. Bancroft, *Human sexuality and its problems* (Edinburgh: Churchill Livingstone, 1989).

66. Here's a story about elephants. Between 1992 and 1997, 17 young, orphaned male elephants, whose parents had been killed in herd cullings, were relocated to a park in Pilanesberg, South Africa. They promptly started acting, well, wild. In particular, they went into musth—a hormonally induced state of heightened sexual and aggressive activity—earlier than is normal, and for longer periods of time than is normal. As a result, the young males stormed around the park, quite out of control and killing about 40 white rhinoceroses in the process. Then, in 1998, the people who run the park relocated six older bull elephants from Kruger Park to Pilanesberg. The "deviant behavior" of the young males, the researchers report, was quickly "rectified." No more rampaging, no more dead rhinoceroses. What happened? Specifically, there occurred a significant reduction in musth in the young males. And why did this occur? It seems clear to the

researchers that the old bulls keep the young bulls in line and that how this happens involves a remarkably complex interaction of social and physiological-hormonal influences. Social contexts influence biological systems! See R. Slotow, G. Van Dyke, J. Poole, B. Page, & A. Klocke, "Older bull elephants control younger males," *Nature, 408* (2000): 425–426.

67. E. Person & L. Ovesey, "Psychoanalytic theory of gender identity," *Journal of the American Academy of Psychoanalysis, 11* (1983): 203–225.

68. Interestingly, as men age, their testosterone levels typically decline significantly, whereas among older women, testosterone levels increase over time relative to estrogen. These physiologic developments help to explain the phenomenon of later-life androgyny—with men becoming less, and women becoming more, assertive—that appears to exist cross-culturally. See D. Gutmann, *Reclaimed powers: Toward a new psychology of men and women in later life* (New York: Basic Books, 1987).

69. L. Miller, "Spirituality and resilience in adolescent girls," Commission on Children at Risk, Working Paper 8 (New York: Institute for American Values, 2002): 9 (chapter 14, this volume).

70. See D. D. Gilmore, *Manhood in the making: Cultural concepts of masculinity* (New Haven, CT: Yale University Press, 1990); D. Gutmann, "Elders and Sons," Commission on Children at Risk, Working Paper 4 (New York: Institute for American Values, 2002) (chapter 13, this volume); Lisa Miller, "Spirituality and resilience in adolescent girls," Commission on Children at Risk, Working Paper 8 (New York: Institute for American Values, 2002) (chapter 14, this volume). Gutmann stresses that, unlike female rites of passage, which tend to celebrate entry into womanhood, male rites of passage are often more grueling, typically involving suffering and endurance. Such rituals seek to help the boy connect with spiritual and mythic meaning and totemic sponsorship from which he will draw strength to control his own aggression and to direct it toward the prosocial goals of his community.

71. National Center on Addiction and Substance Abuse at Columbia University, *The formative years: Pathways to substance abuse among girls and young women ages 8–22* (New York: Author, 2003).

72. S. B. Hrdy, *Mother nature: A history of mothers, infants, and natural selection* (New York: Pantheon, 1999): 393.

73. R. Karen, *Becoming attached: Unfolding the mystery of the infant-mother bond and its impact on later life* (New York: Warner Books, 1994); A. N. Schore, *Affect dysregulation and disorders of the self* (New York: W.W. Norton, 2003).

74. B. M. Stilwell, "The Consolidation of Conscience in Adolescence," Commission on Children at Risk, Working Paper 13 (New York: Institute for American Values, 2002): 2 (chapter 5, this volume). S. B. Hrdy similarly observes that a fundamental human trait "is to develop this unique empathetic component that is the foundation of

all morality"; see Hrdy, *Mother nature: A history of mothers, infants, and natural selection* (New York: Pantheon, 1999): 392–393.

75. R. Karen, "Investing in children and society: What we've learned from seven decades of attachment research," Commission on Children at Risk, Working Paper 7 (New York: Institute for American Values, 2002): 8 (chapter 4, this volume).

76. D. Gutmann, "Adulthood and its discontents," Working Paper 67 (New York: Institute for American Values, 1998): 4.

77. Ibid.

78. B. M. Stilwell, "The consolidation of conscience in adolescence," Commission on Children at Risk, Working Paper 13 (New York: Institute for American Values, 2002): 9 (chapter 5, this volume).

79. M. D. Resnick, "Best bets for improving the odds for optimum youth development," Commission on Children at Risk, Working Paper 10 (New York: Institute for American Values, 2002): 13 (chapter 6, this volume). See also M. D. Resnick, L. J. Harris, & R. W. Blum, "The impact of caring and connectedness on adolescent health and well-being," *Journal of Pediatrics and Child Health*, 29 (1993): s1–9; J. Richmond & W. Beardslee, "Resiliency: Research and practical implications for pediatricians," *Developmental and Behavioral Pediatrics*, 9 (1988): 157–163; M. Rutter, "Psychosocial resilience and protective mechanisms," *American Journal of Orthopsychiatry*, 57 (1987): 316–331; R. E. Sieving et al., "Development of adolescent self-report measures from the National Longitudinal Study of Adolescent Health," *Journal of Adolescent Health*, 28 (2001): 73-81.

80. J. Piaget, *The child's conception of the world* (London: Routledge and Kegan Paul, 1951): 354.

81. Clinical and scholarly work in this area is extensive and dates back many decades. See A.-M. Rizzuto, *The birth of the living God: A psychoanalytic study* (Chicago: University of Chicago Press, 1979); A. Vannesse & P. De Neuter, "The Semantic Differential Parenting Scale," in A. Vergote & A. Tamayo, *Parental figures and the representation of God: A psychological and cross-cultural study* (The Hague: Mouton, 1981): 25–42; K. E. Hyde, *Religion in childhood and adolescence: A comprehensive review of the research* (Birmingham, AL: Religious Education Press, 1990). A somewhat different perspective from the one highlighted in this report—or at least one with a different emphasis— focuses on the role of fathers (as opposed to parental figures more generally) in children's conceptions of God in Western cultures. For example, see D. Bakan, *And they took themselves wives* (San Francisco: Harper & Row, 1979); J. W. Miller, *Calling God father* (New York: Paulist Press, 1999); and Paul C. Vitz, *Faith of the fatherless: The psychology of atheism* (Dallas: Spence, 1999).

82. A. Godin & M. Hallez, "Parental images and divine paternity," in A. Godin (ed.), *From religious experience to religious attitude* (Chicago: Loyola University Press, 1965); M. O. Nelson, "The concept of God and the feeling toward parents," *Journal of Individual Psychology*, 27

(1971): 46–49; D. W. MacKenzie, "The symbolic parent versus actual parent: Approaches in the examination of similarities between a parent and God concept" (Ph.D. thesis, United States International University, 1987).

83. It was Sigmund Freud who first, and famously, theorized that the child's image of God was that of an exalted father, and that religion stemmed in part from the Oedipus complex. See, for example, Freud, *Totem and taboo* (New York: W.W. Norton, 1950). Freud believed that his findings about images of God indicate that God does not exist, but instead is merely a projection of childish fantasies. At the same time, some subsequent researchers and theorists in this field, while building in part on Freud's work, do not conclude that atheism is the necessary or even the most logical philosophical stance to be derived from studying the connections between children's images of parents and their images of God, and have therefore rejected Freud's conclusions about religion as too reductionist. For a concise sociological elaboration of what might be called the trans-Freud interpretation of how human projections may relate to religious experience and phenomena, see P. Berger, *A rumor of angels: Modern society and the rediscovery of the supernatural* (New York: Doubleday, 1990): 50–64, passim. See also P. C. Vitz, *Faith of the fatherless: The psychology of atheism* (Dallas: Spence, 1999).

84. G. Ironson et al., "The Ironson-Woods Spirituality/Religiousness Index is associated with long survival, health behaviors, less stress and low cortisol in people with AIDS," *Annals of Behavioral Medicine*, 24, no. 1 (2002): 34–48.

85. See J. W. Hoffman et al., "Reduced sympathetic nervous system reactivity associated with the relaxation response," *Science*, 215 (1982): 190–192; R. Cooper et al., "Hormonal and biochemical responses to transcendental meditation," *Postgraduate Medical Journal*, 61, no. 714 (1985): 301–304; S. Segerstrom, S. E. Taylor, M. E. Kemeny, & J. L. Fahey, "Optimism is associated with mood, coping, and immune change in response to stress," *Journal of Personality and Social Psychology*, 74, no. 6 (1998): 1646–1655; B. S. Rabin, *Stress, immune function, and health: The connection* (New York: Wiley-Liss, 1999).

86. P. C. Vitz, "Moral and spiritual dimensions of the healthy person: Notes from the founders of modern psychology/psychiatry," Commission on Children at Risk, Working Paper 16 (New York: Institute for American Values, 2002): 14 (chapter 7, this volume).

87. At the same time, it is also worth remembering that throughout history many people, including many who are revered as martyrs, have suffered extreme physical hardships, up to and including death, as a consequence of their religious faith and practice.

88. Hebrews 11:1.

89. J. S. Young, C. S. Cashwell, & J. Shcherbakova, "The moderating relationship of spirituality on negative life events and psychological

adjustment," *Counseling and Values*, 45, no. 1 (2000): 49–57. See also B. R. Johnson, "A tale of two religious effects: Evidence for the protective and prosocial impact of organic religion," Commission on Children at Risk, Working Paper 6 (New York: Institute for American Values, 2002) (chapter 9, this volume); and W. B. Wilcox, "Focused on their families: Religion, parenting, and child well-being," Commission on Children at Risk, Working Paper 17 (New York: Institute for American Values, 2002) (chapter 10, this volume).

90. C. Smith, R. Faris, M. Lundquist Denton, & M. Regnerus, "Mapping American adolescent subjective religiosity and attitudes of alienation toward religion: A research report," *Sociology of Religion*, 64, no. 1 (2003): 111–123.

91. A. Thornton & D. Camburn, "Religious participation and adolescent sexual behavior and attitudes," *Journal of Marriage and the Family*, 51, no. 3 (1989): 641–653.

92. G. H. Gallup Jr., *The religious life of young Americans* (Princeton, NJ: George H. Gallup International Institute, 1992).

93. B. R. Johnson, "A tale of two religious effects: Evidence for the protective and prosocial impact of organic religion," Commission on Children at Risk, Working Paper 6 (New York: Institute for American Values, 2002): 2 (chapter 9, this volume).

94. See W. J. Strawbridge, R. D. Cohen, S. J. Shema, & G. A. Kaplan, "Frequent attendance at religious services and mortality over 28 Years," *American Journal of Public Health*, 87, no. 6 (1997): 957–961; H. G. Koenig et al., "Does religious attendance prolong survival? A six-year follow-up study of 3,968 older adults," *Journal of Gerontology*, 54A (1999): M370–377.

95. B. R. Johnson, "A tale of two religious effects: Evidence for the protective and prosocial impact of organic religion," Commission on Children at Risk, Working Paper 6 (New York: Institute for American Values, 2002): 19 (chapter 9, this volume).

96. J. M. Wallace, *Is religion good for adolescents' health?* (Philadelphia: University of Pennsylvania, Center for Research on Religion and Urban Civil Society, 2002).

97. C. J. Baier & B. E. Wright, " 'If you love me, keep my commandments': A meta-analysis of the effect of religion on crime," *Journal of Research in Crime and Delinquency*, 38, no. 1 (2001): 3–21; H. G. Koenig, M. E. McCullough, & D. B. Larson, *Handbook of religion and health* (New York: Oxford University Press, 2001); B. R. Johnson, S. D. Li, D. B. Larson, & M. McCullough, "Religion and delinquency: A systematic review of the literature," *Journal of Contemporary Criminal Justice*, 16 (2000): 32–52.

98. B. R. Johnson, "A tale of two religious effects: Evidence for the protective and prosocial impact of organic religion," Commission on Children at Risk, Working Paper 6 (New York: Institute for American Values, 2002) (chapter 9, this volume); T. A. Wills, A. M. Yaeger, &

J. M. Sandy, "Buffering effect of religiosity for adolescent substance abuse," *Psychology of Addictive Behaviors, 17*, no. 1 (2003): 24–31.

99. C. Smith & R. Faris, *Religion and American adolescent delinquency, risk behaviors and constructive social activities* (Chapel Hill: University of North Carolina, National Study of Youth and Religion, 2002).

100. Ibid.

101. C. Smith & R. Faris, *Religion and the life attitudes and self-images of American adolescents* (Chapel Hill: University of North Carolina, National Study of Youth and Religion, 2002).

102. For a recent overview of work in this area, see M. Regnerus, C. Smith, & M. Fritsch, *Religion in the lives of American adolescents: A review of the literature* (Chapel Hill: University of North Carolina, National Study of Youth and Religion, 2003).

103. Nor do these findings support the assertion that all aspects of religiosity and spirituality are good for one's health. Scholars are currently working to develop more sophisticated ways to determine which aspects of religiosity and spirituality tend to promote physical well-being, and which may be sources of potential physical harm. Toward that end, scholars have also identified what some have termed *negative religious coping* (such as fatalistic beliefs), which may lead to depression and other deleterious effects on health, in part similar to the effects on health of a harsh or neglectful parent. See K. I. Pargament, B. W. Smith, H. G. Koenig, & L. M. Perez, "Patterns of positive and negative religious coping with major life stressors," *Journal for the Scientific Study of Religion, 37*, no. 4 (1998): 710–724; K. I. Pargament, H. G. Koenig, N. Tarakeshwar, & J. Hahn, "Religious struggle as a predictor of mortality among medically ill elderly patients: A two-year longitudinal study," *Archives of Internal Medicine, 161* (2001): 1881–1885; K. I. Pargament, "The bitter and the sweet: An evaluation of the costs and benefits of religiousness," *Psychological Inquiry, 13*, no. 3 (2002): 168–181.

104. R. A. Emmons & M. E. McCullough, "Counting blessings versus burdens: An experimental investigation of gratitude and subjective well-being in daily life," *Journal of Personality and Social Psychology, 84*, no. 2 (2003): 377–389.

105. J. S. Young, C. S. Cashwell, & J. Shcherbakova, "The moderating relationship of spirituality on negative life events and psychological adjustment," *Counseling & Values, 45*, no. 1 (2000): 49–57. See also L. Miller et al., "Religiosity and depression: Ten-year follow-up of depressed mothers and offspring," *Journal of the American Academy of Child & Adolescent Psychiatry, 36* , vol. 10 (1997): 1416–1425; J. M. Wallace Jr. & T. A. Forman, "Religion's role in promoting health and reducing risk among American youth," *Health Education & Behavior, 25*, no. 6 (1998): 721–741; K. I. Pargament, *The psychology of religion and coping: Theory, research, practice* (New York: Guilford Press, 1997).

106. J. S. Coleman, *Foundations of social theory* (Cambridge, MA: Harvard University Press, 1990): 597–609.
107. W. B. Wilcox, *Good dads: Religion, civic engagement, and paternal involvement in low-income communities* (Philadelphia: University of Pennsylvania, Center for Research on Religion and Urban Civil Society, 2002).
108. W. A. Mason & M. Windel, "Family, religious, school, and peer influences on adolescent alcohol use," *Prevention Researcher, 9*, no. 3 (2002): 6–7.
109. W. B. Wilcox, "Focused on their families: Religion, parenting, and child well-being," Commission on Children at Risk, Working Paper 17 (New York: Institute for American Values, 2002): 22 (chapter 10, this volume). Religious traditions from both East and West exhibit characteristics that tend to promote strong parental investment in children. Julie Thomas of Youngstown State University describes the many ways in which the Buddhist tradition fosters a healthy approach to parenting, including an emphasis on "the importance of parents engaging wholeheartedly in this dance of interconnectedness that in turn is vital to their children's wellbeing." See J. E. Thomas & L. A. Wuyek, "Minding the children with mindfulness: A Buddhist approach to promoting well-being in children," Commission on Children at Risk, Working Paper 15 (New York: Institute for American Values, 2002): 23 (chapter 11, this volume).
110. L. Miller, "Spirituality and resilience in adolescent girls," Commission on Children at Risk, Working Paper 8 (New York: Institute for American Values, 2002): 3 (chapter 14, this volume).
111. S. M. Natal, *Loneliness and spiritual growth* (Birmingham, AL: Religious Education Press, 1986).
112. J. Sobson, "Loneliness and faith," *Journal of Psychological Theology, 61* (1978): 104–109.
113. K. I. Pargament, *The psychology of religion and coping: Theory, research, practice* (New York: Guilford Press, 1997).
114. L. Miller, M. Davies, & S. Greenwald, "Religiosity and substance use and abuse among adolescents in the National Comorbidity Survey," *Journal of the American Academy of Child & Adolescent Psychiatry, 39*, no. 9 (2000): 1190–1197; L. Miller et al., "Religiosity and substance use in children of opiate addicts," *Journal of Substance Abuse, 13* (2001): 323–336.
115. See D. Gutmann, "Elders and sons," Commission on Children at Risk, Working Paper 4 (New York: Institute for American Values, 2002) (chapter 13, this volume); L. Miller, "Spirituality and resilience in adolescent girls," Commission on Children at Risk, Working Paper 8 (New York: Institute for American Values, 2002) (chapter 14, this volume).
116. L. Miller, ibid., 6.
117. This proposition is anything but new. It was developed by Plato and elaborated further by Aristotle and others. At the same time, recent

neuroscientific research has also explored the brain's incessant need to know why. See, e.g., E. d'Aquili & A. B. Newberg, *The mystical mind: Probing the biology of religious experience* (Minneapolis: Fortress Press, 1999).

118. Ibid., 118–119.

119. A. Newberg & E. d'Aquili, *Why God won't go away: Brain science and the biology of belief* (New York: Ballantine Books, 2001): 143.

120. E. d'Aquili & A. B. Newberg, *The mystical mind: Probing the biology of religious experience* (Minneapolis: Fortress Press, 1999): 86. They are using the word *myth* nonpejoratively, defining it as a religious explanation of the world.

121. M. Linehan, *Cognitive-behavioral treatment of borderline personality disorder* (New York: Guilford Press, 1993). See also H. Benson & M. Z. Klipper, *The relaxation response* (New York: Wings Books, 1992).

122. See K. S. Kendler, C. O. Gardner, & C. A. Prescott, "Religion, psychopathology, and substance use and abuse: A multimeasure, genetic-epidemiologic study," *American Journal of Psychiatry*, 154, vol. 3 (1997): 322–329. For rates of religiosity among children of less religious parents, see L. Miller et al., "Religiosity and substance use in children of opiate addicts," *Journal of Substance Abuse*, 13 (2001): 323–336.

123. The concept of the "ideal type" was developed by the German sociologist and political economist Max Weber, who viewed the ideal type as a fundamental conceptualization through which all sociological formulations and definitions should be expressed. See M. Weber, *Basic concepts in sociology* (New York: Carol, 1993): 51–55, and M. Weber, *The Protestant ethic and the spirit of capitalism* (New York: Charles Scribner's Sons, 1958): 71, 98, 200. An ideal type is a simplified, generic description or definition that can be useful in helping us to understand certain aspects of social reality. An ideal type is an abstraction. Empirical reality never corresponds precisely with an ideal type. As an analytical tool, the primary value of ideal types is in helping us to identify the typical, primary, and possibly distinctive features of whatever groups of persons or social institutions are being studied. With respect to what we are calling *authoritative communities*, real-world examples of authoritative communities will almost always reveal more diversity and complexity than is captured by an ideal type.

124. D. Baumrind, "Current patterns of parental authority," *Developmental Psychology Monographs*, 4, no. 1, part 2 (1971).

125. L. Steinberg, "We know some things: Parent-adolescent relationships in retrospect and prospect," *Journal of Research on Adolescence*, 11, no. 1 (2001): 1–19.

126. J. P. Comer, *School power: Implications of an intervention project* (New York: Free Press, 1995). See also J. P. Comer, N. M. Haynes, E. T. Joyner, & M. Ben-Avie (eds.), *Rallying the whole village: The Comer process for reforming education* (New York: Teachers College Press, 1996), and

J. P. Comer, *Child by child: The Comer process for change in education* (New York: Teachers College Press, 1999).

127. M. E. Seligman, *The optimistic child: A proven program to safeguard children from depression and build lifelong resilience* (New York: Perennial, 1996).

128. See P. C. Scales et al., "The role of neighborhood and community in building developmental assets for children and youth: A national study of social norms among American adults," *Journal of Community Psychology*, 29 (2001): 703–727; and P. L. Benson, P. C. Scales, N. Leffert, & E. C. Roehlkepartain, *A fragile foundation: The state of developmental assets among American youth* (Minneapolis: Search Institute, 1999). For an analysis locating Search Institute's 40 development assets within the broader literature on, and various models of, positive child outcomes, see K. A. Moore et al., "What are good child outcomes?," in A. D. Thornton (ed.), *The well-being of children and families: Research and data needs* (Ann Arbor: University of Michigan Press, 2001): 59–84.

129. R. N. Bellah, R. Madsen, W. M. Sullivan, A. Swidler, & S. M. Tipton, *The good society* (New York: Alfred A. Knopf, 1991).

130. P. L. Berger & R. J. Neuhaus, *To empower people: From state to civil society* (Washington, DC: AEI Press, 1996).

131. D. E. Eberly, *America's promise: Civil society and the renewal of American culture* (Lanham, MD: Rowman & Littlefield, 1998); D. E. Eberly and R. Streeter, *The soul of civil society: Voluntary associations and the public value of moral habits* (Lanham, MD: Lexington Books, 2002); and D. E. Eberly (ed.), *The essential civil society reader* (Lanham, MD: Rowman & Littlefield, 2000).

132. A. Etzioni, *The moral dimension: Toward a new economics* (New York: Free Press, 1989); A. Etzioni, *The monochrome society* (Princeton, NJ: Princeton University Press, 2001). Etzioni is the founder and president of the Communitarian Network.

133. F. Fukuyama, *Trust: The social virtues and the creation of prosperity* (New York: Free Press, 1995); and F. Fukuyama, *The great disruption: Human nature and the reconstitution of social order* (New York: Free Press, 1999).

134. R. D. Putnam, *Bowling alone: The collapse and revival of American community* (New York: Simon and Schuster, 2000); and R. D. Putnam (ed.), *Democracies in flux: The evolution of social capital in contemporary society* (New York: Oxford University Press, 2002).

135. See L. M. McClain & J. E. Fleming (eds.), "Symposium on legal and constitutional implications of the calls to revive civil society," *Chicago-Kent Law Review*, 75, no. 2 (2000); and M. A. Glendon & D. Blankenhorn (eds.), *Seedbeds of virtue: Sources of competence, character, and citizenship in American society* (Lanham, MD: Madison Books, 1995).

136. For a summary of a review of more than 1,100 research articles on adolescent development, the basic conclusion of which is that "relationships are key," see Kristin A. Moore & Jonathan F. Zaff, *Building a*

better teenager: A summary of "what works" in adolescent development (Washington, DC: Child Trends, 2002).

137. D. Baumrind, "Current patterns of parental authority," *Developmental Psychology Monographs, 4,* no. 1, part 2 (1971). See also L. Steinberg, "We know some things: Parent-adolescent relationships in retrospect and prospect," *Journal of Research on Adolescence, 11,* no. 1 (2001): 1–19; D. Baumrind, "The influence of parenting style on adolescent competence and substance use," *Journal of Early Adolescence, 11,* no. 1 (1991): 56–95; L. Steinberg, "Youth violence: Do parents and families make a difference?" *National Institute of Justice Journal, 243* (2000): 31–38.

138. See note 128. See also L. Steinberg, *The role of the family in adolescent development: Preventing risk, promoting resilience.* Paper presented at the Children, Youth and Families at Risk Program Initiative, Cooperative Extension Service, U.S. Department of Agriculture, San Diego, March 22, 2001.

139. For a sharp critique focusing on how modern bureaucratic professionalism, unless carefully directed and kept in check, can invade and weaken many institutions of civil society, see J. McKnight, *The careless society: Community and its counterfeits* (New York: Basic Books, 1995).

140. See A. Kornhaber & K. L. Woodward, *Grandparents/grandchildren: The vital connection* (Garden City, NY: Anchor Press, 1981).

141. Alexis de Tocqueville, *Democracy in America,* vol. 2 (New York: Schocken Books, 1961): 120. In the same study (e.g., see vol. 2, 128–133), Tocqueville celebrates the American habit of forming "voluntary associations" as a primary antidote to some of the main dangers of individualism. Indeed, in this respect as in others, much of today's discussion of civil society in the United States amounts essentially to standing on the shoulders of Tocqueville, who wrote *Democracy in America* in the 1830s.

142. For an extended reflection on this theme, see R. T. Gill, *Posterity lost: Progress, ideology, and the decline of the American family* (Lanham, MD: Rowman & Littlefield, 1997).

143. See F. Fukuyama, *Trust: The social virtues and the creation of prosperity* (New York: Free Press, 1995).

144. Quoted in S. Gilbert, "Scientists explore the molding of children's morals," *New York Times,* March 18, 2003, p. F5.

145. In affirming this characteristic as part of the "ideal type" of authoritative communities, we recognize that not all real-life authoritative communities do, or even can or should, formally reflect this dimension. We also recognize here, as we do throughout this report, the distinction between "spiritual" (suggesting personal openness to the transcendent) and "religious" (suggesting the additional dimension of commitment to and participation in formal religious institutions).

146. See J. Wattles, *The golden rule* (New York: Oxford University Press, 1996).

147. I. Kant, *Grounding for the metaphysics of morals* (Indianapolis: Hackett, 1993): 39.

148. Council on Civil Society, *A call to civil society: Why democracy needs moral truths* (New York: Institute for American Values, 1998): 7.

149. For research attempting to place the significant effects of family structure and process within the larger context of the formation of "social capital"—a key concept for students of civil society—see C. L. Bankston & M. Zhou, "Social capital as process: The meanings and problems of a theoretical metaphor," *Sociological Inquiry*, 72 (2002): 285–317.

150. D. Popenoe & B. D. Whitehead, *The state of our unions 2003* (Piscataway, NJ: National Marriage Project of Rutgers University, 2003): 20–22.

151. One of the most significant intellectual shifts of the 1990s, driven in part by new social science research findings, is the growing belief among scholars and leaders from across the political and ideological spectrum that marriage is important for children and that strengthening marriage is an important social goal. Let us give you several illustrations of this by now quite strong consensus. Here are two public policy experts, one a Republican and one a Democrat, writing in 2003 for the Brookings Institution: "Both scholars and politicians now agree that married two-parent families are good for children, and that poverty could be greatly reduced if marriage could be increased" (R. Haskins & P. Offner, *Achieving compromise on welfare reform reauthorization* [Policy brief] [Washington, DC: Brookings Institution, 2003]: 7). From a 2003 statement from the National Council on Family Relations: "A large body of social science research indicates that healthy, married-parent families are an optimal environment for promoting the well-being of children. Children raised by both biological parents are less likely than children raised in single- or step-parent families to be poor, to drop out of school, to have difficulty finding a job, to become teen parents or to experience emotional or behavioral problems. Children living with single mothers are five times as likely to be poor as those in two-parent families" (*Marriage promotion in low-income families* [Fact sheet] [Minneapolis: National Council on Family Relations, 2003]: 1). A 2003 statement from the Center for Law and Social Policy asserted: "The legal basis and public support involved in the institution of marriage help to create the most likely conditions for the development of factors that children need most to thrive—consistent, stable, loving attention from two parents who cooperate and have sufficient resources and support from two extended families, two sets of friends, and society" (M. Parke, *Are married parents really better for children? What research says about the effects of family structure on child well-being* [Washington, DC: Center for Law and Social Policy, 2003]: 7). Here is a 2002 statement from Child Trends: "Marriage is one of the most beneficial resources for adults and children alike" (T. Halle [project director], *Charting parenthood* (Washington, DC: Child Trends, 2002]: 49). And the U.S.

Census Bureau—an agency that rarely reports data in a way suggestive of a clear value judgment about a social institution—stated in a 2003 report on the living arrangements of U.S. children: "Children in two-parent families generally had access to more financial resources and greater amounts of parental time. They also were more likely to participate in extracurricular activities, progress more steadily in school, and have more supervision over their activities such as television watching. The presence of two parents continues to be one of the most important factors in children's lives" (J. Fields, *Children's living arrangements and characteristics: March 2002*, Current Population Reports P20-547 [Washington, DC: U.S. Census Bureau, 2003]: 19).

This new consensus also recognizes that the differences in child outcomes between married-couple and other homes with children are not categorical but instead involve what scholars call overlapping distributions. That is, it is not the case that all (or most) children in one-parent homes experience negative outcomes that in turn are rare or nonexistent among children from married-couple homes. Indeed, some children from one-parent homes do better than some children from two-parent homes. (The distributions overlap.) Instead, the real differences between the two groups center on the odds or the probabilities of negative outcomes. In general, for children growing up in married-couple homes, the odds of experiencing these negative outcomes are significantly lower.

In addition, quantitative studies on child outcomes in married-couple versus other homes often present findings in ways that can obscure some of the actual difference between the two groups, especially when the area being measured is mental and emotional health. For example, say a study finds that 90% of children of marriage score within the "normal" range on a particular measure of mental health, compared with about 75% of children of divorce. Does that mean that the "gap"—the difference in the likelihood of suffering between the two groups—is about 15%? That is one way to put it, and many scholars put it just that way. But the real answer is more complicated. Why? Because it is highly probable that those "normal" scores for the children of divorce are measurably lower than the "normal" scores of the children of marriage. Thus, while both the 75% and the 90% have scored within the "normal" range, there is still a real difference between these two "normal" groups, with the children of divorce being worse off. By the way, this is not a hypothetical case. See E. M. Hetherington & J. Kelly, *For better or for worse: Divorce reconsidered* (New York: W. W. Norton, 2003): 7, 150, 228.

Similarly, this new consensus recognizes that family structure does not by itself determine outcomes for children. In all families, process—the quality of the family relationships—is fundamentally important. At the same time, research shows that family structure is a highly important influence on family process.

152. The United States long had, and probably still has, the world's highest divorce rate, though several other countries (including Sweden, the United Kingdom, and Russia) appear to be approaching the United States in this respect. Although the incidence of divorce in the United States has declined modestly since its historic peak in the early 1980s, the U.S. refined divorce rate (divorces per 1,000 married women age 15 or older) was about 19.5 in 1998, compared with 9.2 in 1960. Of all U.S. persons age 15 or older in 2000, about 8.3% were divorced, more than four times the 1.8% in 1960. Of all recent first marriages in the United States, between 40% and 45% are likely to end in divorce. See *United Nations statistical yearbook* (New York: United Nations Department of Economic and Social Information and Policy Analysis, 1995); see also D. Spain & S. M. Bianchi, *Balancing act: Motherhood, marriage, and employment among American women* (New York: Russell Sage, 1996): 47.

153. In 2002, about 33.8% of all U.S. births occurred to unmarried women. See B. E. Hamilton, J. A. Martin, & P. D. Sutton, "Births: Preliminary data for 2002," *National Vital Statistics Reports*, 51, no. 11 (Hyattsville, MD: National Center for Health Statistics, 2003).

154. In 1996, about 62% of U.S. children under age 18 lived with both of their biological (or adoptive) married-to-each-other parents. See J. Fields, *Living arrangements of U.S. children: Fall 1996*, Current Population Reports (Washington, DC: U.S. Census Bureau, 2001): 70–74. Also, for a critical review of the report's methodology and use of the term *traditional nuclear family*, see D. Blankenhorn & M. Gallagher, *The family "rebound" that wasn't, and the census report that failed* (New York: Institute for American Values, 2001).

155. See K. D. Pruett, "How men and children affect each other's development," *Zero to Three* (August/September 1997): 3–13; K. D. Pruett, *Fatherneed: Why father care is as essential as mother care for your child* (New York: Free Press, 2000); D. Popenoe, *Life without father: Compelling new evidence that fatherhood and marriage are indispensable for the good of children and society* (New York: Free Press, 1996).

156. E. H. Erikson, *Identity: Youth and crisis* (New York: W. W. Norton, 1968): 138. See also J. Snarey, *How fathers care for the next generation: A four-decade study* (Cambridge, MA: Harvard University Press, 1993); S. L. Nock, *Marriage in men's lives* (New York: Oxford University Press, 1998).

157. U.S. Census Bureau, "Families, by presence of own children under 18: 1950 to present," Internet table FM-1 (Internet release date: June 29, 2001), and "Living arrangements of children under 18 years old: 1960 to present," Internet table CH-1 (Internet release date: June 29, 2001). S. Vandivere, K. A. Moore, & M. Zaslow, *Children's family environments: Findings from the National Survey of America's Families* (Washington, DC: Urban Institute, 2001). See also "Births to unmarried women—End of the increase?" *AmeriStat* (Washington, DC: Population Reference

Bureau, 2003); and B. O'Hara, "The rise—and fall?—of single-parent families," *Population Today*, 29, no. 5 (July 2001): 1, 4.

158. A. Dupree & W. Primus, *Declining share of children lived with single mothers in the late 1990s* (Washington, DC: Center on Budget and Policy Priorities, 2001).

159. J. R. Goldstein, "The leveling of divorce in the United States," *Demography*, 36, no. 3 (1999): 409–414.

160. *General social surveys, 1973–2002* (Chicago: National Opinion Research Center, University of Chicago). See also P. R. Amato, D. Johnson, A. Booth, & S. Rogers, "Continuity and change in marital quality between 1980 and 2000," *Journal of Marriage and the Family*, 65 (2003): 1–22.

161. Arland Thornton observes: "Social life [in the United States and numerous other societies] has increasingly shifted from being organized largely around family, kinship, and household structures to being organized by both family and nonfamilial institutions. The proliferation of social organizations in America today means that individual lives intersect with numerous social institutions and settings, including the family, neighborhood, friendship group, church, school, economic bureaucracy, childcare center, protective agency, medical center, restaurants, the mass media, and local, state, and national governments.... Participation in these social organizations helps to define and guide the activities and well-being of individuals and families." See A. Thornton, "Introduction and overview," in A. Thornton (ed.), *The well-being of children and families: Research and data needs* (Ann Arbor: University of Michigan Press, 2001): 20.

162. R. D. Putnam, "Bowling alone: America's declining social capital," *Journal of Democracy*, 6, no. 1 (January 1995): 65–78; and R. D. Putnam, *Bowling alone: The collapse and revival of American community* (New York: Simon & Schuster, 2000).

163. See R. Wuthnow, "The United States: Bridging the privileged and the marginalized?" in R. D. Putnam (ed.), *Democracies in flux: The evolution of social capital in contemporary society* (New York: Oxford University Press, 2002): 59–102.

164. J. M. Twenge, "The age of anxiety? Birth cohort change in anxiety and neuroticism, 1952–1993," *Journal of Personality and Social Psychology*, 79, no. 6 (2000): 1007–1021.

165. G. Ringbäck Weitoft, A. Hjern, B. Haglund, & M. Rosén, "Mortality, severe morbidity, and injury in children living with single parents in Sweden: A population-based study," *Lancet*, 361 (2003): 289–295.

166. Controls are statistical methods by which scholars seek to estimate the causal effects of a particular variable. One benefit of this technique is that it can help scholars avoid the error of suggesting that A is the main or an important cause of something, when in fact the correlation being proposed is partially or wholly spurious. Consider an example. A scholar reports a correlation between height and intelligence. But both height and intelligence are strongly affected by other factors, such

as prenatal and early childhood care and nutrition. Using controls, a scholar can determine that the correlation between height and intelligence is more spurious than causal. More generally, the technique can be used to determine the relative importance of a specific mechanism through which a phenomenon is expressing itself. Consider another example. Flooding the basement damages the furniture, possibly (the scholar believes) through the mechanism of water exposure, but also possibly through knocking the furniture over. When a scholar controls for knocking the furniture over, the scholar is then able to estimate the independent, separate effects of water damage. In the Swedish study, the scholars controlled for socioeconomic status and several demographic variables, because by doing so, they could then estimate the independent, separate effects of family structure on a number of childhood problems. The researchers found that these independent effects of family structure were strong. Just to make matters (even more!) complicated, socioeconomic status and some demographic variables are *themselves* influenced by family structure, so in some cases, the use of scholarly controls of this sort may mean that the reported effects of family structure on child outcomes are in fact underestimated.

167. Numerous other studies confirm this link between family fragmentation and a wide range of childhood problems. To take only one example, one of every three divorces in the United States resulting in the physical separation of a father from his children sends the mother and children into poverty. Father absence due to marital dissolution is thus a primary cause of U.S. child poverty. See S. M. Bianchi, L. Subaiya, & J. R. Kahn, "The gender gap in the economic well-being of nonresident fathers and custodial mothers," *Demography, 35*, no. 2 (1999): 195–203.

168. The term *social capital,* now widely used by economists, sociologists, and others, is based on the proposition that social relationships and social networks can increase, or reduce, the productivity of individuals and groups. It is a term that derives from the field of economics. Accordingly, whereas physical capital refers to the economic value stemming from physical objects, and human capital refers to productive qualities in individuals, social capital refers to those social connections, networks, and relationships that generate traits (such as trustworthiness and honesty) that are valued in the market place, or more broadly, in the society. Some scholars in the fields of child development and public health have criticized the concept of social capital and recommend instead what they view as the better and more specific concepts of *social ecology* and *social efficacy.* See F. Earls & M. Carlson, "The social ecology of child health and well-being," *Annual Review of Public Health, 22* (2001): 143–166.

169. R. D. Putnam, *Bowling alone: The collapse and revival of American community* (New York: Simon & Schuster, 2000): 296–297.

170. See J. E. Korbin & C. J. Coulton, "Understanding neighborhood context for children and families: Combining epidemiological and ethnographic approaches," in J. Brooks-Gunn, G. J. Duncan, & J. L. Aber (eds.), *Neighborhood poverty: Vol. 2. Policy implications in studying neighborhoods* (New York: Russell Sage, 1997): 65–79; D. K. Runyan et al., "Children who prosper in unfavorable environments: The relationship to social capital," *Pediatrics, 101*, no. 1, part 1 (1998): 12–18.

171. Curiously, for reasons perhaps having to do with how different scholarly disciplines define their terrains, many scholars (among them Putnam) have not to date included the family in their definition of civil society or as one of the institutions that foster social connectedness. For us as a commission, a primary advantage of the concept of *authoritative community* is that it transcends this (for many purposes) arbitrary and largely academic division between *private* and *civic*, permitting us instead to look holistically at *all* social institutions that foster connectedness and pass on shared meaning.

172. Many members of this commission voiced particular concern that so many of our children currently do not obtain either the physical or the mental health care that can reduce disability and increase productive function.

173. See, e.g., J. P. Greene & G. Forster, *Sex, drugs, and delinquency in urban and suburban schools* (New York: Manhattan Institute, 2003).

174. See M. R. Warren, *Dry bones rattling: Community building to revitalize American democracy* (Princeton, NJ: Princeton University Press, 2001). See also E. Cortés Jr., "Reweaving the social fabric," *Boston Review, 19*, no. 3–4 (1994): 12–14.

175. E. Cortés Jr., "The broader context of community," *Family Affairs, 7*, no. 1–2 (1996): 6.

176. See J. P. Comer, N. M. Haynes, E. T. Joyner, & M. Ben-Avie (eds.), *Rallying the whole village: The Comer process for reforming education* (New York: Teachers College Press, 1996); and J. P. Comer, *Child by child: The Comer process for change in education* (New York: Teachers College Press, 1999).

177. W. Bradford Wilcox, *Then comes marriage? Religion, race, and marriage in urban America* (Philadelphia: University of Pennsylvania, Center for Research on Religion and Urban Civil Society, 2002); R. A. Cnaan & S. C. Boddie, *Black church outreach: Comparing how black and other congregations serve their needy neighbors* (Philadelphia: University of Pennsylvania, Center for Research on Religion and Urban Civil Society, 2001). See also *Turning the corner on father absence in Black America: A statement from the Morehouse Conference on African American Fathers* (Atlanta, GA: Morehouse Research Institute, 1999).

178. See R. M. Franklin, "Where's Dad? Fatherhood in African American families," remarks delivered at the "Sex, Marriage and Family and the Religions of the Book" conference at the Center for the Interdisciplinary Study of Religion, Emory University School of Law, Atlanta, Georgia,

March 28, 2003. See also R. D. Smith, "Churches and the urban poor: Interaction and social distance," *Sociology of Religion, 62*, no. 3 (2001): 301–313; and R. D. Smith (principal investigator), *Faith-based family support initiatives: Policy implications for the urban poor* (Atlanta, GA: Leadership Center at Morehouse College, 2000).

179. A description of the "Making Connections" program, including "The *Making Connections* Core Results Research Rationale," is available on the Web page of the Annie E. Casey Foundation (www.aecf.org).

180. A. Booth & A. C. Crouter (eds.), *Does it take a village? Community effects on children, adolescents, and families* (Mahwah, NJ: Lawrence Erlbaum, 2001). See also J. Ludwig, "Improving neighborhoods for poor children," in I. V. Sawhill (ed.), *One percent for the kids: New policies, brighter futures for America's children* (Washington, DC: Brookings Institution Press, 2003): 136–155

181. R. D. Putnam, *Bowling alone: The collapse and revival of American community* (New York: Simon & Schuster, 2000): 73, 94.

182. R. I. Lerman, *Impacts of marital status and parental presence on the material hardship of families with children* (Washington, DC: Urban Institute, 2002): 14, 24–25. See also A. Thomas & I. Sawhill, *For richer or for poorer: Marriage as an antipoverty strategy* (Washington, DC: Brookings Institution, 2002); W. Sigle-Rushton & S. McLanahan, "For richer or poorer? Marriage as an antipoverty strategy in the United States," Working Paper 01-17-FF (Princeton, N.J.: Princeton University, Center for Research on Child Wellbeing, 2002). All of these scholars recognize that, as groups, married and unmarried parents differ significantly when it comes to age, education, health status, employment, wage rates, and other factors, and that these differences—much of which constitute what scholars call "selection effects," meaning that they are present *prior to* an individual's entry into marriage—help explain why married couples are typically economically better off and far less likely to experience poverty than both unmarried couples and single parents. Accordingly, none of these studies suggests that marriage is an antipoverty panacea, or that marriage alone would erase the economic differences between married and unmarried couples. At the same time, each of these studies finds that higher marriage rates alone would be likely significantly to reduce child poverty and improve the economic well-being of families in low-income neighborhoods.

Relatedly, it is possible that changes in family structure among low-income Americans in the late 1990s, leading to modest but real increases in the proportion of children living in married-couple homes and in two-parent homes, constitute one (but only one, and probably not the major) explanation for the apparently dramatic decline of *concentrated poverty*—the number of people living in neighborhoods where the poverty rate is 40% or higher—in the 1990s. See P. A. Jargowsky, *Stunning progress, hidden problems: The dramatic decline of concentrated poverty in the 1990s*, Living Cities Census Series

(Washington, DC: The Brookings Institution, May 2003); and G. T. Kingley & K. L. S. Pettit, *Concentrated poverty: A change in course*, Neighborhood Change in Urban America Series, No. 2 (Washington, DC: Urban Institute, May 2003).

183. G. H. Elder Jr., J. S. Eccles, M. Ardelt, & S. Lord, "Inner-city parents under economic pressure: Perspectives on the strategies of parenting," *Journal of Marriage and the Family*, 57, no. 3 (1995): 771–784.

184. L. M. Burton & R. L. Jarrett, "In the mix, yet on the margins: The place of families in urban neighborhood and child development research," *Journal of Marriage and the Family*, 62, no. 4 (2000): 1114–1135; L. M. Burton & T. Price-Spratlen, "Through the eyes of children: An ethnographic perspective on neighborhoods and child development," in A. S. Masten (ed.), *The Minnesota Symposium on Child Psychology: Vol. 29. Cultural processes in child development* (Mahwah, NJ: Lawrence Erlbaum, 1999): 77–96; L. M. Burton & R. Jayakody, "Rethinking family structure and single parenthood: Implications for future studies of African-American families and children," in A. Thornton (ed.), *The well-being of children and families: Research and data needs* (Ann Arbor: University of Michigan Press, 2001): 127–153; A. C. Crouter & R. Larson (eds.), *Temporal rhythms in adolescence: Clocks, calendars, and the coordination of daily life* (San Francisco: Jossey-Bass, 1998); A. Booth & A. C. Crouter (eds.), *Does it take a village? Community effects on children, adolescents, and families* (Mahwah, NJ: Lawrence Erlbaum, 2001).

185. To help achieve this goal, one possible tool is an interactive CD to allow any group to measure itself in light of the 10 characteristics of authoritative communities and help that group to customize a plan for becoming a more authoritative community.

186. M. Resnick, "Best bets for improving the odds for optimum youth development," Commission on Children at Risk, Working Paper 10 (New York: Institute for American Values, 2002), 13 (chapter 6, this volume).

187. I. V. Sawhill (ed.), *One percent for the kids: New policies, brighter futures for America's children* (Washington, DC: Brookings Institution Press, 2003).

188. For example, see L. C. Huffman, S. L. Mehlinger, & A. S. Kerivan, "Risk factors for academic and behavioral problems at the beginning of School," in L. C. Huffman et al., *Off to a good start* (Chapel Hill: University of North Carolina, FPG Child Development Institute, 2000). These researchers do report that parental marital status and family composition may be important factors in school success or failure, but they also assert that these are "fixed markers" that are "not amenable to change" and therefore "not a reasonable basis for structuring targeted interventions."

189. William J. Doherty of the University of Minnesota, whose current work focuses on "family-centered community building," puts it this way: "We have witnessed the erosion of two central forms of human connection in the past forty years: family bonds and civic bonds. These

two trends are usually not addressed together because scholars and others who are concerned about our culture tend to focus on one or the other—either family or community. I maintain that family engagement and civic engagement are two facets of the same phenomenon, and that they are tied to the same social forces. We must therefore transcend the dichotomy between family life and public life that has limited our ability to address the needs of both families and society." See W. J. Doherty, "Renewing our vows," remarks delivered at the Center of the American Experiment, Minneapolis, March 19, 2003; also W. J. Doherty & J. S. Carroll, "The citizen therapist and family-centered community building: Introduction to a new section of the journal," *Family Process, 41*, no. 4 (2002): 561–568; W. J. Doherty & J. S. Carroll, "The Families and Democracy Project," *Family Process, 41*, no. 4 (2002): 579–590.

II
Primal Connections

2 The Biochemistry of Family Commitment and Youth Competence: Lessons from Animal Models

Larry J. Young

Emory University School of Medicine

Darlene D. Francis

University of California, Berkeley

Recent advances in neuroscience are beginning to provide fresh insights into the mechanisms for social interaction, including the molecular and cellular processes involved in the formation of social bonds. Understanding the biochemical factors that contribute to social attachment, as well as the biological consequences of parent–offspring interactions, may contribute to better understanding of normative development. In this chapter, we will review some of the results from studies of nonhuman animals revealing the neurobiological causes and consequences of social bonding and parental care. First, we describe a monogamous rodent that has provided an extensive understanding of the molecular and cellular basis of selective social attachment between mates. This research may serve as a model for understanding social bonding in general as the same mechanisms may contribute to many aspects of social attachments. We will then provide an overview of the underlying neurobiology of parental care. Finally, we will describe studies that examine the enduring consequences of differing parental styles on behavior and neurochemistry and provide a model of how these behaviors may be perpetuated across generations. We must stress that the reader bear in mind that most of the data presented here are from rodent studies, and there is very little evidence at this time that these same underlying mechanisms are similar in humans. However, understanding these processes in animals provides a perspective for thinking about how biological and environmental processes may govern behavioral outcomes in human beings.

Biochemistry of Family Commitment and Attachment in Rodents

The prototype human nuclear family structure consists of a mother, a father, and offspring. Thus, family commitment consists of, first, the bond between the parents, and then, between the parents and the offspring. In contrast with our species, parental care in most mammals is provided entirely by a single parent, the mother. Roughly 5% of mammalian species are socially monogamous, however, with family units consisting of both parents and offspring. One monogamous species, the prairie vole, has been useful in deciphering the neurobiological basis of adult social bonds between mates (Carter, 1998; Insel & Young, 2001). Remarkably, it appears that similar processes that underlie the attachments between mates may also contribute to parental care.

Social Attachment in Adult Voles

Prairie voles (*Microtus ochrogaster*) have become one of the most useful animal models for investigating the biochemistry of social attachment (Insel & Young, 2001; Young, Lim, Gingrich, & Insel, 2001). Prairie voles are hamster-sized rodents found in the Midwestern prairie of the United States. Studies in the field indicate that prairie voles form lifelong bonds with their mates and produce multiple litters together (Carter & Getz, 1993). Prairie vole nests typically consist of a mating pair and multiple generations of offspring, which contribute to the parenting of the youngest litter. The male prairie vole defends the nest and contributes significantly to the rearing of the offspring. Over the past 10 years, a series of laboratory studies has begun to uncover the neurochemical events that cement the bond between the parent voles.

The pair bonding process in voles can be easily studied in the laboratory, making it amenable to pharmacological manipulations. In the lab, pair bonding is assessed using a partner preference paradigm (Figure 1). In this procedure,

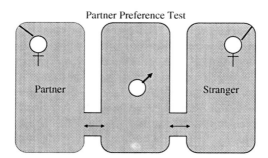

Figure 1. Schematic of the partner preference testing arena used to test for the development of a social bond between two adult voles. In the example, the male is being tested for a social attachment

an adult male and female prairie vole are paired, during which experimental manipulations (i.e., duration of cohabitation, presence or absence of mating, pharmacological treatments, etc.) are performed. After the designated time of cohabitation, the pair is separated and then placed in a partner preference testing arena. The arena consists of three chambers: the "partner" chamber, in which the partner is tethered to restrict its movement; the "stranger" chamber, in which a stimulus animal of equal stimulus value as the partner is tethered; and the neutral chamber, which is connected to the other two chambers by means of tubing. The experimental animal is placed in the neutral chamber and is allowed to roam freely between each chamber for a designated amount of time, typically 3 hours. An animal is said to have developed a partner preference if it spends more than twice as much time in contact with its partner than with the novel female.

Using the partner preference paradigm, some of the parameters of pair bond formation have been examined. The data suggests that while partner preferences can form after long periods of cohabitation, mating facilitates partner preference formation in both male and female prairie voles. For example, in one study, 6 hours of cohabitation without mating was not suffi-cient for the female to develop a partner preference, whereas the same duration of cohabitation with mating was sufficient (Williams, Catania, & Carter, 1992). Similar results have been obtained with males (Insel, Preston, & Winslow, 1995). Thus, it appears that both the quality and quantity of social interactions during the cohabitation contribute to the formation of the pair bond. Mating, while not critical, likely acts to strengthen the pair bond in the monogamous vole. Using the partner preference paradigm in conjunction with pharmaco-logical manipulations, we have begun to understand the chemical triggers and neural circuits underlying this process.

What biochemical processes underlie the pair bonding process? As mentioned earlier, social attachment is fairly rare between adults in mammals, although strong attachments between mother and their offspring are widespread. It is conceivable that similar neural and biochemical systems that are involved in regulating mother–infant relationships have been co-opted to produce the pair bond. This, in fact, appears to be the case. Oxytocin (OT) is a neuropeptide hormone produced in the hypothalamus, which sends projec-

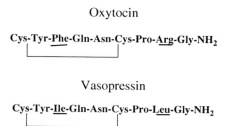

Oxytocin

Cys-Tyr-Phe-Gln-Asn-Cys-Pro-Arg-Gly-NH$_2$

Vasopressin

Cys-Tyr-Ile-Gln-Asn-Cys-Pro-Leu-Gly-NH$_2$

Figure 2. The molecular structures of oxytocin and vasopressin. Note that these peptides differ only at two amino acid residues (underlined)

tions to the posterior pituitary as well as into the brain (Figure 2) (Gainer & Wray, 1994). OT is released into the plasma from the posterior pituitary during labor and is thought to play a role in facilitating parturition through its actions on OT receptors in the uterus. OT is also released into the plasma in a pulsatile manner during nursing where it stimulates the milk ejection reflex, making breast-feeding possible. As will be discussed later in this chapter, studies in both rodents and sheep have suggested that OT released within the brain also plays an important role in initiating maternal behavior as well as facilitating the selective bond between mother and offspring. Several studies have now demonstrated that this same neuropeptide plays a role in the development of the pair bond in the female prairie vole.

Injections directly into the female prairie vole brain of a drug that blocks OT action, prior to cohabitation and mating, inhibits the development of a partner preference (Insel & Hulihan, 1995). Furthermore, infusion of OT into the female prairie vole brain facilitates the formation of the partner preference in the absence of mating (Williams, Insel, Harbaugh, & Carter, 1994). How can a molecule such as OT facilitate a phenomenon as complex as a social bond? First, we must understand how OT exerts its biological action. When released into the brain, OT acts as a neuromodulator, affecting neuronal function and communication. It does this by acting on receptors located in distinct areas of the brain, each of which has a unique function, such as altering perception, motivation, or emotion. Receptors are the molecules on the target cells that transduce the signal of the peptide hormone. Therefore, the first step in understanding the neurobiological mechanisms by which OT might facilitate a pair bond is to determine the location of the receptors in the brain. As it turns out, OT receptors are located in several brain regions known to affect emotionality, including the septum, amygdala, hypothalamus, nucleus accumbens, and prelimbic cortex (Insel & Shapiro, 1992). The first clues as to which particular brain sites are critical for social attachments in voles came from a comparative study in which locations of OT receptors in the prairie vole and that of the montane vole were compared (Insel & Shapiro, 1992). Montane voles, inhabitants of the Rocky Mountain region, are very closely related and similar in appearance to prairie voles, but have a very different family structure (Jannett, 1980). Montane voles do not form pair bonds, and female montane voles raise pups alone until they abandon them after only 2 weeks. The difference in OT receptor distribution in the brain of these closely related species is remarkable. Among other differences, there is a striking difference in OT receptors in the so-called reward circuitry of the brain; the nucleus accumbens and prelimbic cortex. Whereas montane voles have few OT receptors in these regions, prairie voles have high densities of receptors there (Figure 3).

Pharmacological studies have now demonstrated that the activation of OT receptors in these particular sites is critical for partner preference formation. Site-specific injections of an OT receptor blocker into the nucleus accumbens or prelimbic cortex completely disrupt the ability of a female prairie vole to bond with her mate (Young et al., 2001).

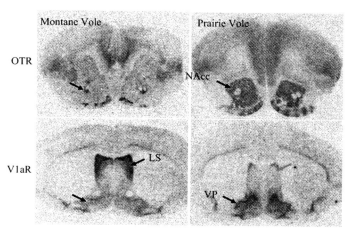

Figure 3. Distribution of oxytocin receptor (OTR; upper) and vasopressin receptor (V1aR; lower) binding in the montane (left) and prairie (right) vole brain. Note the high levels of receptors in the nucleus accumbens (NAcc) and ventral pallidum (VP) in the monogamous prairie vole compared with the montane vole. LS, lateral septum

In a parallel series of studies, it has become clear that when it comes to male prairie voles, a related neuropeptide, arginine vasopressin (AVP), is playing a larger role in the pair bonding process (Winslow, Hastings, Carter, Harbaugh, & Insel, 1993), although OT may also contribute to the process (Cho, DeVries, Williams, & Carter, 1999). AVP is structurally related to OT, a cyclical nonapeptide differing from OT in only two amino acid positions (Figure 2). Like OT, AVP is also synthesized in the hypothalamus and transported to the posterior pituitary (Gainer & Wray, 1994). However, extrahypothalmic AVP neurons from the amygdala project into the forebrain, where they are thought to influence behavior through interactions with the V1a subtype AVP receptor (V1aR). These extrahypothalamic AVP projections are sexually dimorphic, with males producing far more AVP than females (DeVries, 1990). Infusion of a compound that blocks V1aR activation prior to cohabitation and mating prevents male prairie voles from displaying a partner preference (Winslow et al., 1993). Conversely, infusions of AVP during an abbreviated cohabitation without mating facilitate the formation of a partner preference.

How might AVP be facilitating pair bond formation in the male prairie vole? In a study parallel to that described above for OT, the locations of V1aR in the brains of the prairie and montane voles were compared, and several intriguing differences were found (Insel, Wang, & Ferris, 1994). One difference of particular interest is in the ventral pallidum (Figure 3) (Young et al., 2001), which is located very closely to, and is reciprocally connected to, the nucleus accumbens. Like the nucleus accumbens, the ventral pallidum is part of the reward circuitry in the brain (McBride, Murphy, & Ikemoto, 1999). As it turns out, in several unrelated monogamous species, V1aR is abundant in the ventral pallidum compared with nonmonogamous related species. A recent study suggests that the density of V1aR in the ventral pallidum is directly related to the ability to form a pair bond. In this study, viral vector–mediated gene transfer was used to increase the density of V1aR in the ventral pallidum of male prairie voles (Pitkow, Sharer, Ren, Terwilliger, & Young, 2001). Compared with control males injected with an inactive gene, males with increased ventral pallidal receptor density were much more likely to form a partner preference and displayed increased affiliative behavior toward juvenile prairie voles.

It seems that in male and female prairie voles, two closely related molecules facilitate social attachment by activating two separate components of the same reward circuit, namely, the nucleus accumbens for OT and the ventral pallidum for AVP. These regions are rich in another neurotransmitter, dopamine, which has widely been associated with reward. Drugs of abuse, such as amphetamines and cocaine, are thought to produce their euphoric effects by modulating the dopamine system in these regions (McBride et al., 1999). In fact, injections of cocaine into these regions of the rat brain result in the development of a conditioned *place* preference (Gong, Neill, & Justice, 1996). That is, the rat prefers to be in the environment in which it once received an injection of drug into these regions. Perhaps the activation of the OT and AVP receptors in these regions during mating results in the development of a conditioned partner preference in prairie voles. Because montane voles have few receptors in these regions, mating and/or the release of peptide in the brain would not result in the formation of a partner preference but may instead elicit other types of behaviors. If true, social attachment may be mediated, at least in part, by the brain's natural reward systems, which are so often abused by the use of illicit drugs. In addition to facilitating social attachment, both OT and AVP appear to increase nonspecific social interaction, or affiliative behavior (Cho et al., 1999; Witt, Winslow, & Insel, 1992; Young, Nilsen, Waymire, MacGregor, & Insel 1999), as well as social recognition (Englemann & Landgraf, 1994; Ferguson, Young, Hearn, Insel, & Winslow, 2000). Thus, it appears that these molecules may play an important role in modulating many aspects of social relations beyond selective bonding.

There are several caveats to the proposed mechanisms underlying attachment described thus far. First, these data in no way imply that OT and AVP are the only biochemicals involved in social attachment. There is likely a multitude of other factors, dopamine, for instance, that are involved in the chain of events leading to social bonding. Likewise, the reward circuitry is likely not the only brain sites involved in OT- or AVP-facilitated attachments. Other regions, such as the amygdala, hypothalamus, and lateral septum, likely also contribute in the cascade of events that lead to the social bond. Finally, as stated in the outset, one must be careful when making conjecture on the neural basis of human behavior based on rodent studies. Clearly, these neuropeptides or circuitry may be involved in human bonding, but there are very little data at this point, as experimental manipulation of human bonding cannot be performed in the laboratory. However, it should be noted that OT and AVP are released into the plasma during sexual activity in humans. It is plausible that these hormones released during intimate moments serve to strengthen psychological bond between partners.

Biochemistry of Parental Commitment in Mammals

Maternal Responsiveness

In many species, females that have not produced offspring themselves are either indifferent to or avoid young. Then, after delivery of their own young, they become obsessed with caring for them. This nurturing motivation remains strong until the offspring leave the care of their mother. What biochemical changes during pregnancy and delivery promote maternal care? The laboratory rat has provided a great deal of insight into this process. Maternal behavior in rats consists of four basic behaviors: nest building, pup retrieval, nursing, and licking and grooming, each of which emerges around the time of parturition (Figure 4). One of the classic studies of behavioral neuroscience demonstrated that molecules circulating in the blood during pregnancy facilitate the onset of maternal care. In this study, a virgin rat was continuously transfused with the blood of a pregnant rat, such that hormones secreted by the pregnant rat reached the brain of the virgin (Terkel & Rosenblatt, 1972). The virgin rat became maternal precisely coincidental with the onset of parental care of the parturient rat. Several studies have subsequently identified several hormonal molecules that promote maternal responsiveness (Young & Insel, 2002).

As it turns out, many of the same hormones secreted in the body to promote the development and delivery of young also act in the brain to facilitate the nurturing behavior of the mother. First, steroid hormones, such as estrogen and progesterone, are secreted at high levels during pregnancy. Among other things, these hormones serve to maintain the integrity of the uterus to support the implanted embryos. Several studies have now shown that a virgin female rat can be primed to display maternal behavior simply by injecting her with steroid hormones in such a way as to mimic the natural changes of these molecules during pregnancy and labor. Injections of estrogen and progesterone, followed by progesterone withdrawal, facilitate the onset of maternal behavior (Bridges, 1984). These hormones appear to be acting in the preoptic area of the hypothalamus, a brain region that has a high density of estrogen and progesterone receptors and that has been implicated in the expression of maternal behavior. However, these hormones are not acting alone to produce the natural switch toward nurturing behavior, as female rats treated in this way do not display immediate maternal care but require several hours of pup exposure before pup retrieval is observed.

Two neuropeptide hormones, prolactin and OT, appear to be critical for the induction of parental care in rats. Prolactin is a hormone released into the plasma in large amounts from the anterior pituitary just after parturition. As its name suggests, this hormone is involved in the regulation of lactation. Thus, it is not surprising that it also acts as a trigger to facilitate maternal behavior. Drugs that block prolactin release prevent the onset of parental care (Bridges, 1984), and infusions of prolactin into the lateral ventricles of the brain (Bridges, Numan, Ronsheim, Mann, & Lupini, 1990) or directly into the preoptic area facilitate maternal behavior (Bridges et al., 1997). Furthermore, mice with a genetic mutation in the prolactin receptor completely neglect their newborn offspring (Lucas, Ormandy, Binart, Bridges, & Kelly, 1998).

OT, which, as mentioned earlier, promotes uterine contractions and stimulates milk ejection during nursing, also facilitates the onset of maternal behavior in virgin rats within minutes after injection (Pedersen & Prange, 1979). Furthermore, blockade of OT receptors in the medial preoptic area and the ventral tegmental area prevents the onset of parental care in postpartum dams (Pedersen, Caldwell, Walker, Ayers, & Mason, 1994). Interestingly, OT is not required for the maintenance of maternal behavior once it has been established, as blocking OT receptors or destroying the brain's source of OT does not abolish it (Insel & Harbaugh, 1989). In addition to the direct effect on the initiation of maternal behavior, OT probably modulates maternal–offspring interactions through its anxiolytic effects. OT likely produces its anxiolytic

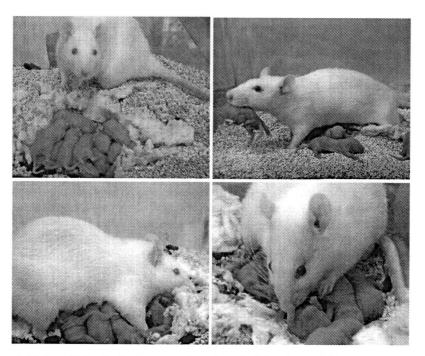

Figure 4. Maternal behavior in the rat consists of nest building (upper left), pup retrieval (upper right), nursing (lower left), and licking and grooming (lower right)

effects through its interactions with receptors in the central nucleus of the amygdala (Bale, Davis, Auger, Dorsa, & McCarthy, 2001).

Rodents typically display promiscuous maternal behavior. That is, they do not discriminate between their own pups and those from other females. Sheep, on the other hand, are selectively maternal and form strong bonds with their own lambs within minutes after they give birth (Kendrick et al., 1997). A series of studies have demonstrated that OT plays a critical role in forming that bond between the ewe and her lamb. For example, injections of OT into the brain of a steroid-primed ewe will cause her to accept a strange lamb as her own (Kendrick, Keverne, & Baldwin, 1987).

Paternal Care

Whereas common laboratory rats have provided most of our knowledge of the neurochemistry of maternal responsiveness, they are useless for examining the biology of paternal care. Again, the monogamous prairie voles have provided some insight. As discussed earlier, AVP plays an important role in facilitating social attachments between mates in male prairie voles. One study has demonstrated that this neuropeptide facilitates paternal care as well (Wang, Ferris, & DeVries, 1994). Infusion of AVP directly into the lateral septum of prairie vole males results in an increase in pup retrieval and time in contact with the pups.

Some studies suggest that prolactin may be involved in paternal care as well. Measurements of prolactin levels in the plasma of expecting father marmosets, which display biparental care, suggested that prolactin levels increase concurrently with the onset of paternal care (Dixson & George, 1982). Furthermore, prolactin levels are elevated in both male and female parentally inexperienced marmosets after carrying infants.

Together, the studies on social attachment and parental care indicate that the peptide hormones OT and AVP play a prominent role in family investment in rodents. Interestingly, species with different family structures display different patterns of receptor localization in the brain. Thus, factors that influence the OT and AVP systems will likely lead to perturbations in social behaviors. As will be discussed in the following section, early life experiences, such as the pattern of parental behavior one experiences during development, alter these neuropeptide systems, thereby possibly providing a biochemical mechanism by which adolescent experience alters adult social competence.

Developmental Influences on Youth Competence in Rodents

It has been known for more than 40 years that neonatal experiences in rats have a powerful effect on emotional reactivity of the offspring. An early handling (infantile stimulation) paradigm was shown to result in reduced emotional reactivity, and a prolonged maternal separation paradigm was found to confer increased emotional reactivity in rats (Plotsky & Meaney, 1993). For example, early handling decreases and prolonged maternal separation increases hypothalamic–pituitary–adrenal activation in response to restraint stress or mild foot shock stress (Ladd, Owens, & Nemeroff, 1996; Liu, Caldji, Sharma, Plotsky, & Meaney, 2000; Plotsky & Meaney, 1993). Not only are there permanent changes in behavioral responses to stressful situations, the underlying neural systems believed to mediate these behaviors are also changed. For example, rats that received more maternal stimulation as pups have altered levels of stress hormone receptors (glucocorticoid receptor) in the hippocampus, a brain region that plays a central role in the regulation of the stress response (Meaney et al., 1996).

Recent studies have begun to examine the mechanisms by which early experience confers these long-term effects. In an important study from Michael Meaney's group at McGill University, researchers discovered that the mothers of handled rat pups showed increased amounts of maternal attention in the form of pup licking compared with mothers of nonhandled pups (Liu et al., 1997). Moreover, there are natural individual differences in the amount of licking that a mother rat spontaneously exhibits toward her pups, and these individual differences in "maternal style" are consistent across litters. More interestingly, these differences in the quality of maternal care translated into differences in stress reactivity and anxiety levels in the offspring (Caldji, Tannenbaum, Sharma, Francis, & Plotsky, 1998). The offspring of mothers with high levels of licking exhibit reduced emotionality and stress responsiveness relative to the offspring of low-licking mothers (Caldji et al., 1998; Liu et al., 1997). Not only do these differences in maternal attention predict emotionality of the offspring, they also predict how the offspring will mother their own pups. That is, the offspring of high-licking mothers also showed high levels of licking toward their own pups in adulthood (Francis, Diorio, Liu, & Meaney, 1999). One important question to ask is whether this variability in maternal care is genetically transmitted to the offspring or somehow "acquired" by the pups. To answer this question, pups from low-licking mothers were cross-fostered to high-licking mothers. In adulthood, these cross-fostered females showed reduced emotional reactivity and anxiety when placed in stressful situations and high levels of licking toward their own offspring (Figure 5).

These various studies of individual differences in maternal style reveal that even natural variations in mothering can result in profound differences not only in the offspring's emotional reactivity but also in the offspring's behavior toward her own infants. This suggests a nongenomic mechanism for the transmission of behavioral traits. Remarkably, these differences in behavioral state are associated with reliable differences in brain chemistry, specifically oxytocin. Females that have received higher levels of maternal stimulation as infants have higher concentrations of oxytocin receptors specifically in the amygdala. Males do not show this difference but have increased levels of vasopressin receptors in the same region (Francis, Young, Meaney, & Insel, 2002).

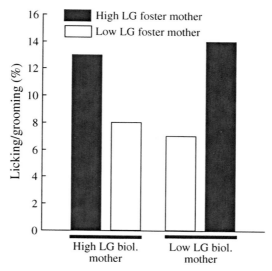

Figure 5. Nongenomic transmission across generations of maternal behavior patterns. Values represent the relative frequency of licking and grooming of pups for mothers that were fostered as pups to either high-licking-grooming (LG) or low-licking-grooming mothers. Pups reared by high-licking-grooming mothers exhibit high levels of licking and grooming as mothers regardless of the behavior of their biological mothers. (Data from Francis, Diorio, Liu, & Meaney, 1999; 286:1155–1158)

These findings suggest that differences in maternal care result in specific changes in the very systems implicated in social bond formation. At a molecular level, it appears that the kind of mothering a rat receives determines the development of the neurochemical systems critical for parental care and social interaction. Although we do not know the mechanisms by which maternal licking determines these neurochemical differences, Champagne, Diorio, Sharma, and Meaney (2001) have discovered an important role for estrogen receptors in this process. They have demonstrated that estrogen administration is effective in promoting maternal responsivity in virgin female rats *only* in the offspring of high-licking mothers. Estrogen was completely ineffective in altering maternal responsivity in offspring of low-licking females. The increase in maternal responsivity in high-licked females was also positively correlated with an increase in OT receptor expression in several maternal brain sites. These results demonstrate a strong interaction between the OT and estrogen systems, and how in concert, they may serve to induce and promote the expression of maternal care.

The studies described thus far are in essence investigating some very old and popular concepts regarding maternal and parental care. We begin to understand how phrases such as "Like mother, like daughter" and "Like begets like" may indeed have very biologically relevant roots. As we have seen, the quality of maternal care one receives regulates the very genes that modulate both coping with stressful stimuli and the quality of social interaction and nurturing provided to one's own offspring (Figure 6). Without interruption,

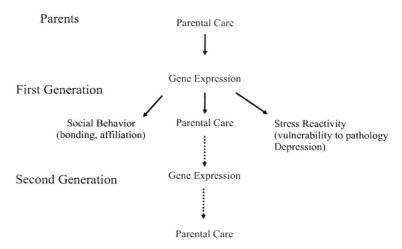

Figure 6. Figure demonstrating early environmental–parental regulation of genes in offspring, which subsequently regulate behavior, stress reactivity, and parental care in the following generation of animals. It is easy to observe how this cycle of transmission can occur ad infinitum without an environmental intervention to disrupt it

the parenting and coping styles are transmitted from generation to generation through this modulation of the brain's biochemistry. Whereas scientists have known for decades about the relationship between quality of early life environments and development, we have only fairly recently begun to address these very "human" questions concerning social bonding and parental care using animal models. Similar to results obtained using rodent and primate models of differing early-life events, it appears as if similar processes may indeed be at work in humans.

Relevancy to Humans

   Two human studies investigating the quality of early-life events in relationship to adult health and well-being demonstrate how successful and effective animal models have been at modeling the human condition. Russek and Schwartz, in 1997, published a follow-up study to an experiment conducted in the early 1950s at Harvard University that investigated the reflections of a sample of healthy, undergraduate Harvard men about their feelings of warmth and closeness to their parents. When these same men were interviewed 35 years later and their medical and psychological histories were taken, a dramatic relationship emerged. Of those men who did not perceive themselves to have had a warm relationship with their parents, 91% had diagnosed diseases (such as coronary artery disease, hypertension, duodenal ulcer, alcoholism), when interviewed. Men who perceived warm relationships with their parents demonstrated only a 45% incidence of disease. This very simple follow-up study reinforces the wealth of animal data that demonstrate that the quality of an organism's early life and environment may play a profound role in the life of that animal later in adulthood

Another more recent study published in the *Journal of the American Medical Association* was the first human report to demonstrate lasting changes in stress reactivity in adult women who had suffered trauma early in life (Heim et al., 2000). The study was modeled after many of the laboratory animal studies described earlier in this chapter. The authors demonstrated that women subjected to early-life stress such as childhood physical or sexual abuse had as adults increased physiologic and hormonal responses to stress. They hypothesized that this increased reactivity may subsequently increase vulnerability to develop stress-related psychiatric disorders later in adulthood.

The results from these two studies suggest that processes at work in voles, rats, and other furry mammals may indeed be directly relevant to humans, underscoring the importance of basic animal models to the study of complex behaviors, including attachment and parental care.

References

Bale, T. L., Davis, A. M., Auger, A. P., Dorsa, D. M., & McCarthy, M. M. (2001). CNS region–specific oxytocin receptor expression: Importance in regulation of anxiety and sex behavior. *Journal of Neuroscience, 21*, 2546–2552.

Bridges, R. S. (1984). A quantitative analysis of the roles of dosage, sequence, and duration of estradiol and progesterone exposure in the regulation of maternal behavior in the rat. *Endocrinology, 114*, 930–940.

Bridges, R. S., Numan, M., Ronsheim, P. M., Mann, P. E., & Lupini, C. E. (1990). Central prolactin infusions stimulate maternal behavior in steroid-treated, nulliparous female rats. *Proceedings of the National Academy of Sciences USA, 87*, 8003–8007.

Bridges, R. S., Robertson, M. C., Shiu, R. P. C., Sturgis, J. J., Henriquez, B. M., & Mann, P. E. (1997). Central lactogenic regulation of maternal behavior in rats: Steroid dependence, hormone specificity, and behavioral potencies of rat prolactin and rat placental lactogen I. *Endocrinology, 138*, 756–763.

Caldji, C., Tannenbaum, B., Sharma, S., Francis, D., & Plotsky, P. M. (1998). Maternal care during infancy regulates the development of neural systems mediating the expression of behavioral fearfulness in adulthood in the rat. *Proceedings of the National Academy of Sciences USA, 95*, 5335–5340.

Carter, C. S. (1998). Neuroendocrine perspectives on social attachment and love. *Psychoneuroendocrinology, 23*, 779–818.

Carter, C. S., & Getz, L. L. (1993). Monogamy and the prairie vole. *Scientific American, 268*, 100–106.

Champagne, F, Diorio, J., Sharma, S., & Meaney, M. J. (2001). Naturally occurring variations in maternal behavior in the rat are associated with differences in estrogen-inducible central oxytocin receptors. *Proceedings of the National Academy of Sciences USA, 98*, 12736–12741.

Cho, M .M., DeVries, A. C., Williams, J. R., & Carter, C. S. (1999). The effects of oxytocin and vasopressin on partner preferences in male and female prairie voles (*Microtus ochrogaster*). *Behavioral Neuroscience, 113*, 1071–1079.

DeVries, G. J. (1990). Sex differences in the brain. *Journal of Neuroendocrinology, 2*, 1–13.

Dixson, A. F., & George, L. (1982). Prolactin and parental behaviour in a male New World primate. *Nature, 299*, 551–553.

Englemann, M., & Landgraf, R. (1994). Microdialysis administration of vasopressin into the septum improves social recognition in Brattleboro rats. *Physiology and Behavior, 55*, 145–149.

Ferguson, J. N., Young, L. J., Hearn, E. F., Insel, T. R., & Winslow, J. T. (2000). Social amnesia in mice lacking the oxytocin gene. *Nature Genetics, 25,* 284–288.

Francis, D., Diorio, J., Liu, D., & Meaney, M. J. (1999). Variations in maternal care form the basis for a non-genomic mechanism of inter-generational transmission of individual differences in behavioral and endocrine responses to stress. *Science, 286,* 1155–1158.

Francis, D. D., Young, L. J., Meaney, M. J., & Insel, T. R. (2002). Naturally occurring differences in maternal care are associated with the expression of oxytocin and vasopressin (V1a) receptors: Gender differences. *Journal of Neuroendocrinology, 14,* 349–353.

Gainer, H., & Wray, W. (1994). Cellular and molecular biology of oxytocin and vasopressin. In E. Knobil & J. D. Neill (Eds.), *The physiology of reproduction* (pp. 1099–1129). New York: Raven Press.

Gong, W., Neill, D., & Justice, J. B. (1996). Conditioned place preference and locomotor activation produced by injection of psychostimulants in ventral pallidum. *Brain Research, 707,* 64–74.

Heim, C., Newport, J., Heit, S., Graham, Y. P., Wilcox, M., Bonsall, R., et al. (2000). Pituitary-adrenal and autonomic responses to stress in women after sexual and physical abuse in childhood. *Journal of the American Medical Association, 284,* 592–597.

Insel, T. R., & Harbaugh, C. R. (1989). Lesions of the hypothalamic paraventricular nucleus disrupt the initiation of maternal behavior. *Physiology and Behavior, 45,* 1033–1041.

Insel, T. R., & Hulihan, T. (1995). A gender-specific mechanism for pair bonding: Oxytocin and partner preference formation in monogamous voles. *Behavioral Neuroscience, 109,* 782-789.

Insel, T. R., Preston, S., & Winslow, J. T. (1995). Mating in the monogamous male: Behavioral consequences. *Physiology and Behavior, 57,* 615–627.

Insel, T. R., & Shapiro, L. E. (1992). Oxytocin receptor distribution reflects social organization in monogamous and polygamous voles. *Proceedings of the National Academy of Sciences USA, 89,* 5981–5985.

Insel, T. R., Wang, Z., & Ferris, C. F. (1994). Patterns of brain vasopressin receptor distribution associated with social organization in microtine rodents. *Journal of Neuroscience, 14,* 5381–5392.

Insel, T. R., & Young, L. J. (2001). Neurobiology of social attachment. *Nature Neuroscience, 2,* 129–136.

Jannett, F. J. (1980). Social dynamics of the montane vole *Microtus montanus,* as a paradigm. *Biologist, 62,* 3–19.

Kendrick, K. M., Costa, A. P. C. D., Broad, K. D., Ohkura, S., Guevara, R., Levy, F., et al. (1997). Neural control of maternal behavior and olfactory recognition of offspring. *Brain Research Bulletin, 44,* 383–395.

Kendrick, K. M., Keverne, E. B., & Baldwin, B. A. (1987). Intracerebroventricular oxytocin stimulates maternal behaviour in sheep. *Neuroendocrinology, 46,* 56–61.

Ladd, C. O., Owens, M. J., & Nemeroff, C. B. (1996). Persistent changes in corticotropin-releasing factor neuronal systems induced by maternal deprivation. *Endocrinology, 137,* 1212–1218.

Liu, D., Caldji, C., Sharma, S., Plotsky, P. M., & Meaney, M. J. (2000). Influence of neonatal rearing conditions on stress-induced adrenocorticotropin responses and norepinepherine release in the hypothalamic paraventricular nucleus. *Journal of Neuroendocrinology, 12,* 5–12.

Liu, D., Tannenbaum, B., Caldji, C., Francis, D., Freedman, A., Sharma, S., et al. (1997). Maternal care, hippocampal glucocorticoid receptro gene expression and hypothalamic-pituitary-adrenal responses to stress. *Science, 277,* 1659–1662.

Lucas, B. K., Ormandy, C. J., Binart, N., Bridges, R. S., & Kelly, P. A. (1998). Null mutation of the prolactin receptor gene produces a defect in maternal behavior. *Endocrinology, 139,* 4102–4107.

McBride, W. J., Murphy, J. M., & Ikemoto, S. (1999). Localization of brain reinforcement mechanims: Intracranial self-administration and intracranial place-conditioning studies. *Behavioural Brain Research, 101,* 129–152.

Meaney, M. J., Diorio, J., Francis, D., Widdowson, J., LaPlante, P., Caldji, C., et al. (1996). Early environmental regulation of forebrain glucocorticoid receptor gene expression: Implications for adrenocortical responses to stress. *Developmental Neuroscience, 18,* 49–72.

Pedersen, C. A., Caldwell, J. D., Walker, C., Ayers, G., & Mason, G. A. (1994). Oxytocin activates the postpartum onset of rat maternal behavior in the ventral tegmental and medial preoptic area. *Behavioral Neuroscience, 108,* 1163–1171.

Pedersen, C. A., & Prange, A. J. (1979). Induction of maternal behavior in virgin rats after intrac-erebroventricular administration of oxytocin. *Proceedings of the National Academy of Sciences USA, 76*, 6661–6665.

Pitkow, L. J., Sharer, C. A., Ren, X., Insel, T. R., Terwilliger, E. F., & Young, L. J. (2001). Facilitation of affiliation and pair-bond formation by vasopressin receptor gene transfer into the ventral forebrain of a monogamous vole. *Journal of Neuroscience, 21*, 7392–7396.

Plotsky, P., & Meaney, M. J. (1993). Early, postnatal experience alters hypothalamic corticotropin-releasing factor (CRF) mRNA, median eminence CRF content and stress-induced release in adult rats. *Molecular Brain Research, 18*, 195–200.

Russek, L., & Schwartz, G. E. (1997). Feelings of parental caring predict health status in midlife: A 35-year follow-up of the Harvard Mastery of Stress Study. *Journal of Behavioral Medicine, 20*, 1–13.

Terkel, J., & Rosenblatt, J. S. (1972). Humoral factors underlying maternal behavior at parturition: Cross transfusion between freely moving rats. *Journal of Comparative Physiology and Psychology, 80*, 365–371.

Wang, Z., Ferris, C. F., & DeVries, G. J. (1994). Role of septal vasopressin innervation in paternal behavior in prairie voles (*Microtus ochrogaster*). *Proceedings of the National Academy of Sciences USA, 91*, 400–404.

Williams, J., Catania, K., & Carter, C. (1992). Development of partner preferences in female prairie voles (*Microtus ochrogaster*): The role of social and sexual experience. *Hormones and Behavior, 26*, 339–349.

Williams, J. R., Insel, T. R., Harbaugh, C. R., & Carter, C. S. (1994). Oxytocin administered centrally facilitates formation of a partner preference in prairie voles (*Microtus ochrogaster*). *Journal of Neuroendocrinology, 6*, 247–250.

Winslow, J., Hastings, N., Carter, C. S., Harbaugh, C., & Insel, T. (1993). A role for central vasopressin in pair bonding in monogamous prairie voles. *Nature, 365*, 545–548.

Witt, D. M., Winslow, J. T., & Insel, T. R. (1992). Enhanced social interactions in rats following chronic, centrally infused oxytocin. *Pharmacology Biochemistry and Behavior, 43*, 855–861.

Young, L. J., & Insel, T. R. (2002). Hormones and parental behavior. In J. B. Becker, S. M. Breedlove, and D. Crews, *Behavioral endocrinology* (2nd ed., pp. 331–368). Cambridge, MA: MIT Press.

Young, L. J., Lim, M. M., Gingrich, B., & Insel, T.R. (2001). Cellular mechanisms of social attachment. *Hormones and Behavior, 40*, 133–138.

Young, L. J., Nilsen, R., Waymire, K. G., MacGregor, G. R.., & Insel, T. R. (1999). Increased affiliative response to vasopressin in mice expressing the vasopressin receptor from a monogamous vole. *Nature, 400*, 766–768.

3 How Mother Nurture Helps Mother Nature: Scientific Evidence for the Protective Effect of Good Nurturing on Genetic Propensity Toward Anxiety and Alcohol Abuse

Stephen J. Suomi

National Institutes of Health

This chapter summarizes a body of research investigating a possible relationship between problems in socioemotional regulation expressed early in life and excessive alcohol consumption in adolescence and early adulthood among group-living rhesus monkeys. A major focus of the research reviewed has been to characterize certain genetic and environmental factors—and their multiple interactions—that consistently predispose some monkeys to consume significantly more alcohol in the same social settings than most others in their social group. Such excessive alcohol consumption is exhibited disproportionately by one subgroup of monkeys who seem unusually fearful in novel or mildly challenging circumstances, as well as by a second subgroup who repeatedly exhibit impulsive and inappropriate aggression. In both cases, difficulties in the regulation of specific emotions evident from early in life onward appear to be linked to a variety of behavioral and physiologic problems that emerge later in development and typically persist thereafter.

By way of background, it is now generally accepted that humans do not have a monopoly on emotionality. Indeed, more than a century ago, Charles Darwin (1872) argued that some mammals are clearly capable of expressing emotions, and an impressive body of recent research has demonstrated that many mammals possess the same basic neural circuitry and exhibit the same general patterns of neurochemical change that have been implicated in human emotional expression (e.g., Panksepp, 1998). Monkeys and apes, in particular, display characteristic patterns of emotional expression that seem strikingly similar to, if not homologous with, those routinely exhibited by infants and young children in virtually every human culture studied to date. To be sure, some complex emotions such as shame are most likely exclusively human, but those apparently require cognitive capabilities well beyond those of human infants and nonhuman primates of any age (cf. Lewis, 1992). Most other emotions are clearly expressed soon after birth by human and nonhuman primate infants alike, and they appear to serve as highly visible and salient social signals to those around them (cf. Suomi, 1997b). Among the most obvious are expressions of fear and those of anger and rage associated with aggression.

Ethologists have long argued that these basic patterns of emotional expression each serve important adaptive functions, having been largely conserved over mammalian evolutionary history. Consider the case of fear: In a world filled with predators and competitors who have the potential to maim or even kill, an individual fully without fear is unlikely to survive very long. On the other hand, excessive or inappropriate fear can essentially paralyze any individual, in effect limiting those very interactions with the environment needed to obtain the physical and social sustenance necessary for survival. Thus, while every human and nonhuman primate is born with the capacity to be fearful, each must learn which particular stimuli merit fearful responses, as well as how to inhibit the expression of fear in nonthreatening situations that present little risk to life or limb (Suomi & Harlow, 1976).

Similarly, the capability to engage in aggressive attack and defense in the service of protecting self, family, and friends from predators and competitors is seemingly crucial for the survival of the individual and the maintenance of any social group of long-term standing. Yet excessive and/or inappropriate aggression by any individual has the potential of destroying the very social fabric that binds the group together. The expression of aggression must therefore be regulated; that is, individual group members must come to know which social stimuli merit an aggressive response and which do not, and for those that do, to what degree, and for how long, if the group is to maintain its social cohesion over time and across generations. Indeed, learning how and when to avoid aggressive encounters and when and how to end those once begun may be at least as important as learning how and when to start or respond to aggression (Suomi, 2000a).

The development of proficiency in socioemotional regulation appears to be especially important for those advanced primate species whose members live in large social groups that are well defined in terms of both kinship relationships and social dominance hierarchies. Among the most complex are those of rhesus monkeys (*Macaca mulatta*), a highly successful species of macaque monkey that lives throughout most of the Indian subcontinent and beyond. In their natural habitats, rhesus monkeys typically reside in large, distinctive social groups ("troops") composed of several female-headed families, each spanning three or more generations of kin, plus numerous immigrant adult males. This form of social group organization derives from the fact that all rhesus monkey females spend their entire life in the troop in which they were born, whereas virtually all males emigrate from their natal troop around the time of puberty and eventually join other troops. Rhesus monkey troops are also characterized by multiple social dominance relationships, including distinctive hierarchies both between and within families, as well as a hierarchy among the immigrant adult males (Lindburg, 1971).

The complex familial and dominance relationships seen in rhesus monkey troops seemingly require that any well-functioning troop member not only be able to regulate its expressions of fear and aggression but also become familiar with the specific kinship and dominance status of other monkeys toward whom those emotions might be expressed. An impressive body of both laboratory and field data strongly suggests that the acquisition of such knowledge represents an emergent property of the species-normative pattern of socialization that rhesus monkey infants experience as they are growing up (Sameroff & Suomi, 1996).

Normative Development of Socioemotional Regulation in Rhesus Monkeys

Rhesus monkey infants begin life highly dependent upon their biological mother for essentially all of their initial biological and psychological needs (in this species, fathers are not active participants in early child care activities). An infant typically spends its first month of life in almost continuous physical contact with its mother, and during this time a strong and enduring social bond between mother and infant emerges naturally (Harlow, 1958). This bond, largely homologous with Bowlby's (1969) characterization of human mother–infant *attachment*, is unique in terms of its exclusivity, constituent behavioral features, and ultimate duration—it is like no other social relationship any monkey will ever experience again in its lifetime, except (in reciprocal form) for females when they grow up to have infants of their own (Suomi, 1999).

Once an infant has become securely attached to its mother, it can use her as an established base from which to begin exploring its immediate social and nonsocial environment. Most infant monkeys soon learn that if they become frightened or otherwise threatened, they can always run back to their mother for immediate safety and comfort through mutual ventral contact—if she hasn't already actively intervened on their behalf. Numerous studies have documented that initiation of ventral contact with the mother promotes rapid decreases in hypothalamic–pituitary–adrenal (HPA) activity, as indexed by lowered plasma cortisol concentrations (e.g., Gunnar, Gonzalez, Goodlin, & Levine, 1981; Mendoza, Smotherman, Miner, Kaplan, & Levine, 1978) and in sympathetic nervous system arousal, as indexed by reductions in heart rate (e.g., Reite, Short, Selier, & Pauley, 1981), along with other physiologic changes commonly associated with soothing. Secure attachment relationships thus help infants learn to manage the fears they will inevitably experience in the course of exploring their ever-expanding world. On the other hand, if a rhesus monkey infant develops an insecure attachment relationship with its mother, both its ability to regulate fear and its willingness to explore may be compromised, consistent with Bowlby's observations regarding human attachment relationships (Bowlby, 1988; Suomi, 1999).

In their second and third months, rhesus infants begin interacting with monkeys other than their mother, and they soon develop distinctive social relationships with specific individuals outside of their immediate family, especially with *peers*—other infants of like age and comparable physical, cognitive, and socioemotional capabilities. After weaning (usually in the fourth and fifth months), play with peers emerges as a predominant social activity for young monkeys and essentially remains so until puberty (Ruppenthal, Harlow, Eisele, Harlow, & Suomi, 1974). During this time, their play interactions become more and more behaviorally and socially complex, increasingly involving patterns of behavior that appear to simulate the full range of adult social activity. By the time they reach puberty, most rhesus monkey juveniles have had ample opportunity to develop, practice, and perfect behavioral routines that will be crucial for functioning as normal adults, especially those involving dominance interactions and aggressive exchanges.

Aggression typically emerges in a rhesus monkey's behavioral repertoire around 6 months of age, and it initially appears in the context of rough-and-tumble play (Symons, 1978). Sham biting, hair pulling, wrestling, and other forms of physical contact are basic components of rough-and-tumble play directed toward peers, occurring with increasing frequency among males in the second half of their first year of life and, in fact, becoming their predominant form of play behavior throughout the juvenile years. Although some form of virtually all of the basic physical components of adult aggressive exchanges can be seen in these rough-and-tumble play bouts, the intensity of such interactions is usually quite controlled and seldom escalates to the point of actual physical injury—if it does, the play bout is almost always terminated immediately, either by adult intervention or by one or more of the participants themselves backing away. The importance of these play bouts with peers for the socialization of aggression becomes apparent when one considers that rhesus monkey infants reared in laboratory environments that deny them regular access to peers during their initial months inevitably exhibit excessive and socially inappropriate aggression later in life (cf. Suomi & Harlow, 1975).

The onset of puberty is associated with major life transitions for both males and females, involving not only major hormonal alterations, pronounced growth spurts, and other obvious physical changes, but also major social changes for both sexes. Males experience the most dramatic and serious social disruptions: When they leave home, they sever all social contact, not only with their mother and other kin but also with all others in their natal social troop. Virtually all of these adolescent males soon join all-male "gangs," and after several months to a year, most of them then attempt to join a different troop, usually composed entirely of individuals largely unfamiliar to the immigrant males (Berard, 1989). The process of natal troop emigration is exceedingly dangerous for adolescent males—the mortality rate from the time they leave their natal troop until they become successfully integrated into another troop can approach 50%, depending on local circumstances (e.g., Dittus, 1979). Recent field studies have identified and characterized striking variability in both the timing of male emigration and the basic strategies followed in attempting to join other established social groups.

Adolescent females, by contrast, never leave their maternal family or natal troop. Puberty for them is instead associated with increases in social activities directed toward maternal kin, especially when these young females begin to have offspring of their own. Indeed, the birth of a new infant (especially to a new mother) often has the effect of "invigorating" the matriline, drawing its members closer both physically and socially and, conversely, providing a buffer from external threats and stressors for mother and infant alike. These females' ties to both family and troop are facilitated throughout adulthood by appropriate regulation of fear and aggression; conversely, these ties can be threatened whenever such socioemotional regulation goes awry (Suomi, 1998).

Individual Differences in the Regulation of Fear

Although the basic sequences of socioemotional development outlined above are typical for most rhesus monkeys growing up both in the wild and in captive social groups, there are nevertheless substantial differences among individuals in the precise timing and relative ease with which they make major developmental transitions, as well as how they manage the day-to-day challenges and stresses that are an inevitable consequence of complex social group life. In particular, recent research has identified two subgroups of monkeys who exhibit specific deficits in socioemotional regulation that can result in increased long-term risk for behavioral pathology, physiologic dysfunction, and even early mortality. Members of one subgroup, comprising approximately 15% to 20% of both wild and captive populations, seem excessively fearful. These monkeys consistently respond to novel and/or mildly challenging situations with extreme behavioral disruption and pronounced physiologic arousal, including significant and often prolonged activation of the HPA axis, sympathetic nervous system arousal, and increased noradrenergic turnover (Suomi, 1986).

These fearful or "uptight" monkeys can usually be readily identified during their first few months of life. Most begin leaving their mothers later chronologically and explore their physical and social environment less than other infants in their birth cohort. Highly fearful youngsters also tend to be shy and withdrawn in their initial encounters with peers: Laboratory studies have shown that they exhibit significantly higher and stabler heart rates and greater secretion of cortisol in such interactions than do their less reactive age-mates. However, when these monkeys are in familiar and stable social settings, they are virtually indistinguishable, both behaviorally and physiologically, from others in their peer group. In contrast, when fearful monkeys encounter extreme and/or prolonged stress, their behavioral and physiologic differences from others in their social group usually become exaggerated (Suomi, 1991a).

For example, young rhesus monkeys growing up in the wild typically experience functional maternal separations during the 2-month-long annual breeding season when their mothers repeatedly leave the troop for brief periods to consort with selected males (Berman, Rasmussen, & Suomi, 1994). The sudden loss of access to its mother is a major social stressor for any young monkey, and, not surprisingly, virtually all youngsters initially react to their mother's departure with short-term behavioral agitation and physiologic arousal, much as Bowlby (1960, 1973) described for human infants experiencing involuntary maternal separation.

However, whereas most youngsters soon begin to adapt to the separation and readily seek out the company of others in their social group until their mother returns, highly fearful individuals typically lapse into a behavioral depression characterized by increasing lethargy, lack of apparent interest in social stimuli, eating and sleeping difficulties, and a characteristic hunched-over, fetal-like posture (Suomi, 1991b). Laboratory studies simulating these naturalistic maternal separations have shown that relative to their like-reared peers, highly fearful monkeys not only are more likely to exhibit depressive-like behavioral reactions to short-term social separation but also tend to show greater and more prolonged HPA activation, more dramatic sympathetic arousal, more rapid central noradrenergic turnover, and greater immunosuppression (Suomi, 1991a). These differential patterns of biobehavioral response to separation tend to remain remarkably stable throughout prepubertal development and may be maintained during adolescence and even into adulthood (Suomi, 1995). There is compelling evidence of significant heritability for at least some components of these differential patterns of response (e.g., Higley, Hasert, Suomi, & Linnoila, 1993).

In naturalistic settings, fearful rhesus juveniles have greater adrenocortical activity, higher parasite loads, and lower antibody titers after tetanus vaccination than do others in their birth cohort (Laudenslager, Rasmussen, Berman, Broussard, & Suomi, 1993; Laudenslager et al., 1999). When they reach adolescence, fearful males tend to emigrate from their natal troop at significantly older ages than the rest of their male cohort, and, when they do finally leave, they typically employ much more conservative strategies for entering a new troop than do their less-reactive peers. Such strategies actually appear to enhance the prospects of surviving the emigration process for these fearful males (Rasmussen, Fellows, & Suomi, 1990). Thus, even though excessive fearfulness apparently puts an individual male at increased risk for adverse biobehavioral reactions to stress throughout development, there may be some circumstances in which this characteristic can actually be adaptive (Suomi, 2000b).

A parallel situation exists for females: Highly fearful young mothers in the wild tend to reject and punish their infants at higher rates around the time of weaning than do other mothers in their troop (Rasmussen, Timme, & Suomi, 1997), and in the absence of social support they appear to be at increased risk for infant neglect and/or abuse (Suomi & Ripp, 1983). Yet, under stable social circumstances, these fearful females not only may turn out to be highly competent mothers but also often achieve relatively high positions of social dominance (Rasmussen et al., 1997; Suomi, 1999). In sum, excessive fearfulness in infancy appears to be associated with increased risk for developing anxious- and depressive-like symptoms and potential problems in parenting in response to stressful circumstances later in life, but such long-term outcomes are far from inevitable.

Recent research has demonstrated that individual differences in biobe- havioral measures of fearfulness obtained during infancy are predictive of differential responses to other situations experienced later in life. One of the most striking of these involves differences in the propensity to consume alcohol in a "happy hour" situation. Over the past decade, Higley and his colleagues have developed an experimental paradigm in which group-living rhesus monkeys are given the opportunity to consume a 7% alcohol aspartame- flavored beverage, a nonalcoholic aspartame-flavored beverage, and/or plain tap water for daily 1-hour periods within their familiar social group (e.g., Higley et al., 1991). Fahlke et al. (2000) found that monkey infants who exhibited high levels of plasma cortisol after brief separations at 6 months of age subsequently consumed significantly more alcohol in this "happy hour" situation when they were 5 years of age than did monkeys whose 6-month cortisol responses were more moderate, independent of gender or rearing background. Indeed, the fearful monkeys seemed to be self-medicating in this situation.

Particularly noteworthy was the finding of Fahlke et al. (2000) that early individual differences in cortisol output were significantly more predictive of differences in alcohol consumption at 5 years than were individual differences in cortisol output obtained contemporaneously with the alcohol paradigm, that is, at 5 years of age. These findings lend additional empirical support to the view that excessive fearfulness during infancy can have significant, long-term consequences for monkeys in other situations experienced later in development.

Individual Differences in the Regulation of Aggression

A second subgroup of rhesus monkeys appears to have problems in regulating their aggressive behavior. These monkeys, comprising approx- imately 5% to 10% of the population, seem unusually impulsive, insen- sitive, and overaggressive in their interactions with other troop members. Impulsive young monkeys, especially males, seem to be unable to moderate their behavioral responses to rough-and-tumble play initiations from peers, often escalating initially benign play bouts into full-blown, tissue-damaging aggressive exchanges (Higley, Suomi, & Linnoila, 1992). Not surprisingly, most of these individuals tend to be avoided by peers during play bouts, and as a result they become increasingly isolated socially. In addition, many of these juvenile males often appear unwilling (or unable) to follow the "rules" inherent in rhesus monkey social dominance hierarchies. For example, they may directly challenge a dominant adult male, a foolhardy act that can result in serious injury, especially when the juvenile refuses to back away or exhibit submissive behavior once defeat becomes obvious. Impulsive juvenile males also show a propensity for making dangerous leaps from treetop to treetop, sometimes with painful outcomes (Mehlman et al., 1994).

Excessively impulsive monkeys, male and female alike, consistently exhibit chronic deficits in central serotonin metabolism, as reflected in unusually low cerebrospinal fluid (CSF) concentrations of the primary central serotonin metabolite 5-hydroxyindoleacetic acid (5-HIAA). Laboratory studies have shown that these deficits in serotonin metabolism appear early in life and tend to persist throughout development, as was the case for HPA responsiveness among highly fearful monkeys. Monkeys who exhibit such deficits are also likely to show poor state control and visual orienting capabilities during early infancy (Champoux, Suomi, & Schneider, 1994), poor performance on delay-of-gratification tasks during childhood (Bennett et al., 1999), and excessive cerebral glucose metabolism under mild isoflurane anesthesia as adults (Doudet et al., 1995). In addition, both laboratory and field studies have reported that individual differences in 5-HIAA concentrations are highly heritable among monkeys of similar age and comparable rearing background (e.g., Higley et al., 1993).

Recent field studies have found that the process of natal troop emigration typically experienced by impulsive males is seemingly the reverse of that shown by fearful males, with a long-term prognosis that is not particularly promising. Ostracized by their peers and frequently attacked by adults of both sexes, most of these excessively aggressive young males are physically driven out of their natal troop prior to 3 years of age, well before the onset of puberty and long before most of their male cohort begins the normal emigration process (Mehlman et al., 1995). These males tend to be grossly incompetent socially and, lacking the requisite social skills necessary for successful entrance into another troop or even to join an all-male gang, most of them become solitary and typically perish within a year (Higley, Mehlman, et al., 1996).

Young females who have chronically low CSF levels of 5-HIAA also tend to be impulsive, aggressive, and generally rather incompetent socially. However, unlike the males, they are not expelled from their natal troop but instead remain with their matriline throughout their lifetime, although studies of captive rhesus monkey groups suggest that these females usually stay at the bottom of their respective dominance hierarchies (Higley, King, et al., 1996). While most soon become mothers, recent research indicates that their maternal behavior often leaves much to be desired (Suomi, 2000a). In sum, rhesus monkeys who exhibit poor socioemotional regulation of impulsive and aggressive behavior and low central serotonin turnover early in life tend to follow developmental trajectories that often result in premature death for males and chronically low social dominance and poor parenting for females.

As was the case for excessively fearful monkeys, overly impulsive and aggressive individuals tend to consume excessive amounts of alcohol when placed in the aforementioned "happy hour" experimental paradigm (Higley, Suomi, & Linnoila, 1996). Interestingly, their pattern of alcohol consumption during the 1-hour sessions appears to be more like "binge drinking" than the "self-medication" pattern typically exhibited by excessively fearful individuals. Recent studies have demonstrated a significant relationship between degree of alcohol intoxication and serotonin transporter availability in these monkeys (Heinz et al, 1998), as well as among alcohol intake, innate tolerance, and serotonin transporter availability (Heinz et al., 2003). Finally, Champoux et al. (2002) have shown that individual differences in alcohol consumption at 5 years of age can be predicted by individual differences in measures of attention and motor maturity obtained as early as 14 days of age, suggesting that certain patterns of infant temperament may be associated with increased risk for substance abuse later in life.

Effects of Early Peer Rearing on the Regulation of Fear and Aggression

Although the findings from both field and laboratory studies cited earlier have consistently shown that differences among rhesus monkeys in their expressions of fearfulness and impulsive aggression tend to be quite stable from infancy to adulthood and are at least in part heritable, this does not mean that they are necessarily fixed at birth or are immune to subsequent environmental influence. To the contrary, an increasing body of evidence from laboratory studies has demonstrated that patterns of emotional expression can be modified substantially by certain early social experiences, especially with respect to early attachment relationships.

Perhaps the most compelling evidence comes from studies of rhesus monkey infants raised with peers instead of their biological mothers. In these studies, infants typically have been permanently separated from their biological mothers at birth, hand-reared in a neonatal nursery for their first month of life, housed with same-aged, like-reared peers for the rest of their first 6 months, and then moved into larger social groups containing both peer-reared and mother-reared age-mates. During their initial months, these infants readily establish strong social bonds with each other, much as mother-reared infants develop attachments to their own mothers (Harlow, 1969). However, because peers are not nearly as effective as typical monkey mothers in reducing fear in the face of novelty or in providing a "secure base" for exploration, the attachment relationships that these peer-reared infants develop are almost always "anxious" in nature (Suomi, 1995). As a result, although peer-reared monkeys show completely normal physical and motor development, most appear to be excessively fearful—their early exploratory behavior tends to be somewhat limited, they seem reluctant to approach novel objects, and they tend to be shy in initial encounters with unfamiliar peers (Suomi, 1997a).

Even when peer-reared youngsters interact with their same-age cagemates in familiar settings, their emerging social play repertoires are usually retarded in both frequency and complexity. One explanation for their relatively poor play performance is that their cagemates have to serve both as attachment figures and playmates, a dual role that neither mothers nor mother-reared peers have to fulfill. Another obstacle to developing sophisticated play repertoires faced by peer-reared monkeys is that all of their early play bouts involve partners who are basically as incompetent socially as they are. Perhaps as a result of these factors, peer-reared youngsters typically drop to the bottom of their respective dominance hierarchies when they are subsequently housed with mother-reared monkeys their own age (Higley, Suomi, et al., 1996).

Several prospective longitudinal studies have found that peer-reared monkeys consistently exhibit more extreme behavioral, adrenocortical, and noradrenergic reactions to social separations than do their mother-reared cohorts, even after they have been living in the same social groups for extended periods (e.g., Higley & Suomi, 1989; Higley et al., 1992). Such differences in prototypical biobehavioral reactions to separation persist from infancy to adolescence, if not beyond. Interestingly, the general nature of the separation reactions exhibited by peer-reared monkeys seems to mirror that shown by "naturally occurring," highly fearful mother-reared subjects. In this sense, early rearing with peers appears to have the effect of making rhesus monkey infants generally more fearful than they might have been if reared by their biological mothers (Suomi, 1997a).

Early peer rearing has another long-term developmental consequence for rhesus monkeys: It tends to make them more impulsive, especially if they are males. Like the previously described impulsive monkeys growing up in the wild, peer-reared males initially exhibit overly aggressive tendencies in the context of juvenile play; as they approach puberty, the frequency and severity of their aggressive episodes typically exceed those of mother-reared group members of similar age. Peer-reared females tend to groom (and be groomed by) others in their social group less frequently and for shorter durations than their mother-reared counterparts, and, as noted earlier, they usually stay at the bottom of their respective dominance hierarchies. These differences between peer-reared and mother-reared age-mates in aggression, grooming, and dominance remain relatively robust throughout the preadolescent and adolescent years (Higley, Suomi, et al., 1996). Peer-reared monkeys also consistently show lower CSF concentrations of 5-HIAA than their mother-reared counterparts. These group differences in 5-HIAA concentrations appear well before 6 months of age, and they remain stable at least throughout adolescence and into early adulthood (Higley & Suomi, 1996). Thus, peer-reared monkeys exhibit the same general tendencies that characterize excessively impulsive wild-living (and mother-reared) rhesus monkeys, not only behaviorally, but also in terms of decreased serotonergic functioning.

Given these findings, it should come as no surprise that peer-reared adolescent monkeys as a group consume larger amounts of alcohol under comparable *ad libitum* conditions than their mother-reared age-mates (Higley et al., 1991). They also rapidly develop a greater tolerance for alcohol, and, as previously noted, this tendency appears to be associated with differences in serotonin turnover rates (Barr et al., 2004) and with differential serotonin transporter availability (Heinz et al., 1998). In sum, early rearing with peers seems to make rhesus monkey infants both more fearful and more impulsive, and their resulting developmental trajectories not only resemble those of naturally occurring subgroups of rhesus monkeys growing up in the wild but also persist long after their period of exclusive exposure to peers has been completed and they have been living in more diverse social groups.

Gene–Environment Interactions

Studies examining the effects of peer rearing and other variations in early rearing history (e.g., Harlow & Harlow, 1969), along with the previously cited heritability findings, clearly provide compelling evidence that *both* genetic and early experiential factors can affect a monkey's capacity to regulate expression of fear and aggression. Do these factors operate independently, or do they interact in some fashion in shaping individual developmental trajectories? Ongoing research capitalizing on the discovery of polymorphisms in one specific gene—the serotonin transporter gene—suggests that gene–environment interactions not only occur but also can be expressed in multiple forms.

The serotonin transporter gene (5-HTT), a candidate gene for impaired serotonergic function (Lesch et al., 1996), has length variation in its promoter region that results in allelic variation in 5-HTT expression. A "short" allele (LS) confers low transcriptional efficiency to the 5-HTT promoter relative to the long allele (LL), raising the possibility that low 5-HTT expression may result in decreased serotonergic function (Heils et al., 1996), although evidence in support of this hypothesis in humans has been decidedly mixed to date (e.g., Furlong et al., 1998). The 5-HTT polymorphism was first characterized in humans, but it also appears in largely homologous form in rhesus monkeys and other simian primates, though interestingly not in other mammalian species (Lesch et al., 1997).

Polymerase chain reaction techniques were used to characterize the genotypic status of monkeys in the studies comparing peer-reared monkeys with mother-reared controls described above with respect to their 5-HTT polymorphic status. The genotypic analyses revealed that the relative frequency of subjects possessing the LS versus the LL allele did not differ significantly between these two rearing groups, an expected finding given that those monkeys had been randomly assigned to their respective rearing conditions at birth. Because extensive observational data and biological samples were previously collected from these monkeys throughout development, it has been possible to examine a wide range of behavioral and physiologic measures for potential 5-HTT polymorphism main effects and interactions with early rearing history. Analyses completed to date suggest that such interactions are widespread and diverse.

For example, Bennett et al. (2002) found that CSF 5-HIAA concentrations did not differ as a function of 5-HTT status for mother-reared subjects, whereas among peer-reared monkeys, individuals with the LS allele had significantly lower CSF 5-HIAA concentrations than those with the LL allele.

One interpretation of this interaction is that rearing by mothers appeared to "buffer" any potentially deleterious effects of the LS allele on serotonin metabolism. A different form of gene–environment interaction was suggested by the analysis of alcohol consumption data: Whereas peer-reared monkeys with the LS allele consumed more alcohol than peer-reared monkeys with the LL allele, the reverse was true for mother-reared subjects, with individuals possessing the LS allele actually consuming *less* alcohol than their LL counterparts. A similar reversal was found for relative levels of alcohol intoxication (Barr et al., 2004). In other words, the LS allele appeared to represent a risk factor for excessive alcohol consumption among peer-reared monkeys but a protective factor for mother-reared subjects. Finally, Champoux et al. (2002) examined the relationship between early rearing history and serotonin transporter gene polymorphic status on measures of neonatal neurobehavioral development during the first month of life and found further evidence of maternal "buffering." Specifically, infants possessing the LS allele who were being reared in the laboratory neonatal nursery showed significant deficits in measures of attention, activity, and motor maturity relative to nursery-reared infants possessing the LL allele, whereas both LS and LL infants who were being reared by competent mothers exhibited normal values for each of these measures.

In sum, the consequences of having the LS allele differed dramatically for peer-reared and mother-reared monkeys: Whereas peer-reared individuals with the LS allele exhibited deficits in measures of neurobehavioral development during their initial weeks of life and reduced serotonin metabolism and excessive alcohol consumption as adolescents, mother-reared subjects with the very same allele showed normal early neurobehavioral development, serotonin metabolism, and reduced risk for excessive alcohol consumption. Indeed, it could be argued on the basis of these findings that having the "short" allele of the 5-HTT gene may well lead to psychopathology among monkeys with poor early rearing histories but might actually be adaptive for monkeys who develop secure early attachment relationship with their mothers.

Implications for Understanding Human Socioemotional Regulation

Earlier in this chapter, it was argued that socioemotional regulation represents a process that is not limited to humans. To what extent can studies of its development and possible biological correlates in rhesus monkeys enhance our understanding of socioemotional regulation in children, particularly those who display debilitating fearfulness or excessive physical aggression as they are growing up? To be sure, rhesus monkeys are clearly *not* furry little humans with tails but rather members of another (albeit closely related) species, and one should be especially cautious when making comparisons between humans and other primate species regarding fearful and aggressive behavior, given that there exist obvious age, gender, and cultural differences in what is considered excessive or abnormal for humans. Nevertheless, there appear to be some general principles emerging from research with rhesus monkeys that are likely to be relevant for the human case.

First, expressions of both fearful and aggressive behavior per se are neither abnormal nor necessarily undesirable but rather represent behavioral capacities present in every individual that usually follow an orderly pattern of ontogenic change. To be adaptive, however, they must be effectively socialized during the childhood years. Indeed, problems in the socialization process may result in alterations of the species-typical developmental trajectories for fear and aggression that can have adverse consequences with respect to long-term morbidity and possibly even mortality. On the other hand, such adverse long-term outcomes are not necessarily inevitable for all individuals who display difficulties in socioemotional regulation early in life, especially if those individuals are able to grow up in stable, supportive social environments (cf. Suomi, 1999).

Second, both excessive fearfulness and excessive physical aggression appear to be associated with specific patterns of physiologic functioning. This is *not* to say that dysregulation of the HPA axis actually causes excessive fearfulness or that deficits in serotonin metabolism directly lead to excessive physical aggression (or vice versa), but rather that each of these behavioral propensities seems to be closely linked to nonnormative patterns of biological activity for both males and females throughout development. In particular, the inverse relationship between CSF 5-HIAA concentrations and excessive physical aggression is exceedingly robust, such that factors that can alter the expression of physical aggression also typically alter CSF 5-HIAA concentrations. Moreover, individual differences in CSF 5-HIAA concentrations appear to be relatively stable throughout development, despite major normative ontogenic changes in the concentrations themselves, and they also tend to be stable across situations. These trait-like characteristics make it possible to predict individual differences in physical aggression throughout development on the basis of CSF 5-HIAA values obtained early in life. The same general principles also seem to apply to the relationship between HPA axis hyper-responsiveness and excessive fearfulness, albeit to a somewhat less robust degree.

A third basic principle is that deficits in physiologic functioning and abnormalities in socioemotional regulation at the behavioral level are the exclusive product of neither nature nor nurture but rather reflect the interaction of both. For example, it is possible to demonstrate significant heritability for individual differences in 5-HIAA concentrations, and it is also clear that certain rearing experiences often result in deficits in serotonin metabolism. However, the recent findings that specific polymorphisms in the serotonin transporter gene are associated with different behavioral and biological outcomes for rhesus monkeys as a function of their early social rearing histories suggest that more complex gene–environment interactions actually are responsible for the phenomenon. It is hard to imagine that the situation would be any less complex for humans.

References

Barr, C., Newman, T., Lindell, S., Shannon, C., Champoux, M., Lesch, K. P., et al. (2004). Interaction between serotonin transporter gene variation and rearing condition in alcohol preference and consumption in female primates. *Archives of General Psychiatry, 61*, 1146–1152.

Bennett, A. J., Lesch, K. P., Heils, A., & Linnoila, M. (1998). Serotonin transporter gene variation, CSF 5-HIAA concentrations, and alcohol-related aggression in rhesus monkeys (*Macaca mulatta*). *American Journal of Primatology, 45*, 168–169.

Bennett, A. J., Lesch, K. P., Heils, A., Long, J., Lorenz, J., Shoaf, S. E., et al. (2002). Early experience and serotonin transporter gene variation interact to influence primate CNS function. *Molecular Psychiatry, 17*, 118–122.

Bennett, A. J., Tsai, T., Hopkins, W. D., Lindell, S. G., Pierre, P. J., Champoux, M., et al. (1999). Early social rearing environment influences acquisition of a computerized joystick task in rhesus monkeys (*Macaca mulatta*). *American Journal of Primatology, 49*, 33–34.

Berard, J. (1989). Male life histories. *Puerto Rican Health Sciences Journal, 8*, 47–58.

Berman, C. M., Rasmussen, K. L. R., & Suomi, S. J. (1994). Responses of free-ranging rhesus monkeys to a natural form of maternal separation: I. Parallels with mother-infant separation in captivity. *Child Development, 65*, 1028–1041.

Bowlby, J. (1960). Separation anxiety. *International Journal of Psycho-Analysis, 51*, 1–25.

Bowlby, J. (1969). *Attachment*. New York: Basic Books.

Bowlby, J. (1973). *Separation*. New York: Basic Books.

Bowlby, J. (1988). *A secure base*. New York: Basic Books.

Champoux, M., Bennett, A., Shannon, C., Higley, J., Lesch, K., Soumi, S. (2002). Serotonin transporter gene polymorphism, differential early rearing, and behavior in rhesus monkey neonates. *Molecular Psychiatry, 7*, 1058–1063.

Champoux, M., Suomi, S. J., & Schneider, M. L. (1994). Temperamental differences between captive Indian and Chinese-Indian hybrid rhesus macaque infants. *Laboratory Animal Science, 44*, 351–357.

Darwin, C. (1872). *The expression of emotions in man and animals*. New York: Appleton.

Dittus, W. P. J. (1979). The evolution of behaviours regulating density and age-specific sex ratios in a primate population. *Behaviour, 69*, 265–302.

Doudet, D., Hommer, D., Higley, J. D., Andreason, P. J., Moneman, R., Suomi, S. J., et al. (1995). Cerebral glucose metabolism, CSF 5-HIAA, and aggressive behavior in rhesus monkeys. *American Journal of Psychiatry, 152*, 1782–1787.

Fahlke, C., Lorenz, J. G., Long, J., Champoux, M., Suomi, S. J., & Higley, J. D. (2000). Rearing experiences and stress-induced plasma cortisol as early risk factors for excessive alcohol consumption in nonhuman primates. *Alcoholism: Clinical and Experimental Research, 24*, 644–650.

Furlong, R. A., Ho, L., Walsh, C., Rubinsztein, J. S., Jain, S., Pazkil, E. S., et al. (1998). Analysis and meta-analysis of two serotonin transporter gene polymorphisms in bipolar and unipolar affective disorders. *American Journal of Medical Genetics, 81*, 58–63.

Gunnar, M. R., Gonzalez, C. A., Goodlin, B. L., & Levine, S. (1981). Behavioral and pituitary-adrenal responses during a prolonged separation period in rhesus monkeys. *Psychoneuroendocrinology, 6*, 65–75.

Harlow, H. F. (1958). The nature of love. *American Psychologist, 13*, 673–685.

Harlow, H. F. (1969). Age-mate or peer affectional system. In D. S. Lehrman, R. A. Hinde, & E. Shaw (Eds.), *Advances in the study of behavior* (Vol. 2, pp. 333–383). New York: Academic Press.

Harlow, H. F., & Harlow, M. K. (1969). Effects of various mother-infant relationships on rhesus monkey behaviors. In B. M. Foss (Ed.), *Determinants of infant behaviour* (Vol. 4, pp. 15–36). London: Metheun.

Heils, A. Teufel, A., Petri, S., Stober, G., Riederer, P. Bengel, B., et al. (1996). Allelic variation of human serotonin transporter gene expression. *Journal of Neurochemistry, 6*, 2621–2624.

Heinz, A., Higley, J. D., Gorey, J. G., Saunders, R. C., Jones, D. W., Hommer, D., et al. (1998). In vivo association between alcohol intoxication, aggression, and serotonin transporter availability in nonhuman primates. *American Journal of Psychiatry, 155*, 1023–1028.

Heinz, A., Jones, D. W., Gorey, J. G., Bennet, A., Suomi, S.J., Weinberger, D. R., et al. (2003). Serotonin transporter availability correlates with alcohol intake in non-human primates. *Molecular Psychiatry, 8*, 231–234.

Higley, J. D., Hasert, M. L., Suomi, S. J., & Linnoila, M. (1991). A new nonhuman primate model of alcohol abuse: Effects of early experience, personality, and stress on alcohol consumption. *Proceedings of the National Academy of Sciences USA, 88*, 7261–7265.

Higley, J. D., King, S. T., Hasert, M. F., Champoux, M., Suomi, S. J., & Linnoila, M. (1996). Stability of individual differences in serotonin function and its relationship to severe aggression and competent social behavior in rhesus macaque females. *Neuropsychopharmacology, 14*, 67–76.

Higley, J. D., Mehlman, P. T., Taub, D. M., Higley, S., Fernald, B., Vickers, J. H., et al. (1996). Excessive mortality in young free-ranging male nonhuman primates with low CSF 5-HIAA concentrations. *Archives of General Psychiatry, 53*, 537–543.

Higley, J. D., & Suomi, S. J. (1989). Temperamental reactivity in nonhuman primates. In G. A. Kohnstamm, J. E. Bates, & M. K. Rothbard (Eds.), *Handbook of temperament in children* (pp. 153–167). New York: Wiley.

Higley, J. D., & Suomi, S. J. (1996). Reactivity and social competence affect individual differences in reaction to severe stress in children: Investigations using nonhuman primates. In C. R. Pfeffer (Ed.), *Intense stress and mental disturbance in children* (pp. 3–58). Washington, DC: American Psychiatric Press.

Higley, J. D., Suomi, S. J., & Linnoila, M. (1992). A longitudinal assessment of CSF monoamine metabolite and plasma cortisol concentrations in young rhesus monkeys. *Biological Psychiatry, 32*, 127–145.

Higley, J. D., Suomi, S. J., & Linnoila, M. (1996). A nonhuman primate model of Type II alcoholism? Part 2. Diminished social competence and excessive aggression correlates with low CSF 5-HIAA concentrations. *Alcoholism: Clinical and Experimental Research, 20*, 643–650.

Higley, J. D., Thompson, W. T., Champoux, M., Goldman, D., Hasert, M. F., Kraemer, G. W., et al. (1993). Paternal and maternal genetic and environmental contributions to CSF monoamine metabolites in rhesus monkeys (*Macaca mulatta*). *Archives of General Psychiatry, 50*, 615–623.

Laudenslager, M. L., Rasmussen, K. L. R., Berman, C. M., Broussard, C. L., & Suomi, S. J. (1993). Specific antibody levels in free-ranging rhesus monkeys: Relationship to plasma hormones, cardiac parameters, and early behavior. *Development Psychobiology, 26*, 407–420.

Laudenslager, M. L., Rasmussen, K. L. R., Berman, C. J., Lilly, A., Shelton, S. E., Kalin, N. H., et al. (1999). A preliminary analysis of individual differences in rhesus monkeys following brief capture experiences: Endocrine, immune, and health indicators. *Brain, Behavior, & Immunology, 13*, 124–137.

Lesch, K. P., Bengel, D., Heils, A., Sabol, S. Z., Greenberg, B. D., Petri, S., et al. (1996). Association of anxiety-related traits with a polymorphism in the serotonin transporter gene regulatory region. *Science, 274*, 1527–1531.

Lesch, L. P., Meyer, J., Glatz, K., Flugge, G., Hinney, A., Hebebrand, J., et al. (1997). The 5-HT transporter gene-linked polymorphic region (5-HTTLPR) in evolutionary perspective: Alternative biallelic variation in rhesus monkeys. *Journal of Neural Transmission, 104*, 1259–1266.

Lewis, M. (1992). *Shame: The exposed self*. New York: Free Press.

Lindburg, D. G. (1971). The rhesus monkey in north India: An ecological and behavioral study. In L. A. Rosenblum (Ed.), *Primate behavior: Developments in field and laboratory research* (Vol. 2, pp. 1–106). New York: Academic Press.

Mehlman, P. T., Higley, J. D., Faucher, I., Lilly, A. A., Taub, D. M., Vickers, J. H., et al. (1994). Low cerebrospinal fluid 5 hydroxyindoleacetic acid concentrations are correlated with severe aggression and reduced impulse control in free-ranging primates. *American Journal of Psychiatry, 151*, 1485–1491.

Mehlman, P. T., Higley, J. D., Faucher, I., Lilly, A. A., Taub, D. M., Vickers, J. H., et al. (1995). CSF 5-HIAA concentrations are correlated with sociality and the timing of emigration in free-ranging primates. *American Journal of Psychiatry, 152*, 901–913.

Mendoza, S. P., Smotherman, W. P., Miner, M., Kaplan, J., & Levine, S. (1978). Pituitary-adrenal response to separation in mother and infant squirrel monkeys. *Developmental Psychobiology, 11*, 169–175.

Panksepp, J. (1998). *Affective neuroscience: The foundations of human and animal emotions.* New York: Oxford University Press.

Rasmussen, K. L. R., Fellows, J. R., & Suomi, S. J. (1990). Physiological correlates of emigration behavior and mortalitry in adolescent male rhesus monkeys on Cayo Santiago. *American Journal of Primatology, 20,* 224–225.

Rasmussen, K. L. R., Timme, A., & Suomi, S. J. (1997). Comparison of physiological measures of Cayo Santiago rhesus monkey females within and between social groups. *Primate Reports, 47,* 49–55.

Reite, M., Short, R., Selier, C., & Pauley, J. D. (1981). Attachment, loss, and depression. *Journal of Child Psychology and Psychiatry, 22,* 141–169.

Ruppenthal, G. C., Harlow, M. K., Eisele, C. D., Harlow, H. F., & Suomi, S. J. (1974). Development of peer interactions of monkeys reared in a nuclear family environment. *Child Development, 45,* 670–682.

Sameroff, A. J., & Suomi, S. J. (1996). Primates and persons: a comparative developmental understanding of social organization. In R. B. Cairns, G. H. Elder, & E. J. Costello (Eds.), *Developmental science* (pp. 97–120). Cambridge, UK: Cambridge University Press.

Suomi, S. J. (1986). Anxiety-like disorders in young primates. In R. Gittelman (Ed.), *Anxiety disorders of childhood* (pp. 1–23). New York: Guilford Press.

Suomi, S. J. (1991a). Up-tight and laid-back monkeys: Individual differences in the response to social challenges. In S. Brauth, W. Hall, & R. Dooling (Eds.), *Plasticity of development* (pp. 27–56). Cambridge, MA: MIT Press.

Suomi, S. J. (1991b). Primate separation models of affective disorders. In J. Madden (Ed.), *Neurobiology of learning, emotion, and affect* (pp. 195–214). New York: Raven Press.

Suomi, S. J. (1995). Influence of Bowlby's attachment theory on research on nonhuman primate biobehavioral development. In S. Goldberg, R. Muir, & J. Kerr (Eds.), *Attachment theory: Social, developmental, and clinical perspectives* (pp. 185–201). Hillsdale, NJ: Analytic Press.

Suomi, S. J. (1997a). Early determinants of behaviour: Evidence from primate studies. *British Medical Bulletin, 53,* 170–184.

Suomi, S. J. (1997b). Nonverbal communication in nohuman primates: Implications for the emergence of culture. In P. Molnar & U. Segerstrale (Eds.), *Where nature meets culture: Nonverbal communication in social interaction* (pp. 131–150). Hillsdale, NJ: Erlbaum.

Suomi, S. J. (1998). Conflict and cohesion in rhesus monkey family life. In M. Cox & J. Brooks-Gunn (Eds.), *Conflict and cohesion in families* (pp. 283–296). Mahwah, NJ: Erlbaum.

Suomi, S. J. (1999). Attachment in rhesus monkeys. In J. Cassidy & P. R. Shaver (Eds.), *Handbook of attachment: Theory, research, and clinical applications* (pp. 181–197). New York: Guilford Press.

Suomi, S. J. (2000a). A biobehavioral perspective on developmental psychopathology: Excessive aggression and serotonergic dysfunction in monkeys. In A. J. Sameroff, M. Lewis, & S. Miller (Eds.), *Handbook of developmental psychopathology* (pp. 237–256). New York: Plenum.

Suomi, S. J. (2000b). Behavioral inhibition and impulsive aggressiveness: Insights from studies with rhesus monkeys. In L. Balter & C. Tamis-Lamode (Eds.), *Child psychology: A handbook of contemporary issues* (pp. 510–525). New York: Taylor & Francis.

Suomi, S. J., & Harlow, H. F. (1975). The role and reason of peer friendships. In M. Lewis & L. A. Rosenblum (Eds.), *Friendships and peer relations* (pp. 310–334). New York: Basic Books.

Suomi, S. J., & Harlow, H. F. (1976). The facts and functions of fear. In M. Zuckerman & C. D. Spielberger (Eds.), *Emotions and anxiety: New concepts, methods, and applications* (pp. 3–34). Hillsdale, NJ: Erlbaum.

Suomi, S. J., & Ripp, C. (1983). A history of motherless mother monkey mothering at the University of Wisconsin Primate Laboratory. In M. Reite & N. Caine (Eds.), *Child abuse: The nonhuman primate data* (pp. 49–77). New York: Alan R. Liss.

Symons, D. (1978). *Play and aggression: A study of rhesus monkeys.* New York: Columbia University Press.

4 Investing in Children and Society: What We Have Learned from Seven Decades of Attachment Research

Robert Karen

Psychoanalyst and Author

A woman drags a child onto a crowded subway train. She throws the little girl onto a seat and tells her to stay put. The girl fidgets and the mother gets cross, starts telling her off, and finally shouts her into submission with a soul-piercing indictment. This is her own child, a child who we know, virtually by definition, loves her mother more than life itself. We can only imagine the agony of this little girl and the scar tissue she must be laying down.

A witness to such an event will have dreams of retaliation and rescue. But whether there is retaliation or not, there will be no rescue for this child. Unless we could magically put another loving adult in her home, a father, a grandmother, an aunt, a stepfather, there is probably nothing preferable for her than what she has right now. As important as foster care is for children suffering dangerous abuse or neglect, to take a child who is even minimally loved and cared for away from a parent with a brutal anger problem would, in most cases, amount to replacing a bad situation with a worse one. If there is to be a solution for this child, it will have to lie in getting help to her mother: social (in the sense of practical support in child rearing), financial (because many parents cannot be sensitive caregivers when they're weighed down by economic worry), and psychological (so that the mother will be less likely to act out her own demons in this relationship). As we sit on the train and our hearts go out to this child, we might feel that no price is too high to get such help to the mother. And, if we think of the kind of citizen this child is likely to become, the kind of neighbor, the kind of parent, we might redouble such thinking. Providing emotional security to children is in the end not just a matter of caring for the most vulnerable souls among us but of making an investment in the kind of society we wish to build for ourselves and for our own children.

In the 1930s, when child psychiatry was coming into being, the professionals who were concerned with child welfare knew precious little about what children needed, at a minimum, in order to feel that the world of people was a positive place and that they had value. There was little knowledge about what experiences in infancy would enable them to feel confident enough to explore, to develop healthy peer relations, or to rebound from adversity. No one could say with any confidence whether having a loving parent truly mattered one way or another, and there were many who asserted that it did not. This was the period in which the British psychoanalyst John Bowlby began developing his thoughts regarding what would eventually become attachment theory, a body of research, thinking, and clinical work that would come to answer many of these questions.

In those days, certain obvious things were focused on when a child was brought into a guidance center with behavior problems: Did she come from a broken home? Was the house well kept? Was there enough to eat? Was either of the parents a drinker? Did the parents establish a proper moral environment? And so on. But as far as Bowlby was concerned, such questions were almost entirely irrelevant, often reflecting no more than the prejudices of the day. He argued in his first professional paper that in concerning themselves with such issues, child care workers overlooked critical factors of psychological importance. Their reports frequently concluded, "The environment appears satisfactory," when from Bowlby's point of view it was not satisfactory at all: "It is surprising what vital facts can be overlooked in a perfunctory interview," he wrote: "the mother being in a T.B. sanatorium for six months when the child was two, the grandmother dying in tragic circumstances in the child's home, the fact that a child was illegitimate and attempts had been made to abort the pregnancy" (1940, p. 155). Intentionally or not, he said, parents often conceal such unhappy experiences, and an interviewer must probe for them.

The standard concerns that had come to occupy some child psychiatrists—finances, housing, diet, schooling, religious training—all missed the point, said Bowlby. What mattered was not the physical or religious but the emotional quality of the home. And not just the emotional quality at the moment when the child was brought in for treatment, but going back to birth and even before. He pointed to a recent study of criminals in which the authors found in one case that delinquency had "no relationship to early or later unsatisfactory environment" (East & Hubert, cited in Bowlby, 1940, p. 156), when, in fact, the child was illegitimate and had been born in a Salvation Army home, facts that begged further investigation.

Two environmental factors were paramount in early childhood, Bowlby wrote. One was the death of the mother or a prolonged separation from her. To buttress this point, he offered examples of children who had lengthy separations from their mothers when very young and who subsequently became cunning, unfeeling, thieving, and deceptive—qualities that were similar to what a number of child psychiatrists in New York City and elsewhere had begun reporting.

The second factor was the mother's emotional attitude toward the child, an attitude that becomes apparent in how she handles feeding, weaning, toilet training, and the other mundane aspects of maternal care. One group of mothers demonstrate an unconscious hostility toward the child, he said, which often shows up in "minor pin-pricks and signs of dislike." Such mothers often compensate for their hostility with an overprotecting attitude: "being afraid to let the child out of their sight, fussing over minor illness, worrying lest something terrible should happen to their darlings" (Bowlby, 1940, p. 164). The underlying hostility emerges, however, "in unnecessary deprivations and frustrations, in impatience over naughtiness, in odd words of bad temper, in a lack of the sympathy and understanding which the usually loving mother intuitively has" (p. 169). Another group of mothers are neurotically guilty and cannot withstand a child's hostility or criticism. "Such mothers will go to endless lengths to wheedle affection from their children and to rebuke in a pained way any show of what they call ingratitude" (p. 169). In either case, the results for the child are lasting emotional damage.

One problem that Bowlby had personal experience of was the old-fashioned, very British style of parenting, which was impatient with the child's emotional demands; which held that the greatest sin was to spoil children by showing too much concern for their outbursts, protests, or plaints; which was insensitive to the harm done by separating the child from its primary caregiver (Bowlby himself was sent away to boarding school at age 8); and which held that strict discipline was the surest route to maturity. All of these approaches he vehemently opposed, advocating in their stead a warmer, more tolerant household, whose hallmark was the ability of the parents to accept the expression of negative emotions:

> Nothing helps a child more than being able to express hostile and jealous feelings candidly, directly, and spontaneously, and there is no parental task more valuable, I believe, than being able to accept with equanimity such expressions of filial piety as, "I hate you, Mummy," or "Daddy, you're a beast." By putting up with these outbursts we show our children that we are not afraid of hatred and that we are confident it can be controlled; moreover, we provide for the child the tolerant atmosphere in which self-control can grow. (Bowlby, 1979, p. 12)

What many parents do, however, is just the opposite. Believing that feelings like hatred and jealousy are dangerous and must be stamped out, they either punish any expression of them or demonstrate their disapproval by shaming the child and exploiting his guilt. How can he be such an ingrate? How can he cause so much pain to his devoted parents? The effect is to drive the unacceptable feelings underground, creating a guilty and fearful child. What's more, both methods, Bowlby argued, "tend to create difficult personalities, the first—punishment—promoting rebels and, if very severe, delinquents; the second—shame—guilty and anxiety-ridden neurotics" (1979, p. 12).

In the child welfare clinic where Bowlby worked as a young analyst in the late 1930s, he came across a number of juvenile thieves. In trying to understand those children, Bowlby did not make a simple equation between bad mothering and bad behavior. Rather, he wanted to show how mistreatment was filtered through the child's inevitable fantasies and distortions to produce the unhappy behavioral outcome. He argued that when a mother is irritable, nagging, and critical, when she unnecessarily interferes with and frustrates the child, he will become not only angry and aggressive but also greedy, both for affection and for the things that represent affection to him, such as sweets. In such aggression and greed lie the roots of theft. The child's hostility and avarice will at first be directed at the frustrating mother, which will make her all the more irritable, nagging, and critical. And thus an early vicious circle is established that will be incorporated into the child's view of the world and later relationships.

Having disturbed and emotionally abusive parents was not, however, unique to the young thieves. Indeed, there was very little difference in this respect between the 44 thieves Bowlby collected for his study and the 44 nonthieving disturbed children who also attended the clinic and constituted his control group. Bowlby was thus unable to say anything conclusive about the etiology of thievery. But he was relatively certain that if he were to look at a third set of 44 normal children, children who clearly did not need psychiatric care, he would not find these gross parental failings. In the problem parents he believed he had located a clear, if general, source of child emotional disturbance. But he did not have a third set of children, and so even this aspect of his analysis remained speculative.

Bowlby sensed that such a study was beyond his reach in any case. While it is easy enough to get anecdotal evidence of parental neglect and abuse, making a comparison that has any claim to scientific validity is difficult. How do you rate neglect, mistreatment, unkindness, unresponsiveness, abuse, not to mention subtler and more manipulative forms of bad parenting? How can you be sure that the people who do the ratings are looking at the same things in the same way? What's more, in interviews, some parents are more forthcoming, some more concealed; and observing parents in the home over a long period of time is a costly proposition, which can also be skewed by inevitable parental deception and their efforts to stay on good behavior in front of researchers. In this respect, Bowlby's entire goal of creating a developmental psychopathology based on a scientific evaluation of the environment seemed doomed from the start. It would be 40 years before his colleague Mary Ainsworth would find a way around this conundrum.

But Bowlby found one environmental factor that was easy to document and not open to misinterpretation—namely, prolonged early separations of child and mother, and this was where he turned his attention.

Derek B. was the first young thief Bowlby met at the clinic. He had been referred for persistent stealing, truancy, and staying out late. He appeared to come from a normal, happy family, with sensible, affectionate parents and an older brother who seemed perfectly well adjusted. Derek's infancy was unremarkable. But at 18 months he contracted diphtheria and was sent to the hospital. He remained hospitalized for 9 months without ever seeing his parents, which was the standard procedure at the time. The hospital staff adored him, but when he came home, he seemed a stranger. He called his mother "nurse" and showed no affection; "it seemed like looking after someone else's baby," his mother said (Bowlby, 1944, p. 40). Derek so stubbornly refused to eat that he was finally allowed to starve for a time. After a year and a half, he seemed to settle down, but he remained strangely detached, unmoved by either affection or punishment. His mother described him as hard-boiled.

Derek's play was often violent and destructive, and he frequently stole toys. In fact, he seemed to care for no one, except perhaps his brother. He preferred to play alone, fought frequently with other children, destroyed his and their toys, lied to his teachers, and stole from everyone. He spent the money he stole on sweets, which he shared with his brother and other children. He was repeatedly beaten, both by his parents and by the school authorities, but such punishment seemed to have no impact, except to make him cry for a few moments.

Bowlby diagnosed Derek as an "affectionless character" (1944, p. 40), but he might just as easily have used Bellevue psychiatrist Loretta Bender's diagnosis of psychopathic personality disorder. Fourteen of Bowlby's 44 thieves fell into this affectionless category. Of those 14, fully 12 had, like Derek, suffered prolonged, early separations. This struck Bowlby as a stunning finding. Only 5 of the remaining 30 young thieves, who were not affectionless, had experienced such separations, and only 2 of the 44 controls. This discovery—this association between prolonged early separation and affectionless character—would determine the future course of Bowlby's career, placing him in the forefront of the small group of mental health workers who were attempting to warn their peers about the dangers of maternal deprivation.

The World Health Organization Report

In 1948, the Social Commission of the United Nations decided to launch a study of the problems and needs of homeless children, a major concern in postwar Europe. Bowlby was chosen for the job. In 1950, he moved to Geneva for 6 months to investigate and write a report that would have ramifications in the field of psychiatry, in adoption procedures, and in ordinary home life around the world.

Bowlby spent 6 weeks gathering data on the continent—in France, Sweden, Switzerland, Holland—and then 5 weeks in the United States, using the opportunity to communicate with social workers and child psychiatrists, including David Levy, Loretta Bender, William Goldfarb, Harry Bakwin, and René Spitz, and to become acquainted with the literature. He found an unexpected gold mine: Levy writing about adopted children who were deceitful and eerily detached; Bender reporting on psychopathic children who had been in a series of foster care and adoptive homes; Bakwin, Goldfarb, and Spitz warning about the psychiatric damage done to institutionalized babies; and a number of European clinicians with similar, if less conclusive, findings. Bowlby quickly assimilated this and a related mass of material and 6 months later produced *Maternal Care and Mental Health* , which finally united and gave a single voice to the solitary figures who had been urging modern society to see the suffering of its children.

Bowlby emphasized that all of the researchers, though unaware of one another's work, had unanimously found the same symptoms in children who'd been deprived of their mothers—the superficial relationships, the poverty of feeling for others, the inaccessibility, the lack of emotional response, the often pointless deceitfulness and theft, and the inability to concentrate in school. "So similar are the observations and the conclusions—even the very words—that each might have written the others' papers" (1951, p. 31).

Wartime experience in England rounded out the picture. In Hampstead, Dorothy Burlingham and Anna Freud ran a residential nursery for children whose families' lives had been disrupted by the war, some of the mothers living in shelters because their homes had been bombed out in the Blitz. The two analysts found that only infants in the first months of life adjusted easily to such an environment. They struggled to make the separation for the other young children in their care easier by doing it in slow stages, but while this process worked for children over 3 or 4 years of age, for children between 1.5 and 2.5 years, it proved a catastrophe. A typical case was Bobby, a 24-month-old boy who, despite being looked after by a mother substitute and visited daily by his mother during the first week, started deteriorating when her visits tapered off, becoming listless, incontinent, aggressive, and unwilling to eat.

Anna Freud told Bowlby that nothing they did could prevent the severe deterioration of the very young children placed in their care. She and Burlingham felt the problems inherent in the situation were so grave and would take so many workers to correct that they concluded "it would be preferred to arrange for each helper to take a couple of children home with her and close the nursery" (Bowlby, 1951, p. 132).

All this naturally proved to be an opportunity for Bowlby to argue that the mother–infant relationship was an extremely important one, that it was not a pleasant amenity for the child but an absolute necessity for its developing humanity, and that significant early separations were perilous to the child and ultimately to society as well. Many professionals were resistant to accepting these findings. But Bowlby forcefully argued that they and their policies must change. He insisted that families, especially poor families, needed greater assistance if they were to stay intact. He advocated that large numbers of people be trained in marriage and child guidance and in work with parents of the very young. He said the large outlays of funds required would be far less than the later costs of institutional care and delinquency.

While noting that certain researchers were hopeful that, given extraordinary care, maternally deprived youngsters were capable of being rehabilitated, Bowlby warned that others had found such children damaged beyond repair (1951). He also acknowledged that some children do seem to escape the ravages of early separation. But, in a typical Bowlby flourish, he added, "The same is true of the consumption of tubercular-infected milk or exposure to the virus of infantile paralysis. In both these cases a sufficient proportion of children is so severely damaged that no one would dream of intentionally exposing a child to such hazards" (1951, p. 47).

At this time, social workers in many countries typically separated children from their mothers because of unsatisfactory home conditions—which often meant untidiness or material want—or because the mother was unwed. To Bowlby, this was madness. He argued that those responsible for child welfare had been so preoccupied with physical health and, often, physical appearance, that they at times took expensive steps "to convert a physically neglected but psychologically well-provided child into a physically well-provided but emotionally starved one" (1951, p. 76). Bowlby believed that, unless a mother (or a foster mother) was cruel or abusive, an untidy, disorganized, and unwed mother was often better equipped to emotionally care for a child than a tidy and well-run institution.

The impact of the World Health Organization report can scarcely be overstated. Most immediate was the effect on public policy, particularly adoption, social work, and hospital practices worldwide. The report caused new thinking about the causes and prevention of delinquency and the training of young women for motherhood. It stimulated an extraordinary flood of research, including experimental work with animals. Shortly afterward, Bowlby hired James Robertson to study the tragic effects of the widespread policy of hospitalizing very young children with only minimal if any visitation allowed from parents. The result, a documentary film called *A Two-Year-Old Goes to Hospital* (see Karen, 1994), revolutionized the treatment of children in hospitals.

Given Bowlby's concerns and the directions they would eventually take, one recommendation in his World Health Organization report stands out with special resonance to anyone reading it some 50 years later: "The partial forms of maternal deprivation, due sometimes to ignorance but more often to unconscious hostility on the part of the mother deriving from experiences in her own childhood, could well form the subject of another report" (1951, p. 71). A third member of his team, Mary Ainsworth, would soon address this issue.

Ainsworth's Discovery: Quality of Attachment

Inspired by her work with Bowlby and Robertson, and curious about Bowlby's newfound interest in ethology, which showed the critical importance of warm, consistent, and dependable parenting among lower mammals, and of attachment behaviors, such as clinging, crying, and following among their young, the Canadian psychologist Mary Ainsworth decided to study babies in the home environment.

In 1954, in Uganda, where she had recently moved with her husband, Ainsworth launched what would prove to be one of the pioneering studies in infant research. With no lab, with meager institutional support, with no help collecting or analyzing the data, and with no one but her interpreter, she rounded up 28 unweaned babies from several villages near Kampala and began observing them in the home, using the careful, naturalistic techniques that the ethologists had applied to goslings and stickleback fish. Ainsworth was able to observe the development of a whole array of attachment behaviors in these children, their use of their mothers as what she would call a "secure base," their ability to differentiate attachment figures from other friendly people, and differences in the security of their attachments (Ainsworth, 1967).

When Ainsworth moved to Johns Hopkins University several years later, she replicated her African study with some stunning new results. This time she employed several associates to carefully code parental behavior in a way that ingeniously circumvented the traditional limitations involved in such evaluations (Karen, 1994). In a technique that was extremely unusual at the time, Ainsworth and her fellow researchers closely observed real mothers and children in their homes, paying careful attention to the mother's style of responding to the infant in a number of fundamental areas: feeding, crying, cuddling, eye contact, smiling. At 12 months the infant and mother were taken to the lab and observed as the mother was separated from the baby. During two intervals, a stranger was left behind in the room; during another the baby was entirely alone (Ainsworth, Blehar, Waters, & Wall, 1978).

Ainsworth spotted three distinct patterns in the babies' reactions. One group of infants protested or cried on separation, but when the mother returned they gave her a positive greeting, frequently stretched out their arms to get picked up, and molded to her body. They were relatively easy to console. Ainsworth labeled this group "securely attached."

She labeled the other two groups "insecurely" or "anxiously attached." The first of these tended to be clingy from the beginning and afraid to explore the room on their own, only to become terribly anxious and agitated upon separation, often crying profusely and trying desperately to follow and find their missing mothers. These children typically sought contact with the mother when she returned and simultaneously arched away from her angrily, resisting all efforts to be soothed. Ainsworth called them "ambivalent."

The second insecure group gave the impression of independence. They explored the new environment without using mother as a base; they didn't turn around to be certain of her presence, as those labeled "securely attached" did; and when she left, many of them didn't seem affected. Upon the mother's return, however, they snubbed or avoided her. Ainsworth called them "avoidant," and she assumed what would be established by further research: that they, too, were agitated and angry, but had learned to suppress it. She had caught them, at age 1, in the first stages of dissociation.

Without the painstaking observation that came before, Ainsworth's findings would have been relatively meaningless, no more than a demonstration that children reacted differently when separated from and reunited with their mothers. But because Ainsworth's team had observed these mother–child pairs for a total of 72 hours over the course of the prior year, they were able to describe specific associations between the babies' attachment style and the mothers' style of parenting. Mothers of securely attached children were found to be more responsive to the infant's feeding signals, readily returned the infant's smile, and were quicker to respond to its crying. Mothers of anxiously attached children were either unresponsive, inconsistent, or rejecting. The three patterns seen in the laboratory observation proved directly related to how the babies were being raised (Karen, 1994).

In subsequent studies, attachment researchers found that, without intervention or changes in family circumstances, attachment patterns formed in infancy persist. At age 2, anxiously attached children often lack self-reliance and show less enthusiasm for problem solving than the securely attached. At 3.5 to 5 years, their teachers often find them to be problem kids with poor peer relations and little resilience. At 6, they are more likely to display hopelessness in reaction to imagined separations. The ambivalent children were frequently fretful and less able to focus in school; the avoidants often unpopular, aggressive, and unable to take comfort from an adult when hurt. Reliable, statistically verifiable information like this—about what infants need in order to feel secure and how they are likely to feel and behave in later years if they don't get it—had never before been available.

Parents, too, were examined, and former Ainsworth student, Mary Main, now a professor at the University of California, Berkeley, found that the way parents remember and organize their own childhood experiences—how reflective they are, how much understanding they've achieved, how much denial they use, whether they value or dismiss the importance of love and connectedness in relationships—is a powerful predictor of which attachment group their own children will fall into. This was the beginning of a second flood of attachment research, showing intergenerational transmission of secure and insecure patterns.

Questions about child rearing that had only been speculated about could now be answered with greater authority. For years, mothers had been warned against picking up their babies when they cried. It seemed contrary to nature and intuition, but behavioral theory asserted that picking up the kid reinforced the crying, and if you did it enough you'd have a monstrous crybaby on your hands. Attachment research seems to have disproved this, at least as a general principle.

Ainsworth's central premise was that the responsive mother provides a "secure base." The infant needs to know that his primary caregiver is steady, dependable, there for him. Fortified with the knowledge of his mother's availability, the child is able to go forth and explore the world. Lacking it, he is insecure and anxious, and his exploratory behavior stunted. Warm, sensitive care, Ainsworth insisted, does not create dependency; it liberates and enables autonomy. "It's a good thing to give a baby and a young child physical contact," she says, "especially when they want it and seek it. It doesn't spoil them. It doesn't make them clingy. It doesn't make them addicted to being held" (quoted in Karen, 1994, p. 173).

In almost 40 years of Strange Situation research, stable, middle-class American homes consistently produce about two-thirds securely attached babies and one-third anxiously attached. As these numbers suggest, being securely attached hardly ensures that these babies will be free of neurosis or even of insecurities, only that they have been given the confidence that someone will be there for them and that they are thus minimally capable of forming satisfying relationships and passing on that ability to their children. But in unstable homes, where parents, often single, are under great stress, and where neglect or abuse is more common, this minimal bulwark is often missing and the numbers of anxiously attached babies swell. Meanwhile, researchers have found a fourth attachment pattern, called disorganized, made up of more deeply compromised children with especially disturbed parents.

Ainsworth's discovery of attachment patterns would prove a bonanza to Bowlby. Bowlby had wanted to show the world that early parenting was crucial in emotional development. He studied separations, not because he considered them more important than other damaging experiences of early childhood, but because they were easy to research. The big game in Bowlby's mind, however, had always been the parent's attitude toward the child, the parent's everyday behavior, be it loving, rejecting, or some odd mixture of the two. Ainsworth had now made this, too, researchable. For the first time, something could be said with scientific accuracy about the emotional impact of parents' everyday behavior on their young.

Throughout their early years, insecurely attached children are believed to be relatively amenable to change. Avoidant children, for example, will seek attachments with teachers and other adults, and, if they are lucky, they will find a special person who will provide them with an alternative model of relatedness. Research has shown that secure attachment to the father (or to a secondary caregiver, like a grandmother or a nanny) will be the best insurance in helping to overcome insecure attachment to the mother. But even if it's only an uncle they see occasionally, the knowledge that he cares will keep a different model of relatedness alive in them. Indeed, studies of resiliency indicate that a child's having had such a person in her life can make a significant difference in her ability to believe in herself and to overcome adversity (see, e.g., Egeland, Jacobvitz, & Sroufe, 1988).

But it is often hard for the insecurely attached youngster to find such an alternate attachment figure outside the home, because the strategies that he has adopted for getting along with his parents and the distorted patterns of interaction he's gotten into with them form a relationship template that he takes with him elsewhere and that tends to alienate him from the very people who might otherwise be able to help. The behavior of the insecurely attached child—whether aggressive or cloying, all puffed up or easily deflated—often tries the patience of peers and adults alike. It elicits reactions that repeatedly reconfirm the child's distorted view of the world. People will never love me; they treat me like an irritation; they don't trust me; or, I always feel that I need them more than they need me.

Psychologist Alicia Lieberman, a former student of Ainsworth's, has applied attachment thinking to psychotherapy with mothers and their babies who had been earlier assessed as anxiously attached. Lieberman reported the case of a mother who often provoked her 18-month-old by teasing him and taking away his favorite toys. Typically, the baby threw a tantrum on such occasions, but the mother did nothing to alleviate his distress, explaining her apparent indifference by saying he should be able to take care of himself. Lieberman was eventually able to ask the mother if that was the way it had been for her as a child. The mother gradually recalled that throughout her childhood she had been "mercilessly teased and physically abused by her psychotic older sister." If she asked for help, her mother would say, "You girls work it out yourselves."

Lieberman spoke to her tenderly about "a young child's needs to be believed and protected when she asks for help." At this the mother began to cry profusely: "Nobody listened to me. I was so scared and I had to take care of myself." Lieberman asked, "Do you think that is why you feel that Andy should get out of his tantrum all by himself?" The mother seemed surprised and thoughtful. She said, "Maybe. I need to think about it." She then became considerably more tender toward her son. During the next session another tantrum occurred. The mother, for the first time, embraced Andy while he cried (Lieberman, 1991, pp. 268–269).

In a study of 100 mother–infant pairs who had been assessed in the Strange Situation at 12 months, Lieberman found that after 1 year of this type of treatment, the anxious pairs were virtually indistinguishable from those who had been rated secure (Lieberman, Weston, & Paul, 1991).

The Day-Care Debate

To many mothers, Ainsworth's prescriptions seem as natural as maternity itself (of course a baby needs a warm, dependable mom!). But as pleasing as it is for people to discover that psychology is catching up to what has always seemed intuitively correct to them, it is equally displeasing to come face-to-face with a body of evidence that suggests that you yourself didn't or aren't or won't be doing it right. Attachment theory, which has seemed at times to advocate a more traditional, stay-at-home role for the mother, at least in the first year, has thus had the capacity to enrage as well as enchant. And it hasn't had to go outside the field to achieve this.

The day-care issue has been most explosive, with attachment studies continuously finding that extensive out-of-home care in the first year can threaten secure attachment—and, therefore, skew the child's subsequent efforts to relate to the outside world. Results are even worse in low-quality day-care centers that are typically available to most Americans, with poorly trained staff, frequent staff turnover, and a high child-to-staff ratio (Karen, 1994). Such findings have drawn tremendous fire and bristle with political implications.

Rather than go into the day-care data further, I will summarize what I believe is the best way to understand it. First, there's much to consider for both sides in the day-care debate. For those who are wary of infant day care, it should be kept in mind that although the statistics may be on their side—the risks are indeed higher—statistics do not determine the fate of any individual baby. Babies, on the whole, do best with parental care, next best with nanny care, then a high-quality day-care institution, and worst in the typical day-care center. Nevertheless, some do fine in alternate care, while still others do better in day care than they would have done at home. Not every baby has the option of a willing, nurturing mom. To be home with a depressed mother who'd rather be elsewhere is not a great thing, and studies have shown that a mother's satisfaction with what she's doing is a key variable in determining how well children do (Karen, 1994). If her baby is taken off her hands for 30 or 40 hours a week, it may free her to be a better mother when they're together.

Parents need to know that it is possible for both of them to work, that they can put their baby in some form of high-quality nonparental care and still have an emotionally sound child. There does not seem to be a hard-and-fast rule, written into our genetic code, requiring that a baby be cared for full-time by its mother or father until it is a year old. Many parents, especially if they are at ease with themselves and their decisions, and many babies, especially if they have an easy temperament and an alternate caregiver who loves them and makes them feel secure, can maintain a solid relationship despite beginning extensive nonparental care at some point during the first year. Even in studies of run-of-the-mill out-of-home care, 50% of the children seem to be doing all right.

But those who prefer not to worry about infant day care need to face some facts as well. Most infants, in order to feel that their love is reciprocated, that they are valued and accepted, and that they are secure enough to happily explore the world—the foundation of emotional well-being—seem to need a lot of unhurried time with at least one person who is steadily there for them, preferably with someone who's completely and utterly in love with them. And for many babies that need may not diminish as quickly as we might hope. Because so much gets established in that early period, most developmentalists, regardless of their public stance on day care, recommend that one parent spend some months at home after birth, and the number of months they recommend is often far less than what they would want for their own child.

Even under what might be considered normal conditions, it can take a lot of relaxed, deep-time familiarity to understand a baby's quirks and preferences—to know, for instance, that he's only rejecting his bottle because he wants his blanket first, or that he's willing to nap only if held in a tight, rocking embrace until he stops his struggling and cranky crying and drops off to sleep. If the child has a difficult temperament or the mother, for whatever reason, has a hard time adjusting to the baby and reading its signals, or if she is simply slow to develop her confidence, the two will need long periods of time to get in sync with each other and become a secure pair.

It has been argued that anxious attachment to a mother or father might not be the worst thing for a young child, especially if she forms secure attachments elsewhere. But it is certainly not a happy development for the parent–child relationship itself. And because anxiously attached children have a way of pushing their parents' buttons and resisting overtures toward change, a vicious circle may set in that keeps the relationship from getting righted. What's more, in our primitive state of knowledge, we cannot be at all sure that anxious attachment is the only outcome to be feared.

Given these considerations, no parent can afford to listen to generalizations or make a decision based on ideological preference.

Investing in the Social Environment

It should be remembered that the driving force behind attachment thinking has been a quest to discover what children need, and hundreds, if not thousands, of attachment studies over the past four decades have been designed to show what happens if they get it and what happens if they don't. Bowlby, Ainsworth, and their followers have had a huge and steady influence on child-care practices around the world. Adoption policies, hospital policies, social work policies, not to mention the everyday behaviors of parents, have all been affected. That infants become profoundly attached to parents or parental figures, that they love them with every ounce of their being, that they need to be loved and affirmed by them and are wounded by losses and lengthy separations are perhaps better understood now than ever before.

But this enlightenment has been patchy, inconsistent, and often conflicting with other social needs or wants, such as the importance of careers to mothers, businesses' wish not to be disrupted by lengthy parental leaves, and the general reluctance to spend lavishly to assure high-quality child-care programs. That a U.S. court in 1993 could order a 2½-year-old child (the famous "Baby Jessica") returned to biological parents she did not know, thereby severing her ties to the adoptive parents who raised her, without consideration for the child's feelings, suggests that our courts and our laws remain ignorant of child development.

In his 1951 report for the World Health Organization, Bowlby stated optimistically that, having conquered most of the diseases caused by malnutrition and infection, society was now free to turn its attention to mental health. He advocated supporting families with a helping hand or financial assistance in times of need, with psychotherapy, and with other services, so that children would not have to suffer the deprivations and other torments that are so harmful and preventable, and so that they would not grow up to be the sorts of parents and fellow citizens one would not wish to have in one's midst. In the post–World War II period, many industrialized countries have developed supportive services for families. But more needs to be done, especially in the United States, which has lagged significantly behind on all fronts.

That social policy and social interventions can make a society more humane and give parents a better chance to raise secure children has been demonstrated in numerous studies. People respond in remarkable ways when they feel that someone is there to help them, that they are not isolated and hopeless. A series of studies have now found that when mothers have solid social supports—whether from the extended family or an outside helper—the likelihood of secure attachment is enhanced, particularly, one study found, when the infant has a trying temperament (Crockenberg, 1981; Jacobson

& Frye, 1991). Even 6 hours of helpful instruction over the course of several months to poor Dutch mothers of temperamentally difficult children seems to have been a godsend to them, enabling them to form secure attachments where avoidance would otherwise have been predicted (van den Boom, 1988).

Alicia Lieberman's therapeutic work with troubled mother–infant pairs, in which the mother learns not so much better techniques of child care but how her own emotions, based on her own childhood experience, may be getting in the way of providing responsive care, has also been shown to make a huge difference in the development of secure attachment. Studies of women giving birth in a Guatemala hospital—where they had previously been left alone for much of the time—demonstrated that the constant friendly support of an untrained female helper enabled them to have a much shorter labor (8.7 hours on average as opposed to 19.3), to have half the perinatal complications, and to be better able to enjoy the early hours of their baby's life (Sosa, Kennell, Klaus, Robertson, & Urrutia, 1980). Such support—educative, therapeutic, and warmly attentive—if provided to children and parents (as well as to the sick and the dying, who have been found to have soaring attachment needs) could help relieve the sense of isolation, alienation, and insecurity that pervades our society.

In Syracuse, New York, an extensive program of child care and family support was offered to a group of low-income families until their children reached the age of 5. A follow-up study when the children were 15 found them doing much better than a control group of children from similar backgrounds. They performed better in school and were more apt to report liking their teachers. Adolescent boys from similar families who did not have access to the program during their early years committed four times as many offenses, and the offenses were more severe. A similar program in Connecticut provided health and social services to poor families with infants and toddlers. Ten years later, the children and their mothers were doing far better than those who had not received such early support. The other families were costing the state an average of almost $3,000 more each year in welfare and special education (Zero to Three/National Center for Infant Programs, 1993).

Most parents have social support. It takes the form of friends; close relatives, including brothers and sisters who may also be parents and can give them hand-me-downs and advice; and their own parents, who may be in the position to help out with child care and to support them financially. They may not have a lot of support, but it's enough to get by and to give their children the kind of care they need. Other parents lack these supports entirely. Many would benefit from community assistance of the sort offered in the Syracuse and Connecticut programs. But when it comes to providing such services, the United States—the only industrialized country that has not instituted a system of child care for working parents, a guaranteed minimum family income, and national health care for families with small children—is particularly impoverished. While we now have a parental leave law, it is small in comparison with that of Sweden, where mothers can take a year off with full pay and the guarantee that their job will be there for them when they return. A report in the *New York Times* on the Australian health care system offers one small example of the routine support other nations provide: "When a baby is born ..., the hospital notifies an infant health center in the family's neighborhood. Within days, the parents are visited by a highly trained nurse. Typically these 'sisters' try to get to know the mother, offer a phone number where they can be reached for advice on everything from bathing to breast-feeding, and make an appointment for the baby at the health center. These nurses take care of all the baby's routine health needs" (Rodell, 1993, p. 16).

In such an environment, parents feel more secure and are less likely to let anxieties impinge upon their relationships with their children.

If parents are poor, have themselves suffered early maltreatment or neglect, and are isolated as well from sources of support, then the chances of their children becoming securely attached and well functioning decline. Even the ability to learn is impaired by such conditions. According to a Zero to Three report, which echoes two decades of attachment research and other studies in early development, students do well in school if they arrive having already developed in their early years confidence, curiosity, self-control, a sense of effectiveness, the ability to relate well to others, the capacity to communicate, and the ability to cooperate. Children from overstressed homes, with few resources and little social support, often fail to develop these qualities, leaving them with bad feelings about themselves and little hope of success later.

And this is not a marginal issue. According to Cornell psychologist Urie Bronfenbrenner, who believes that children are at risk all over the world due to a dearth of stable, loving relationships, in the United States, unique among developed nations, a quarter of all young children, from newborns to 5-year-olds, have the added burden of poverty. Studies like Glen Elder's *Children of the Great Depression*, as well as a host of more recent investigations, have documented the toll that poverty and family instability can take on the lives of such children. (Paternal unemployment alone has been associated with unstable, unhappy, unproductive lives among sons; Bronfenbrenner, 1986.) The deprivation experienced by many poor families in our society results in serious medical, psychological, and social problems that could have been prevented. They include disturbed family relationships; child abuse; lonely children coming home to empty houses, being kept company for hours on end by television, and coalescing into destructive groups with similarly deprived youngsters; and eventually, of course, more alienated, dysfunctional adults who have little stake in society—who, it could be said, lack a secure attachment to society and act out their anger by being uncaring, uninvolved citizens, or worse.

Developmentalists have made numerous proposals for correcting these conditions. Zero to Three, whose board of directors includes many of the nation's leading child development experts, advocates that every parent have the opportunity to take at least 6 months off from work after the birth of a child to help promote responsive caregiving; that the government establish strong, meaningful standards for day care, mandating appropriate staff ratios and training and including family subsidies to close the gap between what families can afford to pay and what day care really costs if the staff gets adequate pay (Zero to Three/National Center for Clinical Infant Programs, 1993); and that comprehensive health care be available to all families, as well as decent affordable housing and income support for families below the poverty line. Equally important, Zero to Three recommends an integrated network of services that would enable parents—including foster parents, some of whom are caring for babies handicapped by traumatic early experiences, such as being born addicted to cocaine—to benefit from all that we have learned about what children need in their early years. Such services would provide easy access to parenting education; to a developmental specialist who works with their pediatrician and could help them understand what their baby is experiencing or why it behaves as it does; to treatment of the kind Alicia Lieberman provides to disturbed mother–infant pairs; and to a friendly person who is familiar with their circumstances and can point them in the direction of the various social services that are available to them.

Teachers could also be given better training in the meaning of the disturbing, sometimes maddening, behavior they see in their classrooms. They could work more closely with school psychologists so that anxiously attached children don't get driven more deeply into their early attachment models, as is now typically the case, but are encouraged to open up and see the world of people anew. Having additional lay adults in the schools, hired on the basis of their ability to relate to children, to serve as potential attachment figures to the children who need them could facilitate this process and take a huge burden off teachers. The school years are a unique opportunity for troubled children to be redirected emotionally, but that opportunity has not been seized.

Foster care, too, needs to be treated with greater respect, concern, and urgency. For more than one-half million American children, it represents a last chance to internalize some sense of love, self-worth, stability, and belonging. Various governmental entities spend, in aggregate, some $22 billion a year on foster care, but most systems are haphazard, ill thought out, and unnourished by attention and care. No effort has been made to establish a national policy on foster care or to locate and replicate the programs that work. Foster parents are not paid enough to give them a real stake in this important job or to hold them accountable for doing it right. And foster families are not provided with adequate services—psychological, educational, medical, or just generally supportive, a helping hand in dealing with internal and external conflicts or navigating the maze of governmental agencies. Instead of weaving a strong bottom net in our child-care security system, we've created a virtual cesspool of chaos and neglect where the average child can expect to bounce from one foster family to another and come out the end dazed and alone with no guidance for taking his next steps in the world. (See, for example, "Foster Care: A Call to Action," from ABC news: abcnews.go.com/Primetime/FosterCare/.)

Implementing programs that take attachment needs seriously would be very expensive—a lot more than a supercollider, though perhaps less than the savings and loan bailout of 1989 and far less than the wars in Iraq and Afghanistan. There would be savings, too, just as there always are when preventive programs are instituted, especially where children are concerned. The bills for later welfare services would probably be reduced, as would the destruction caused by alienated youths and the cost of expensive incarcerations. But, most important, it would offer us a different quality of life, one in which we would be taking care of human needs that all societies attended to before the current era. Sadly, we are nowhere near making any of these commitments.

Americans tend to be livid about crime, infuriated by homeless beggars, and indignant at the antisocial behavior of minority or poverty youth. But our response to these social ills is like that of Aladdin's uncle, who, you may recall, sent the boy into the underground chamber in search of the magic lamp. With Aladdin struggling back up the stairs, the uncle made louder and louder demands that he hand up the lamp while refusing to give Aladdin the hand he needed to emerge from the cramped stone stairwell. When Aladdin could not produce the lamp because he was too weighed down, his uncle, oblivious to the obvious solution and incensed at being thwarted, slammed shut the overhead door, thereby abandoning his nephew and the lamp in one swat. This is America today, stubbornly committed to threats and punishments (and moralistic exhortations regarding family values) as the only method to bring about changes in problems whose causes are in large part social, economic, and psychological. Although police action and criminal justice are always important, no amount of threats and punishments can reverse the alienation and hostility of those who have paranoid or infantile character structures, who are overwhelmed by feelings of being cheated and deprived, who have no faith in their ability to nourish or be nourished, and who face every encounter with a lover, a child, or society itself with the expectation that they will exploit or be exploited. People like this will cost their communities a bundle, whether or not they are handled in an enlightened way. But at least by providing psychiatric and social supports, we can hope to improve their behavior, lessen future damage, especially to their children, and perhaps give them some release from their inner demons. Meanwhile, nothing would serve us better than to pay *whatever it costs* to help families give their children adequate, loving care so that such personalities will be less prevalent in the next generation—and to keep doing so even if some unworthies take advantage. Investing in secure attachment is not a cure-all by any means, but it is a win–win proposition for everyone involved. Unfortunately, like Aladdin's uncle, for the present time, we would rather pay through the nose by punishing.

References

Ainsworth, M. (1967). *Infancy in Uganda: Infant care and the growth of love.* Baltimore: The Johns Hopkins University Press.
Ainsworth, M. D. S., Blehar, M. C., Waters, E., & Wall, S. (1978). *Patterns of attachment: A psychological study of the strange situation.* Hillsdale, NJ: Erlbaum.
Bowlby, J. (1940). The influence of early environment in the development of neurosis and neurotic character. *International Journal of Psycho-Analysis, 21,* 1–25.

Bowlby, J. (1944). Forty-four juvenile thieves: Their characters and home life. *International Journal of Psychoanalysis, 25*, 19–52, 107–127. Reprinted (1946) as monograph. London: Bailiere, Tindall and Cox.

Bowlby, J. (1951). *Maternal care and mental health*. Geneva: World Health Organization.

Bowlby, J. (1979). *The making and breaking of affectional bonds*. New York: Routledge.

Bronfenbrenner, U. (1986, Fall). A generation in jeopardy: America's hidden family policy. *Developmental Psychology Newsletter*, 47–54.

Crockenberg, S. (1981). Infant irritability, mother responsiveness, and social support influences on the security of infant-mother attachment. *Child Development, 7*, 169–176.

Egeland, B., Jacobvitz, D., & Sroufe, L. A. (1988). Breaking the cycle of abuse: Relationship predictions. *Child Development, 59*, 1080–1088.

Jacobson, S. W., & Frye, K. F. (1991). Effect of maternal social support on attachment: Experimental evidence. *Child Development, 62*, 572–582.

Karen, R. (1994). *Becoming attached: First relationships and how they shape our capacity to love*. New York: Oxford University Press.

Lieberman, A. (1991). Attachment theory and infant-parent psychotherapy: Some conceptual, clinical and research considerations. In D. Cicchetti & S. Toth (Eds.), *Models and integrations: Rochester Symposium on Developmental Psychopathology*. Rochester, NY: University of Rochester Press.

Lieberman, A., Weston, D., & Paul, J. H. (1991). Preventive intervention and outcome with anxiously attached dyads. *Child Development, 62*, 199–209.

Rodell, S. (1993, July 25). Memo to Hillary: Please have a look at Australia's system [Editorial notebook]. *New York Times*, p. 16.

Sosa, R., Kennell, J., Klaus, M., Robertson, S., & Urrutia, J. (1980). The effect of a supportive companion on perinatal problems, length of labor, and mother-infant interaction. *New England Journal of Medicine, 303*, 597–600.

van den Boom, D. C. (1988). *Neonatal irritability and the development of attachment: Observation and intervention*. Unpublished doctoral dissertation. University of Leiden, The Netherlands.

Zero to Three/National Center for Clinical Infant Programs. (1993). *Heart Start: The emotional foundations of school readiness*. Arlington, VA. [Booklet in two parts.]

III
Meaning and Morality

5 The Consolidation of Conscience in Adolescence

Barbara M. Stilwell

Indiana University School of Medicine

The end product of moral development is the conscience. Similar to John Bowlby's ideas about how attachment relationships result in mental representations or internal working models (Bowlby, 1988), the conscience is also a mental representation—an internal working model of what an individual believes to be morally good or bad, morally right or wrong (Stilwell & Galvin, 1985; Stilwell, Galvin, & Kopta, 1991). The conscience functions as a dynamic entity within the self, continuously prompting responses to moral issues. By the end of adolescence, the impact of conscience on an individual is reciprocal with that individual's impact on conscience. A moral working alliance is formed between them, modification constantly subject to new experience, maturation, or regression. That alliance may be strong or weak, openly accepted or ignored. It may operate as a collision, a collusion, or a collaboration. It may be experienced as an ongoing war or a peacekeeping process.

Moralization of Attachment

Moralization is a process whereby a value-driven sense of *oughtness* emerges within specific human behavioral systems, namely, the systems governing attachment, emotional regulation, cognitive processing, and volition. Biological substrates prepare us to moralize experience under the tutelage of available morally attuned support systems. Very early in development, infant attachment and parent bonding interact to form a *security–empathy–oughtness* representation within the child's mind (Stilwell, Galvin, Kopta, Padgett, & Holt, 1997). Physiologic feelings associated with security and insecurity combine with intuitively perceived, emotionally toned messages that certain behaviors are parent-pleasing or nonpleasing; prohibited, permitted, or encouraged; whereas other behaviors gain no attention at all. A bedrock value for human connectedness guides the child's readiness to behave in response to parent wishes and attentiveness. Seeking parent approval is at the heart of the conscience domain *moralization of attachment*.

Just like scientific hypotheses, children's working models exist to be tested. A child's biologically prepared value for autonomy makes this so. So does her inherent desire to be fun-loving and imaginative. Thus, children will test the consequences of compliance and noncompliance time and time again. It is as though they are continuously asking the question, "How does doing what is permitted/prohibited or pleasing/displeasing affect the well-being of my most important relationships, my emotional equilibrium, my sense making, and the confidence of my self-directions?" Testing implicit or explicit rules involving right and wrong builds a stronger working model of conscience. Testing allows a child to claim ownership of internalized rules. It satisfies his needs for connectedness and autonomy simultaneously.

In adolescence, testing the working model of conscience accelerates and elaborates. The process goes on internally—between self and the "old authority" of the childhood conscience. It also goes on externally—between self and newfound authority, including authority within the peer community and popular culture.

Other Domains of Conscience

Moral–Emotional Responsiveness

Moral–emotional responsiveness is a domain of conscience closely linked to the moralization of attachment (Stilwell, Galvin, Kopta, & Norton, 1994). Discrete emotions, aroused in the context of situations that invite moral judgment, motivate moral responsiveness. Early in normal development, an internal representation of "am good" becomes linked to "feel good" and desire to "do good." Using the terminology of psychologist Carroll Izard (1977), for discrete emotions (the terminology includes words designating a range of intensity), we find that certain emotions group together in the moralization process. The positive emotions—*interest to excitement* and *enjoyment to joy*—become aroused in children when significant adult figures respond to their behavior with pleasure, approval, humor, or encouragement. These are the moral "go-ahead" emotions (Stilwell, Galvin, & Kopta, 2000, pp. 52–56). They urge us to do more of the same or to build on prior pleasing and approval experiences. In a mischievous or possibly deviant developmental trajectory, positive emotions can also be aroused when we get away with something we were not supposed to have gotten away with.

A second grouping and range of discrete emotions—*surprise to astonishment, shyness to embarrassment,* and *fear to terror* —become moralized as the "stop, look, listen, and be careful emotions." These emotions arouse us to evaluate situations in terms of potential harm to self, others, objects, or the planet that supports us. Moral judgments connect past, current, or anticipated harm to rules about goodness and badness. Cautiousness and courage become connected to actions felt to be morally mandated. When negatively moralized, cautiousness and courage are exercised in behalf of successfully carrying out wrongful actions.

A third grouping and range of discrete emotions—*dismell to disgust, anger to rage,* and *contempt to hatred*—become moralized as the "danger zone emotions." When positively moralized, these emotions help us stay away from situations that are morally offensive; to become angrily protective or protestant in the face of wrongdoing in the world; or to become hotly contemptuous in the pursuit of justice. When negatively moralized, these emotions solidify around justifications for wrongdoing as in revenge, harm toward self, or harm toward the earth's bounty.

A fourth grouping and range of discrete emotions—*sadness to anguish, shame to humiliation,* and *guilt to more guilt*—become moralized as the "slow down, go inside, and think about it emotions." These feelings invite moral self-examination. Self-examination prepares us to take on the tasks of reparation after wrongdoing in order to reinstate moral–emotional equilibrium. Moral healing restores the connection between "am good," "feel good," and the desire to "do good." When negatively moralized, these emotions can be particularly destructive to self and others.

Moral Valuation

Moral valuation is the domain of conscience wherein we use all of our cognitive capacities to examine personally held values about good or bad, right or wrong (Stilwell, Galvin, Kopta, & Padgett, 1996). Moral values exist within a *valuational triangle* in which obligations to self are always being balanced with obligations to authority and to peers. Tension always exists within the valuational triangle. This is the domain of conscience that prompts our memories to search for moral precedents; prompts us to actively formulate rules to live by; prompts us to be alert to new issues and complexities needing moralization; prompts us to logically weigh moral dilemmas; and prompts us to hide behind justifications when we feel inadequate or uncertain about responding to moral complexity. Processing issues in terms of the valuational triangle becomes particularly active during midadolescence.

Moral Volition

Moral volition is the domain of conscience wherein we use autonomy and will to follow through on the values we hold (Stilwell, Galvin, Kopta, & Padgett, 1998). Moral volition channels our ability to focus and concentrate; to curtail impulsiveness; to override competing desires; to transform courageous feelings into action. Moral volition is impaired in psychopathologic syndromes in which impulsiveness and impairment in self-control play a major role.

The domains of moral attachment, moral–emotional responsiveness, moral valuation, and moral volition are the supporting pillars of conscience. They interact in forming the dynamic overarching domain, *conceptualization of conscience* (Stilwell et al., 1991). Conscience is our internal working model for addressing moral complexity in the world. Bringing into consciousness what is psychologically at work when we semiautomatically or deliberately respond to moral issues is the task of moral education or morally focused psychotherapy. Moral psychoeducation is integral to many services for adolescent youth. Or if it isn't, it ought to be.

Conceptualizing the Conscience in Adolescence

Childhood Building Blocks

The conscience is always a work in progress. Influenced by the concepts of Jean Piaget (1932/1965) and Lawrence Kohlberg (1984), we found that, in normal development, conceptual understanding of conscience progresses through five invariant, hierarchically organized stages before the age of 18. Prior to adolescence, we speak of the External conscience and the Brain–Heart conscience. Before the age of 7, understanding of morality is reflected in children's reports of what happens to their sense of well-being when they behave in ways deemed by those in authority to be good or bad, right or wrong. Thus the name External conscience.

Between the ages of 7 and 11, children put great energy into codifying rules of conscience absorbed from both morally directed life routines and morally evocative personal experiences. The Brain–Heart conscience is a repository of these governing and self-governing rules. The Brain–Heart conscience tends to be straightforward, legalistic, sometimes immutable.

The Personified Conscience of the Young Adolescent

At the dawn of adolescence, biological maturation renders understanding of conscience ready for further elaboration. Around the ages of 12 or 13, the emerging adolescent begins to conceptualize her conscience in personal, anthropomorphic terms (Stilwell et al., 1991). The authority of real persons who have heretofore directed her moral life—showing their pleasure, disapproval, or scorn—as well as rules of oughtness solidified from autobiographical memories, begin to coalesce into a dynamic entity within herself. The conscience becomes a presence available for internal dialogue. Like memory, it is never an exact duplication of real persons and experiences. Rather, it is a composite working model of moral obligation derived from prior experiences, present challenges, and anticipations about the future. For the most part, that moral obligation is expressed in dialogues between conscience and self. Hence the name Personified conscience.

The emerging adolescent, then, is influenced by three sources of moral authority: the ongoing influence of real authority figures; the ongoing influence of internalized rules; and the new influence of actively processing moral issues with her Personified conscience.

Self-questioning is part of moral processing. Typical moral questions that a young adolescent asks himself are: "What kind of person do I want to be? What kind of a reputation do I want to have? What will my conscience think of what I'm doing?" Intuitively realizing that marching strictly to the moral drumbeat of childhood authority or following rules of conscience with exactitude is humanly impossible, the emerging adolescent begins to reconceptualize moral rules as virtues and rule-following as striving. "I try to be [honest, a good friend, a good student]." Reformulating immutable rules of authority into statements of striving introduces moral flexibility to the emerging adolescent. This means that he can begin to think in terms of human fallibility, tolerance, and forgiveness toward self and others.

If a young adolescent's family life becomes a battle zone with authoritarianism and rigidity pitted against her motivation for moral self-discovery, further development of her conscience may be seriously hampered. She may rigidly wall off moral dialogue with important adults in her life. She may become defensive in moral dialogues with herself. Her moral self-esteem may plummet. In contrast, if authority figures in her life ease the way by fostering dialogue centered on questions such as "What kind of a person do you want to be? What qualities of goodness do you want to pursue? What can we do to understand each other better?," both interpersonal relationships and conscience development will be enhanced. When authority figures encourage responsible but flexible moral processing, the young adolescent learns to be tolerant and forgiving toward herself and others, including the adults who are rearing her.

The Confused Conscience of the Midadolescent: Dealing with New Sources of Power

Expanded Sources of Authority

Around the ages of 14 and 15, newly recognized sources of social power prompt the midadolescent to again equilibrate the conceptualization of his conscience and how he uses it in everyday life. These newly found sources include the power of "other" adults in the community beyond those who have reared him; the power of peer groups that either accept or reject him; and newly discovered personal power that he either finds he has or wishes he had.

No longer a "good little boy" or even a "young man striving to be good," the midadolescent discovers new forces that must be integrated into his moral life. If biologically blessed, he is sexually appealing and has the power to attract. Or he wishes he did. If biologically blessed, he is more quick witted and sharp tongued and, therefore, can win more arguments ...or be more deceptive. Or he wishes he could. If biologically blessed, he is more physically powerful and, therefore, can be more protective or more intimidating. Or he wishes he could be. If lucky, he has more opportunities for adventure and, therefore, can take more risks. Or he wishes he could. Both biological and social evolutionary forces push him toward finding a place among peers separate from his place in his family. Or, to wish that he had such a place.

The midadolescent looks for moral authority in new places. Her accelerating interests in self-discovery, adventure, freedom, independence, and learning what makes other people tick (i.e., what their values and beliefs are) are all admirable characteristics for a young person growing up in a multicultural democracy. She shows an interest in observing and evaluating adults other than those who have been rearing her. Often, she finds them more intriguing than her own family. Even her best friends' parents have "cool" ideas that she thinks her own parents lack. Parents find this phenomenon intriguing, also, and even acceptable—as long as those other adults honor the moral foundation they have been struggling to establish. This means that those "other" adults strictly adhere to generational boundaries and responsibilities. It means that they respect the midadolescent's dependent status even when she decks herself out in pseudomaturity. It also means that, if she is growing up in a deviant household or culture, "other" adults may have the power to influence her to follow a more positive moral pathway.

Adults who do not fully understand the moral need for them to be responsible authority figures with other parents' teenagers include the teacher with sexual seduction in mind; the overly demanding or cruel coach; the neighbor willing to set the teenager up in a drug-dealing business; the Internet companion ready to offer all kinds of immoral and psychologically costly adventures. In less blatant form, moral nurturance is also deficient when adults, failing to understand their obligation to be persons of authority with other parents' teenagers, ignore or avoid young people; dismiss teenagers' wrongdoing as expectable mischief; fail to be authoritative models; treat teenagers contemptuously; fail to inform more powerful authorities in the community when adolescent antisocial behavior deems it necessary; fail to be involved in community groups that support the moral development of youth; or avoid ongoing moral dialogue because it is too time-consuming or heated as teenagers grope to find words and concepts.

The adult community also influences the midadolescent's conscience through its institutions, especially those connected to free enterprise. It is in the market arena that the conscience of the midadolescent meets the commercial conscience of the community. Value dissonance is rampant. The entertainment industry offers sensationalism and vulgarity. Advertising offers products that promise enhancement of sexuality, physical power, thrill seeking, and unhealthy feel-good behavior. Violent and sexually demeaning graphics may be used to sell the most innocent of products. Malls, the Internet, and credit card industries offer infinite opportunities to override thrift. The media offer at least momentary fame for infamous behavior.

Each one of these institutions, on its own, or with the assistance of government regulation, also offers some conscientious protection in the way of guidelines, barriers, advertising and marketing curtailment, or forums for dialogue. Public service announcements and some advertising offer health-oriented education. A few business–religious–community alliances offer incentive programs for influencing youth to delay gratification or to seek a more enduring goodness. Nonetheless, the longing of adolescents for the status and buying power of the adult community that they either live in or imagine makes self-acceptance, modesty, frugality, industriousness, healthy living, and delayed or curtailed gratification difficult values to internalize.

The contributions of market self-monitoring, government regulation, and private incentive programs are helpful but limited in nurturing adolescent conscience development. What really holds potential for making a moral impact on a midadolescent is a powerful connection with individual adults whom he comes to admire or even idealize. It is that teacher, coach, counselor, religious youth worker, Big Brother, neighbor, stepparent, grandparent, police officer, or other individual in the community who can inspire him to make personal moral sense out of the social confusion of his surroundings. These adults can provide inspiration and opportunities for the adolescent to express moral aspirations in the larger community—in spite of or because of its many imperfections. Learning that his participation in social health-promoting activities or service projects can have a moral impact within the larger community gives the midadolescent and his conscience a new sense of allied power, a vision beyond social confusion, a feeling of moral hope.

Expanded Peer Power

Trying to be "an individual" is a taxing experience for the midadolescent. Differentiating herself from her parents' generation can be done, at least superficially, through dress, hairstyle, language, music, and entertainment preferences. But that leaves her looking and acting more or less like everyone else. Finding her place in the peer community—figuring out what power and impact she has on it as well as what power and impact it has on her—is a challenging task in searching for meaning. Moralizing that meaning is even more challenging.

A midadolescent's consciousness of his peer community invariably leads to assessing all of the groupings of power within it. Labels change from decade to decade, but, in general, group distinctions are repeatedly made between those who attain status and power mainly through exercising their academic, athletic, or popularity/political abilities. Some enviable individuals achieve status and power by excelling in all of these arenas. Equally eager for status and power are the groups known for their antisocial strivings—those who tout their risk-taking escapades and mutualize so-called friendship through health-impairing or intimidating behaviors. Some teenagers are both accomplished and deviantly directed.

A youth who is disenfranchised from the more empowered segments of his peer community owing to race, ethnicity, religious affiliation, or poverty may nonetheless seek status and power through accomplishment—following the American dream—or through deviancy, which is also part of the American dream if it is eventually transcended. On the other hand, a youth who comes from a background of abuse and neglect, made even more painful by peer scorn or rejection, is continuously at risk for being traumatized in social encounters. It is the abused, rejected, and traumatized midadolescent who may isolate himself with powerful fantasies of revenge enhanced by deviancy-promoting ideas from the world of so-called infotainment. It is this teenager who may acquire weapons and be intent on using them. Similarly isolated, bullied, and revenge-oriented peers may join him. Feeding off of each other's hurts and hurtful ideas, they may mutually destroy any goodness-seeking remnants that existed in their childhood conscience. Was this scenario possibly true for Dylan Klebold and Eric Harris, the perpetrators of the Columbine High School shootings?

Social complexities prompt the midadolescent to upgrade her understanding of the Golden Rule. Interpreting the Golden Rule involves balancing fairness with caring. Her childhood understanding of this ubiquitous rule was mostly focused on dyadic relationships—how to treat and how to expect to be treated in relationship to siblings, classmates, or playmates. Up to this point in development, her moral reasoning generally led her to one or more of these interpretations: (1) return kindness with kindness; (2) return harm with limited harm in order to prompt an empathic response in the other person; (3) curtail returning harm with harm in order to establish a personal reputation of goodness regardless of consequences; or (4) initiate and maintain kindness without expectation of return, satisfied by the approval of conscience.

Applying the Golden Rule within a group of look-alike, think-alike, do-alike teenagers is relatively easy. It is merely an extension of dyadic moral processing within a chosen peer group. Members of that group probably have many values in common. But how does one individual treat another who is engaging in an activity that adversely affects a whole group—as in classroom cheating? How does one individual maintain a friendship with another who has joined a deviant group? What are the moral issues when an individual from one group allies with an individual from another group and the groups have competing loyalties, even clashing values? And how does a whole group of teenagers treat another whole group in the face of power and status conflicts between the groups?

These thorny issues are really lifespan issues. It is in midadolescence, however, that they first strike home, particularly in large, consolidated high schools. Efforts by school personnel to mandate cooperation and structure competition generally favor students who excel. Furthermore, adult solutions to peer-centered problems, although authoritatively constructive, do not get at the peer-centered core of the Golden Rule: how to treat others as I would want to be treated when egalitarian status is skewed. Inside of school or out, midadolescents face the problem of generating peer-based solutions to the peer-based social problems of inclusion, exclusion, ridicule, intimidation, and so forth. Outside of school, the romanticized high school tragedy of *West Side Story* symbolizes real clashes on streets and in alleys around the world where status and power are defined by ethnic, religious, economic, or political membership. Midadolescence is a time when direct or vicarious experience with these problems brings Golden Rule complexities into consciousness and contributes to conscience confusion. The only way out of the confusion is to learn how to confidently take a personal stand, situation by situation.

Expanded Power of the Self

Moral individuation parallels psychological individuation from early to late adolescence in a two-step progression. The first step involves achieving a sense of separateness from family while taking on a sense of membership in the peer community. The second step involves individuating one's place in the peer community, particularly with regard to moral values. Conscience development does not leap from one stage to the next. Autobiographical memories retain the best of old working models while searching for a more complex model, situation by situation.

There will always be times when we look toward an authority figure for "the answer," reminiscent of the External stage of conscience. There will always be times when we look for an applicable rule, reminiscent of the Brain–Heart stage. There will always be times when virtuous striving appears adequate in meeting the demands of the Personified conscience. The midadolescent would be content with these older models of moral order if his social life would just remain simple. Instead, the social complexities of new sources of moral authority (i.e., adults outside of the family, peers, and the popular culture) drive him to search for a more complex model. Making sense out of new input while honoring the old is particularly stressful in midadolescence. Similar challenges will occur time and time again in adulthood. If all goes well the first time through this passage, the adolescent transitions to the Integrated stage of conscience conceptualization.

The Integrated Conscience of the Older Adolescent

Sometime during the last 2 years of high school, around the age of 16 or after, the older adolescent and her conscience begin to form a new kind of alliance. With regard to authority-centered values she starts to envision herself as part of authority—a responsible link in various chains of command. This viewpoint may occur to her when she is placed in charge of younger children at home, while babysitting, or when doing volunteer work. It may occur to her when she is asked to assume a leadership role in a classroom activity or in a youth group in the community. It may occur to her when she is made team captain in a work setting. If she is a person prone to decline leadership roles, observing her peers in positions of command still stimulates moral processing about the responsibilities of leadership.

Precipitous experiences may demand precipitous acceptance of responsibility. Learning that a girlfriend is pregnant or imagining what it would be like to be in that situation may suddenly awaken an adolescent to the responsibilities of being a grown-up. Family adversities such as the death of a parent, illness, realignment, or economic crisis may similarly awaken him. A community disaster may bring forth a strong sense of responsibility. Less dramatically, the simple vicarious experience of watching one of his peers manage a crisis may bring the older adolescent's values of personal responsibility into focus, stimulating him to think about how people in authority ought to behave. These mental exercises prepare him to take charge when his turn comes. Moralizing these experiences enriches all domains of conscience.

Sometime after the age of 16, the older adolescent begins to examine anew the relationship she has with her peer group. She may comfortably maintain a social alliance with a close group of friends she has known since grade school. Or, she may spend less time with them as she increasingly spends more time with a boyfriend. She may realize that she has become different from or has outgrown her old group—which usually means that she is more carefully differentiating her values from theirs. She may confront an individual's or a whole group's behavior over a moral issue, or she may just become "too busy" to do things with them anymore. If she chooses confrontation, she may find that she has more moral courage than she formerly imagined. She may find herself increasingly articulate when speaking to others. If she is basically shy, yet not a loner, she may make these judgments silently. If she is despairing, she may label certain people or groups as hopeless.

The older adolescent begins to make more careful evaluations when choosing friends. Or, he may make silent judgments of character while socially retreating to individual pursuits, or, miracle of miracles, he may show interest in family activities on occasion. He may consider his peers in more generalized categories, focusing on groups that are disenfranchised. He may be part of or identify with one of those groups. Experiencing disenfranchisement may arouse sociopolitical interests. He may envision idealistic goals about making the world a fairer place. Or, he may be overwhelmed by such complexities and retreat in dismay.

Long-term goal setting comes into focus for the older adolescent. The moral dimensions of goal setting deserve consideration. The emerging adolescent asked herself, "What kind of person do I want to be?" She focuses on virtuous striving within her family, school, and peer group. Now, as an older adolescent, she contextualizes moral striving in terms of "What do I want to do or become in adulthood?" Without the foundation of setting goals in terms of virtuous striving in early adolescence and working through the confusing input from peer and popular culture in midadolescence, the older adolescent may address questions about the future only in terms of "What will bring me the most status, power, and financial success possible?" Moralization of the question may be weak or nonexistent. Vocational counseling, therefore, needs to incorporate moral dimensions. Vocational counselors have great opportunities to foster conscience development.

Taxing Issues

Although this excursion through the consolidation of conscience in adolescence is presented as a chronological saga, using the landmark of age is only relevant for adolescents who have had certain advantages while growing up. These advantages include a normal unfolding of biological readiness for moral development; stage-appropriate moral nurturance from parents, school, and community; a constitutional capacity for surmounting adversity; and a consciousness of moral processing.

Adolescents who have not been so advantaged—those who suffer from biological limitations, deficient moral nurturance, overwhelming life adversities, or deviant cultural influences—may demonstrate conscience functioning that is delayed, regressed, stymied, or deviantly directed. Occasionally, moral development may be accelerated. A conscience-sensitive interview with a teenager with numerous disadvantages may sound very confusing to the listener. In normal development, confusion resolves on behalf of further development. In impaired moral development, confusion may signify psychopathologic interference to conscience functioning (Goenjian et al., 1998). Evidence of adequacy and inadequacy may exist side by side. Autobiographical memories may consolidate prohibitions excessively and prosocial strivings minimally. Rules of conscience may only be rules for survival, reflecting primitive or continuously frightening life circumstances. Revengeful justifications for avoiding moral responsibility may abound. The supporting domains of conscience may fail to integrate in lockstep progression. Consciousness of a moral working model within the self may even be hidden from awareness.

Anchoring normally progressive stages in a multidomain conscience model generates a framework for measuring strengths and weaknesses in adolescents whose conscience functioning is weak or deviantly directed. However, demonstrating the absence of normal development insufficiently describes impaired conscience functioning. Criteria must also be developed to demonstrate conscience regression, deviancy, or disintegration. Such criteria will be useful in measuring the effects of psychopathology and treatment on conscience functioning.

Taxing Solutions

In the broader social and cultural arena, what policies can youth-service organizations adopt to improve conscience functioning among youth? How can schools, religious and community youth groups, treatment facilities, and other organizations develop criteria for measuring how they impact conscience development among the youth they serve? We suggest that broadly framing policy questions in terms of domains of conscience is a starting point.

1. How can the organization help adolescents strengthen their moralization of attachment? How can it strengthen their security–empathy–oughtness bond? What programming will honor the strength of "old" authority in a teenager's conscience while fostering morally sensitive bonding to "new" adult authority and peer affiliations?
2. How can the organization help adolescents strengthen moral–emotional responsiveness? How can it strengthen the bond between "am good–feel good" and the motivation to "do good"? How can prosocial opportunities be presented in ways that will strengthen the moral "go-ahead" emotions, "interest to excitement and enjoyment to joy"? How can desire to inhibit antisocial impulses be strengthened by attending to the "stop, look, listen, and be careful emotions" of surprise to astonishment, shyness to embarrassment, and fear to terror? How can violent reactivity be curtailed by helping adolescents heed the dangerousness of emotions of dismell to disgust, anger to rage, and contempt to hatred? How can moral introspection be promoted by attending to the "slow down, go inside, and think about it" emotions of sadness to anguish, shame to humiliation, and guilt? How can the organization help adolescents process their self-identified or society-identified wrongdoing in ways that will promote reparation, healing, and resolution?
3. How can the organization help adolescents use their cognitive capacities to identify, process, and adopt values that respect authority, self, and peers? How can it help them more adequately understand their justifications for inaction or wrongful action; deal with moral uncertainties and dilemmas; identify new moral issues? How can it help them more carefully critique the moral impact of the popular culture that continuously bombards them?
4. How can the organization help adolescents develop moral volition? How can it help them become persons of conscience within their own community? How can it help them identify forces that interfere with their moral volition, including problems with attention, anxiety, depression, and impulsivity?
5. How can the organization help adolescents develop and maintain awareness of moral issues in the world around them and their capacity for moral processing and action? How can it strengthen the bedrock values of connection, harmony, goodness seeking, and autonomy in the youth it serves?

Acknowledgment

This chapter is based on research supported, in part, by the Association for the Advancement of Mental Health Research and Education, Indianapolis, Indiana.

References

Bowlby, J. (1988). *A secure base: Parent-child attachment and healthy human development.* New York: Basic Books.

Goenjian, A., Stilwell, B. M., Steinberg, A. M., Fairbanks, L. A., Galvin, M. R., Karayan, I., et al. (1998). Moral development and psychopathological interference in conscience functioning among adolescents after trauma. *Journal of the American Academy of Child and Adolescent Psychiatry, 38,* 376–384.

Izard, C. E. (1977). *Human emotion.* New York & London: Plenum.

Kohlberg, L. (1984). *Essays on moral development: Vol. 2. The psychology of moral development.* San Francisco: Harper & Row.

Piaget, J. (1965). *The moral judgment of the child.* New York: Free Press. [Original work published 1932]

Stilwell, B., & Galvin, M. (1985). Conceptualization of conscience in 11-12 year olds. *Journal of the American Academy of Child and Adolescent Psychiatry, 24,* 630–636.

Stilwell, B., Galvin, M., & Kopta, S. M. (1991). Conceptualization of conscience in normal children and adolescents, ages 5 to 17. *Journal of the American Academy of Child and Adolescent Psychiatry, 30,* 16–21.

Stilwell, B., Galvin, M., Kopta, S., & Norton, J. (1994). Moral-emotional responsiveness, a two factor domain of conscience functioning. *Journal of the American Academy of Child and Adolescent Psychiatry, 33,* 130–139.

Stilwell, B., Galvin, M., Kopta, S., & Padgett, R. (1996). Moral valuation, a third domain of conscience functioning. *Journal of the American Academy of Child and Adolescent Psychiatry, 35,* 230–239.

Stilwell, B., Galvin, M., Kopta, S., & Padgett, R. (1998). Moral volition: The fifth and final domain leading to an integrated theory of conscience understanding. *Journal of the American Academy of Child and Adolescent Psychiatry, 37,* 202–210.

Stilwell, B., Galvin, M., Kopta, S., Padgett, R., & Holt, J. (1997). Moralization of attachment, a fourth domain of conscience functioning. *Journal of the American Academy of Child and Adolescent Psychiatry, 36,* 1140–1147.

Stilwell, B., Galvin, M., & Kopta, S. (2000). *Right vs. wrong: Raising a child with a conscience.* Bloomington: Indiana University Press.

6 Best Bets for Improving the Odds for Optimum Youth Development

Michael D. Resnick

University of Minnesota

Research on Resiliency and Protective Factors in the Lives of Youth

Academics have long lamented the gap between research knowledge and its use in programs, policies, and practices. The frequent refrain "If only they would listen!" reflects frustration over the complexity of moving new knowledge into the realm of implementation as well as the highly unrealistic expectation that adoption of innovation will occur based on the sheer and obvious merit of the findings being unveiled (obvious, at least, in the eyes of the scientist).

On the other hand, we now find ourselves in a fascinating period in the adolescent health field when programmatic and policy adoption of innovative ideas may be outpacing the scientific bases to support them. What is still being regarded as innovative in some scientific circles is already achieving the status of commonsense understanding in numerous community settings. Specifically, from the mid-1990s onward, we have witnessed a dramatic acceleration of interest in the concepts of resiliency, protective factors, and healthy youth development. Fueled by an urgent interest in the questions "What works? What must be done?," the concept of a *dual strategy* of protecting young people from harm through a combination of risk reduction and the promotion of protective factors has gained currency across numerous health disciplines and among educators, social service providers, and youth workers—among, in short, a wide array of adult advocates and practitioners working with and on behalf of young people (Catalano & Hawkins, 1996; Matsen & Coatsworth, 1998; Resnick, 2000; Resnick, Bearman, & Blum, 1997).

Across the United States, many of these community-centered initiatives that seek to boost protective factors while reducing risk factors are focused on such domains as teen pregnancy, youth suicide, interpersonal violence, juvenile delinquency, substance use, and mental health. These efforts, usually spearheaded by intersectoral community coalitions, often spring from awareness and understanding of relevant scientific literatures. They are also inspired by popularization of the core constructs of *resiliency, risk factors,* and *protective factors* through widespread discussions of assets in the lives of young people associated with prosocial behaviors (Benson & Saito, 2000). As a result of these efforts, there are a growing number of adults across communities and regions of the United States who are discussing and debating venues and methods for increased youth participation, youth leadership, and creative engagement in community building through service-learning and volunteerism.

This surge in interest in reducing risky behaviors among adolescents while cultivating prosocial attitudes and behaviors is hardly restricted to the United States. In some respects, domestic initiatives in the United States are dwarfed by internationally organized efforts to move the scientific knowledge base and rhetoric of youth development into programmatic and policy arenas. Recent efforts by the World Health Organization (WHO) reflect a commitment to the strategy of "enhancing protective factors, in addition to reducing risk [as] equally important. Programming strategies need to strike a balance, addressing both risk and protective factors" (World Health Organization, 2002). The WHO's commitment to the dual strategy is derived from its examination of data from more than 50 countries, bolstered by national initiatives for healthy youth development in developing as well as developed countries. The WHO seeks to deepen the scientific basis for its actions by sponsoring systematic evaluations of these national initiatives. The organization has also commissioned scientists to develop, test, and disseminate valid and reliable measures that will (1) capture the key constructs that drive the logic models behind these initiatives and (2) document progress in attaining the goals of risk reduction and enhancement of protection among youth.

At the national level, outside of the efforts of the WHO, individual nations are using the repository of scholarly knowledge to promulgate national plans for the promotion of healthy youth development. Unlike the United States, which has not articulated a national youth policy, nations such as New Zealand have commissioned extensive syntheses of scientific literature on risk, protective factors, resiliency, and youth development (Ministry of Youth Affairs, 2002a) as an underpinning to accompanying policy documents that are meant to guide legislative priority setting and resource allocation.

In the midst of this flurry of activity, ranging from the actions of small-town community task forces to national initiatives, the output of scientific inquiry and dissemination of new research on protective factors among young people has markedly accelerated across adolescent health disciplines in the past few years (Blum, Kelly, & Ireland, 2001; Brook, Brook, Arencibia-Mireles, Richter, & Whiteman, 2001; Magnani et al., 2002; Rew, Taylor-Seehafer, Thomas, & Yockey, 2001; Vance, Bowen, Fernandez, & Thompson, 2002; Wolkow & Ferguson, 2001).

The legitimacy of this domain of scientific inquiry has received an enormous boost from the publication of a report from the prestigious National

Research Council and Institute of Medicine (2002) focused on the current status of community efforts to promote healthy youth development. Tellingly, the description of individual and contextual protective factors includes discussions of measurement strategies, theoretical underpinnings, empirical evidence, and practice wisdom. Yet, the quest to understand the interplay between risk and protective factors within the major social systems in young people's lives became a central component of scientific investigation well over a quarter century ago (Masten & Garmezy, 1988). It has subsequently become essential to identifying intervenable factors relevant to clinical practice, the further development of the scientific underpinnings of prevention research, and health promotion programming (Atkins, Oman, Vesely, Aspy, & McLeroy, 2002; Borowsky, Ireland, & Resnick, 2001; French et al., 2001; Matsen & Coatsworth, 1998; Resnick, Harris, & Blum, 1993; Sieving et al., 2006).

The seminal works on youth adolescent resiliency from the 1970s and 1980s (Anthony & Cohler, 1987; Garmezy & Rutter, 1983; Murphy & Moriarty, 1976; Werner, 1989) focused on young people who lived in stressful contexts predictive of poor social and psychological outcomes. Because of a variety of adverse circumstances, such as poverty, familial conflict, and parental mental illness, young people reared in such settings were considered to be at heightened risk for a variety of outcomes familiar to youth-focused practitioners, including substance use, interpersonal and self-directed violence, emotional distress, and school failure. So while the starting point of investigations into resiliency was the examination of youthful populations at high risk (i.e., with a heightened probability of multiple, adverse outcomes), primary interest was in the identification of variables that enabled some not merely to survive but to thrive under conditions of seeming adversity. Accordingly, questions for research and practice focused on the identification of protective factors: events, circumstances, experiences, and other factors that buffered young people from involvement in behaviors and outcomes damaging to themselves and/or to others (Hawkins, Catalano, & Miller, 1992; Rutter, 1979).

Research into protective factors against the major threats to adolescent health and well-being has evolved from descriptive identification of those factors to the disentangling of complex, interactive processes over time (Luthar, 1991; Masten, Best, & Garmezy, 1990). Both theoretical and empirical work has focused on the braided processes that affect the well-being of young people and their capacity to function effectively in everyday life (Garmezy, 1993; Sameroff & Seifer, 1989). From a developmental perspective, effective functioning means achievement of the developmental tasks associated with an era of life. In adolescence, these tasks include engagement in school and academic achievement, participation in extracurricular activities, development of close friendships, and crystallization of a cohesive sense of self (Matsen & Coatsworth, 1998).

In developmental psychology (Egeland, Jacobvitz, & Sroufe, 1998), nursing (Calvert, 1997; Killien, 1982), social work (Chandy, Harris, & Blum, 1994; Turner, Norman, & Zunz, 1995), and medicine (Blum, 1998; Weist, Freedman, & Paskewitz, 1995), as well as in legislative testimony and policy documents

(Ministry of Youth Affairs, 2002a, 2002b; Pittman & Fleming, 1991), different definitions and categorizations are used to express similar understandings as to the kinds of experiences, assets, and events that are protective among high-risk young people, and among youth in general. In one such characterization (Chase-Lansdale, Wakschlag, & Brooks-Gunn, 1995), protective factors are characterized as emanating from the complex interplay of *extrafamilial environmental processes* (neighborhood, school, peer group, community groups, community institutions), *familial processes* (family resources, parental characteristics, parental behavior/parenting), *self-system processes* (competence, nurturing, connectedness, social responsibility), and *individual characteristics* (self-beliefs, health, development, cognition). Individual characteristics reflect both genetic predisposition and social-developmental variables (Quinton & Rutter, 1998; Werner & Smith, 1992). Self-system processes repeatedly identified in studies of resilient young people include the development of a close relationship with at least one caring, competent, reliable adult who recognizes, values, and rewards prosocial behaviors (Garmezy, 1993; Neiman, 1988; Werner, 1989). Numerous researchers (Resnick, Harris & Blum, 1993; Rutter, 1987; Sieving et al., 2001) have demonstrated the protective impact of extrafamilial adult relationships for young people, including other adult relatives, friends' parents, teachers, or adults in health and social service settings. This sense of connectedness to adults is salient as a protective factor against an array of health-jeopardizing behaviors of adolescents (Resnick et al., 1993; Sieving et al., 2001) and has protective effects for both girls and boys across various ethnic, racial, and social class groups (Resnick et al., 1997). Such connectedness is enhanced by opportunities for social skill development and other competencies (such as those developed through service-learning and other extracurricular activities) that provide a substantive basis for the nurturance of self-confidence and a sense of well-being in young people (Dinges & Duong-Tran, 1993; Dryfoos, 1990). The development of these self-system processes has received increasing attention from such diverse perspectives as youth work, program evaluation, juvenile justice, education, and social legislation, seeking to improve adolescent well-being through the use of adult mentorship programs, social skills training, volunteerism, and community service (Schorr, 1997; Schorr & Schorr, 1988; U.S. Congress, 1988, 1991a, 1991b).

Probably of greatest interest to practitioners and program-based youth-serving professionals is the accumulating body of evidence suggesting that individual attributes, while important, coexist with other factors that are amenable to intervention and that can reduce the likelihood of adverse outcomes for youth. To be sure, as summarized by several investigators (Barnard, 1994; Brooks, 1994; Turner et al., 1995), individual characteristics such as strong verbal and communication skills, an easy temperament, problem-solving capacities, humor, empathy, perspective-taking skills, and spirituality are critical components of resiliency and resistance to involvement in health-jeopardizing behaviors. But a synthesis of "lessons learned" from a generation of research on successful, high-functioning children and youth also under-scores the role of deliberate interventions at the familial and extrafamilial levels, designed to enhance protective factors in the lives of young people (Atkins et al., 2002; Borowsky et al., 2001; Sieving et al., 2002). Numerous recent reports indicate successes in enhancing young people's well-being and diminishing involvement in risky behaviors by strengthening family functioning and family communication (Batavick, 1997; Blum et al., 2001; Call et al., 2002; Emshoff, Avery, Raduka, Anderson, & Calvert, 1996; Hawkins, Catalano, Kosterman, Abbott, & Hill, 1999; O'Sullivan, 2001; Scales, 1997; Vakalahi, 2001). Many of these interventions have adopted the dual approach of reducing risks in the environments of young people whenever possible, while also enhancing multiple protective factors at the individual, familial, and extrafamilial levels, such as social skills, academic competence, family relationships, and relationships with adults and institutions outside of the family (Hawkins et al., 1999; Matsen & Coatsworth, 1998;).

To summarize, the resiliency paradigm seeks to identify protective, nurturing factors in the lives of young people who would otherwise be expected to be characterized by a variety of adverse outcomes (French et al., 2001; Rutter, 1979; Sameroff & Seifer, 1989). It explores positive prospects for *adolescents at risk*, a term used to describe a segment of the population that under current conditions has a low probability of growing into responsible, effective, high-functioning adulthood (Fischhoff, Nightingale, & Iannotta, 2001). This explication of protective factors in the lives of young people draws from a research perspective that has turned the traditional pursuit of pathology in the social and behavioral sciences into a quest for understanding successes, resistance, and resilience. It now frames the preeminent health and human services delivery questions for the foreseeable future: To what extent and under what circumstances can protective factors be *transplanted* into the lives of young people who have been socialized in a stressful climate of uncertainty and fear? For adolescents whose lives have been bereft of protective, resiliency-promoting factors, at what point in the life trajectory is it simply too late to remedy serious threats to health and well-being (Neiman, 1988; Richmond & Beardslee, 1988)? This urgent agenda underscores the central role of clinical and programmatic research in identifying modifiable factors and the interventions that can successfully nurture resilience in populations of high-risk adolescents. And as a further challenge to academic researchers and the consumers of that research, it also demands the effective translation of that research into best programs, policies, and practices that benefit young people (Neiman, 1988; Resnick, 2000).

Very significant for practice, research, and the dissemination of best practices with ethnic and racial minorities, the resiliency paradigm is grounded in a perspective that repudiates the traditional focus on problems that has characterized much of the research on social groups that have long experienced social oppression (Attneave, 1989; Blum, Harmon, Harris, Bergeisen, & Resnick, 1992). By emphasizing strengths, capacities, and possibilities, rather than the restatement of pathology (Yates, 1987), this theory-guided, solution-oriented approach finds increasing acceptance among minority constituents precisely because it emphasizes hope and potential (Hunter, 2001; Makini et al.,

2001; Neuman, Mason, & Chase, 1991; Price, Dake, & Kucharewski, 2001; Rew, Thomas, Horner, Resnick, & Beuhring, 2001; Wilson, 2001).

Whereas much of the earlier literature examined resilience and social competence in at-risk populations, much of the recent adolescent research guided by a resiliency perspective has sought to understand how to prevent or minimize adolescents' involvement in the major health-risking behaviors. Particular attention has been directed at prevention or reduction of adolescent substance use (Belcher & Shinitzky, 1998; Brown, Schulenberg, Bachman, O'Malley, & Johnston, 2001; French et al., 2001; Johnson, Strander, & Berbaum, 1996; Patton, 1995; Scheier, Botvin, & Baker, 1997; Vakalahi, 2001), interpersonal violence perpetration and the effects of exposure to violence (Edari & McManus, 1998; Fitzpatrick, 1997; Gabriel, Hopson, Haskins, & Powell, 1996; Howard, 1996), and self-directed violence (Borowsky et al., 2001; Borowsky, Resnick & Ireland, 1999; Price et al., 2001). Common to these studies is a focus on factors amenable to intervention at the individual, family, school, and community levels. Of greatest interest is the fact that across an array of adverse outcomes, researchers have identified recurring, crosscutting protective factors that show promise for application across varied populations of youth. In antithesis to narrow, focused categorical programming that directs specific interventions at targeted, specific groups of adolescents, the results of these studies suggest that across gender, racial, and ethnic groups, certain protective factors have great potential for reductions or prevention of many kinds of health-jeopardizing behaviors (Bernat & Resnick, 2006).

Building upon factors emanating from a resiliency framework, some of these most commonly cited crosscutting protective factors include a strong sense of connectedness to parents, family, school, community institutions, and adults outside of the family; the development and enhancement of academic and social competence; involvement in extracurricular activities that create multiple friendship networks and promote the experience of being in service to others; and activities that deepen young people's sense of confidence and competence (National Research Council and Institute of Medicine, 2002; Resnick et al., 1993, 1997).

The Interweave with Youth Development

Some of the most interesting and innovative applications of resiliency-based programmatic and clinical research are evident in programs that are grounded in a youth development perspective. Paralleling the burgeoning interest in resiliency and protective factors, the youth development framework assumes that young people have fundamental, underlying needs for healthy development, some of which are unique to adolescence as a time of life. These building blocks for healthy development are not necessarily synonymous with what is described as the developmental tasks of adolescence. Many of these building blocks constitute experiences or circumstances that permit the achievement of developmental tasks. They are also highly congruent with the list of key protective factors identified by resiliency researchers.

What, then, are these building blocks for healthy development? One of the most fascinating and imaginative explorations of fundamental requirements for healthy human development is found in the work of Stephen Boyden, professor of human ecology at the Australian National University. In his book *Western Civilization in Biological Perspective: Patterns in Biohistory* (1987), Boyden described the universal, underlying psychosocial needs of human beings that are conducive to happiness and good health. He used as evidence everything that had been learned about hunter-gatherer societies, the social form in which human beings have spent the greatest amount of time in evolutionary history. He suggested that this set of needs for healthy development provides clues as to the basic health needs of the human species. These needs include an environment and lifestyle that provide a sense of:

- Personal involvement
- Responsibility
- Satisfaction
- Love
- Confidence
- Belonging
- Challenge
- Comradeship
- Pleasure
- Security

The absence of these elements in the lives of many young people is viewed as an enormous threat to adolescents' health, well-being, and life chances (Eckersley, 1993; Resnick et al., 1997).

While expressing an intergenerational understanding of essential needs for human development, what Boyden's list lacks is an orientation to adolescence as a unique developmental period in the human experience. Perhaps the most elegant articulation of this comes from a paper commissioned more than 30 years ago by (what was then called) the U.S. Department of Health, Education, and Welfare, which requested a position paper articulating the fundamental requirements for healthy adolescent development (Konopka, 1973). This request came at a time of tumultuous social change, intense dissatisfaction over U.S. involvement in Vietnam, political scandal, and heightened concern over issues of adolescent substance use, violence, sexual behavior, and alienation. Drawing upon her decades of youth work and pioneering efforts in the field of social group work with adjudicated adolescents, Dr. Gisela Konopka of the University of Minnesota described eight elements as the *sine qua non* of developmental requirements. These included the need for every young person to:

- Participate as a citizen, a household member, a worker, and a responsible member of society;
- Gain experience in decision making;

- Interact with peers and acquire a sense of belonging;
- Reflect on self, in relation to others, and to discover self by looking outward as well as inward;
- Discuss conflicting values and formulate his or her own value system;
- Experiment with his or her own identity, with relationships to other people, with ideas; to try out various roles without having to commit himself or herself irrevocably;
- Develop a feeling of accountability in the context of a relationship among equals; and
- Cultivate a capacity to enjoy life. (It should be added that at age 92, Konopka suggested a ninth element for the list: the need to participate in the creative arts and learn the skills of self-expression; personal communication, 2002.)

In local, regional, and national studies, a growing body of evaluation evidence points to the successes of programs that are grounded in a youth development perspective (Jarvis, Shear, & Hughes, 1997; Kirby, 1997; Oden, 1995; Resnick, 2000). Integral to their successes is the incorporation of many of the elements Konopka articulated. These are experiences that develop and deepen social competencies, reinforce prosocial attitudes and values, and set high expectations of the individual while providing pathways to experiences of success, mastery, and achievement. Critical to these efforts is the sustained involvement of caring adults in the context of individual and group-based relationships (Roth, Brooks-Gunn, Murray, & Foster, 1998). Critical reviews and syntheses of scientific and programmatic literature demonstrate that using a variety of programmatic formats, a youth-development perspective and strategy hold great promise for prevention and reductions of specific risk behaviors, such as teen pregnancy, substance use, and violence, as well as the longer term outcome of helping young people move forward in life on a positive and effective developmental trajectory (Catalano & Hawkins, 1996; Dryfoos, 1990; Hawkins et al., 1999; Kirby, 1997, 2001; Luthar, 1991; McLaughlin, Irby, & Langman, 1994; O'Sullivan, 2001; Roth et al., 1998).

Paralleling the growth of research in international contexts on protective factors and resilience, interest in youth development as a fundamental principle of youth-serving programs is evident in numerous developed and developing nations throughout the world. Some of these programs provide the world's foremost examples of youth engagement and leadership in both the design and control of such programs. As described in recent reviews (Blum, 1998; Burt, 1998; Ministry of Youth Affairs, 2002a, 2002b), these programs in Latin America, Africa, Asia, and Europe often blend educational, health, and social empowerment, decision making, and control within the program. Some combine educational programs with job training, life skills development, sports and recreation, community service, and skills in micro entrepreneurship.

Integral to these efforts is a philosophical commitment to the principle that young people are resources to be developed, not problems to be solved (McLaughlin et al., 1994). Concomitantly, there is an understanding that developing capacities and competencies in young people, through the involvement of caring, compassionate adults, is essential. This belief stands in marked contrast with a strategy of only providing services to adolescents, as the role of adults in this context is to expand capacities and to open doors of possibility.

The Need for Advocacy

Despite the growth of scholarly and programmatic work grounded in the concepts of resiliency and protective factors, the appeal of a youth development framework is neither automatic nor universal. As a challenge to academic researchers and program-focused individuals, advocates for healthy youth development must be prepared to use evidence-based research to demonstrate the utility of a youth development framework and strategies that simultaneously seek to reduce risk factors while enhancing protective factors (Resnick, 2005).

To this end, Martha Burt and colleagues at the Urban Institute (Burt, 1998) persuasively underscored the consequences of failing to make investments in healthy youth development. Citing data for the 1990s from the Carnegie Council on Adolescent Development, they noted that each year's class of high school dropouts, over the course of their lifetime, will cost the nation $260 billion in lost earnings and foregone taxes, and that each additional year of secondary education reduced the probability of public welfare dependency in adulthood by 35%, with associated reductions in public costs. Burt also noted that when all direct and indirect costs to society were factored in, ranging from criminal justice costs to foregone earnings, the monetary value of "saving" one high-risk youth ranged from $1.5 to $2.0 million. Even if the economic assumptions underpinning this analysis inflated the estimate by a factor of 10, Burt concluded, these savings would still justify considerable investment in high-risk youth. Whether the focus of programs, policy, and practice in this area will assume a primary focus on high-risk young people or seek to heighten protection while reducing risk among all youth, it is clear that advocacy for this approach will remain an enduring requirement as competing priorities battle for primacy in domestic and international political agendas.

Conclusions

From both current and forthcoming scholarly work and program evaluation efforts, the empirical evidence that documents the effectiveness of enhancing protective factors and actively nurturing healthy youth development will continue to accumulate. This information will provide guidelines for best practices when the weight of evidence is sufficiently developed and ideas about "best bets" when strategies show particular promise. Advocates will need to translate this research into formats that are readily accessible across disciplines, with particular emphasis on those in positions to make resource allocation decisions affecting young people in schools, in community settings, and within health care systems. Without question, the health and social indicators on adolescents will continue to present a mixed picture of the status of young people in U.S. society (Resnick et al., 1997). Critical to the advancement of youth health and well-being is the assurance that those who would persuasively argue that nothing can be done to reverse the prospects of high-risk youth are superseded by practitioners, researchers, and advocates who can demonstrate, at multiple points of action, that there is an ambitious and effective agenda for young people ahead.

Author's Note

This chapter expands on M. D. Resnick (2000), Protective factors, resiliency and healthy youth development. *Adolescent Medicine: State of the Art Reviews*, *11*(1), 157–164.

References

Anthony, E., & Cohler, B. (1987). *The invulnerable child*. New York: Guilford.
Atkins, L., Oman, R. F., Vesely, S. K., Aspy, C. B., & McLeroy, K. (2002). Adolescent tobacco use: The protective effects of developmental assets. *American Journal of Health Promotion, 16*(4), 198–205.
Attneave, C. (1989). Who has the responsibility? An evolving model to resolve ethical problems in intercultural research. *American Indian and Alaska Native Mental Health Research, 2*, 18–24.
Barnard, C. (1994). Resiliency: A shift in our perception? *American Journal of Family Therapy, 22*, 135–144.
Batavick, L. (1997). Community-based family support and youth development: Two movements, one philosophy. *Child Welfare, 76*, 639–663.
Belcher, H., & Shinitzky, H. (1998). Substance abuse in children. *Archives of Pediatric and Adolescent Medicine, 192*, 952–960.
Benson, P. L., & Saito, R. N. (2000). The scientific foundations of youth development. In *Youth Development: Issues, Challenges and Directions* (pp. 125–148). Philadelphia: Public/Private Ventures.
Bernat, D., & Resnick, M. D. (2006). Healthy youth development: Science and practice. *Journal of Public Health Management and Practice*, Suppl. (November), s10–16.
Blum, R. W. (1998). Healthy youth development as a model for youth health promotion: A review. *Journal of Adolescence Health, 22*(5), 368–375.
Blum, R. W., Harmon, B., Harris, L., Bergeisen, L., & Resnick, M. D. (1992). American Indian–Alaska Native youth health. *Journal of the American Medical Association, 267*, 1637–1644.
Blum, R. W., Kelly, A., &. Ireland, M. (2001). Health-risk behaviors and protective factors among adolescents with mobility impairments and learning and emotional disabilities. *Journal of Adolescent Health, 28*(6), 481–490.
Borowsky, I. W., Ireland, M., & Resnick, M. D. (2001). Adolescent suicide attempts: Risks and protectors. *Pediatrics, 107*, 485–493.
Borowsky, I., Resnick, M., & Ireland, M. (1999). Suicide attempts among Indian-Alaska native youth: Risk and protective factors. *Archives of Pediatrics and Adolescent Medicine, 153*, 573–580.
Boyden, S. (1987). *Western civilization in biological perspective: Patterns in biohistory*. Oxford: Clarendon Press.
Brook, J. S., Brook, D. W., Arencibia-Mireles, O., Richter, L., & Whiteman, M. (2001). Risk factors for adolescent marijuana use across cultures and across time. *Journal of Genetic Psychology, 162*(3), 357–374.

Brooks, R. (1994). Children at risk: Fostering resilience and hope. *American Journal of Orthopsychiatry, 64,* 545–553.

Brown, T., Schulenberg, J., Bachman, J. G., O'Malley, P. M., & Johnston, L. D. (2001). Are risk and protective factors for substance use consistent across historical time? National data from the high school classes of 1976 through 1997. *Prevention Science, 2*(1), 29–43.

Burt, M. R. (1998). *Reasons to invest in adolescents.* Paper prepared for the Health Futures of Youth II: Pathways to Adolescent Health Conference. Washington, DC: Maternal and Child Health Bureau.

Call, K., Riedel, A. A., Hein, K., McLoyd, V., Peterson, A., & Kipke, M. (2002). Adolescent health and well-being in the twenty-first century: A global perspective. *Journal of Research on Adolescence, 12*(1), 69–98.

Calvert, W. (1997). Protective factors within the family, and their role in fostering resiliency in African American adolescents. *Journal of Cultural Diversity, 4,* 110–117.

Catalano, R., & Hawkins, J. D. (1996). The social development model: A theory of antisocial behavior. In J. D Hawkins (Ed.), *Delinquency and crime: Current theories* (pp. 149–197). Cambridge: Cambridge University Press.

Chandy, J., Harris, L. J., & Blum, R. W. (1994). Risk and protective factors for disordered eating among children of substance abusing parents. *International Journal of the Addictions, 25,* 27–36.

Chase-Lansdale, P. L., Wakschlag, L. S., & Brooks-Gunn, J. (1995). A psychological perspective on the development of caring in children and youth: The role of the family. *Journal of Adolescence, 18,* 515–556.

Dinges, N., & Duong-Tran, Q. (1993). Stress life events and co-occurring depression, substance abuse, and suicidality among American Indians and Alaska Native adolescents. *Culture, Medicine, and Psychiatry, 16,* 487–502.

Dryfoos, J. G. (1990). *Adolescents at risk: Prevalence and prevention.* New York: Oxford University Press.

Eckersley, R. (1993). Failing a generation: The impact of culture on the health and well-being of youth. *Journal of Pediatrics and Child Health, 29,* 216–219.

Edari, R., & McManus, P. (1998). Risk and resiliency factors for violence. *Pediatric Clinics of North America, 45,* 293–305.

Egeland, B., Jacobvitz, D., & Sroufe, L. A. (1998). Breaking the cycle of abuse. *Child Development, 59,* 1080–1088.

Emshoff, J., Avery, E., Raduka, G., Anderson, D. J., & Calvert, C. (1993). Findings from SUPER STARS: A health promotion program for families to enhance multiple protective factors. *Journal of Adolescent Research, 11,* 68–96.

Fischhoff, B., Nightingale, E., & Iannotta, J. E. (2001). *Adolescent risk and vulnerability: Concepts and measurement.* Washington, DC: National Academy Press.

Fitzpatrick, K. (1997). Fighting among America's youth: A risk and protective factors approach. *Journal of Health and Social Behavior, 38,* 131–148.

French, S. A., Leffert, N., Story, M., Neumark-Sztainer, D., Hannan, P., & Benson, P. L. (2001). Adolescent binge/purge and weight loss behaviors: Associations with developmental assets. *Journal of Adolescent Health, 28*(3), 211–221.

Gabriel, R., Hopson, T., & Haskins, M., & Powell, K. E. (1996). Building relationships and resilience in the prevention of youth violence. *American Journal of Preventive Medicine, 12*(Suppl. 5), 48–55.

Garmezy, N. (1993). Children in poverty: Resilience despite risk. *Psychiatry, 56,* 127–136.

Garmezy, N., & Rutter, M. (1983). *Stress, coping, and development in children.* New York: McGraw-Hill.

Hawkins, J. D., Catalano, R. F., Kosterman, R., Abbott, R., & Hill, K. G. (1999). Preventing adolescent health-risk behaviors by strengthening protection during childhood. *Archives of Pediatric and Adolescent Medicine, 153,* 226–234.

Hawkins, J., Catalano, R., & Miller, J. (1992). Risk and protective factors for alcohol and other drug problems in adolescence and early adulthood: Implications for substance abuse prevention. *Psychological Bulletin, 112,* 64–105.

Howard, D. (1996). Searching for resilience among African-American youth exposed to community violence: Theoretical issues. *Journal of Adolescent Health, 18,* 254–262.

Hunter, A. J. (2001). A cross-cultural comparison of resilience in adolescents. *Journal of Pediatric Nursing, 16*(3), 172–179.

Jarvis, S., Shear, L., & Hughes, D. (1997). Community youth development: Learning the new story. *Child Welfare, 76,* 719–741.

Johnson, K., Strander, T., & Berbaum, M. (1996). Reducing alcohol and other drug use by strengthening community, family, and youth resiliency: An evaluation of the Creating Lasting Connections program. *Journal of Adolescent Research, 11,* 36–67.

Kirby, D. (1997). *No easy answers: Research findings on programs to reduce teen pregnancy.* Washington, DC: National Campaign to Prevent Teen Pregnancy.

Kirby, D. (2001). *Emerging answers: Research findings on programs to reduce teen pregnancy.* Washington, DC: National Campaign to Prevent Teen Pregnancy.

Konopka, G. (1973). Requirements for healthy development of adolescent youth. *Adolescence, 8,* 1–26.

Luthar, S. (1991). Vulnerability and resilience: A study of high-risk adolescents. *Child Development, 62,* 600–616.

Magnani, R. J., Karim, A. M., Weiss, L. A., Bond, K. C., Lemba, M., & Morgan, G. T. (2002). Reproductive health risk and protective factors among youth in Lusaka, Zambia. *Journal of Adolescent Health, 30*(1), 76–86.

Makini, G. J., Hishinuma, E. S., Kim, S. P., Carlton, B. S., Miyamoto, R. H., Nahulu, L. B., et al. (2001). Risk and protective factors related to native Hawaiian adolescent alcohol use. *Alcohol and Alcoholism, 36*(3), 235–242.

Masten, A. S., Best, K. M., & Garmezy, N. (1990). Resilience and development: Contributions from the study of children who overcome adversity. *Development and Psychopathology, 2,* 425–444.

Matsen, A., & Coatsworth, J. D. (1998). The development of competence in favorable and unfavorable environments. *American Psychologist, 53,* 205–220.

Masten, A., & Garmezy, N. (1988). Risk, vulnerability and protective factors in developmental psychopathology. In B. B. Lahey & A. E. Kazddin (Eds.), *Advances in clinical child psychology* (pp. 1–52). New York: Plenum.

McLaughlin, M., Irby, M., & Langman, J. (1994). *Urban sanctuaries: Futures of inner-city youth.* San Francisco: Jossey-Bass.

Ministry of Youth Affairs. (2002a). *Building strength: A review of research on how young people can achieve the best outcomes across families, peer groups, schools and the community.* Wellington, New Zealand: Author.

Ministry of Youth Affairs. (2002b). *Youth development strategy Aotearoa: Action for child and youth development.* Wellington, New Zealand: Author.

Murphy, L., & Moriarty, A. (1976). *Vulnerability, coping, and growth: From infancy to adolescence.* New Haven, CT: Yale University Press.

National Research Council and Institute of Medicine. (2002). *Community programs to promote youth development.* Washington, DC: National Academy Press.

Neuman, A. K., Mason, V., & Chase, E. (1991). Factors associated with success among Southern Cheyenne and Arapaho Indians. *Journal of Community Health, 16,* 103–115.

Neiman, L. (1988). A critical review of resiliency literature and its relevance to homeless children. *Children's Environments Quarterly, 5,* 17–25.

Oden, S. (1995). Studying youth programs to assess influences on youth development: New roles for researchers. *Journal of Adolescent Research, 10,* 173–186.

O'Sullivan, A. (2001). The family as a protective asset in adolescent development. *Journal of Holistic Nursing, 19*(2), 102–126.

Patton, L. (1995). Adolescent substance abuse: Risk factors and protective factors. *Pediatric Clinics of North America, 42,* 283–293.

Pittman, K. J., & Fleming, W. E. (1991). *A new vision: Promoting youth development.* Testimony before the House Select Committee on Children, Youth and Families.

Price, J., Dake, J., & Kucharewski, R. (2001). Assets as predictors of suicide attempts in African American inner-city youths. *American Journal of Health Behavior, 25*(4), 367–375.

Quinton, D., & Rutter, M. (1998). *Parental breakdown: The making and breaking of intergenerational links.* Aldershot, UK: Avebury.

Resnick, M. D. (2000). Resilience and protective factors in the lives of adolescents. *Journal of Adolescent Health, 27*(1), 1–2.

Resnick, M. (2005). Healthy youth development: Getting our priorities right. *Medical Journal of Australia, 183,* 398–400.

Resnick, M., Bearman, P., & Blum, R. (1997). Protecting young people from harm: Findings from the National Longitudinal Study of Adolescent Health. *Journal of the American Medical Association, 278,* 823–832.

Resnick, M. D., Harris, L. J., & Blum, R. W. (1993). The impact of caring and connectedness on adolescent health and well-being. *Journal of Pediatrics and Child Health, 29,* s1–s9.

Rew, L., Taylor-Seehafer, M., Thomas, N. Y., & Yockey, R. D. (2001). Correlates of resilience in homeless adolescents. *Journal of Nursing Scholarship, 33*(1), 33–40.

Rew, L., Thomas, N., Horner, S., Resnick, M. D., & Beuhring, T. (2001). Correlates of recent suicide attempts in a triethnic group of adolescents. *Journal of Nursing Scholarship, 33*(4), 361–367.

Richmond, J., & Beardslee, W. (1988). Resiliency: Research and practical implications for pediatricians. *Developmental and Behavioral Pediatrics, 9,* 157–163.

Rose, M., & Killien, M. (1982). Risk and vulnerability: A case for differentiation. *Advances in Nursing Science, 5,* 227–240.

Roth, J., Brooks-Gunn, J., Murray, L., & Foster, W. (1998). Promoting healthy adolescents: Synthesis of youth development program evaluations. *Journal of Research on Adolescence, 8,* 423–459.

Rutter, M. (1979). Protective factors in children's responses to stress and disadvantage. In M. Kent & J. Rolf (Eds.), *Primary prevention of psychopathology: Social competence in children* (pp. 49–74). Hanover, NH: University Press of New England.

Rutter, M. (1987). Psychosocial resilience and protective mechanisms. *American Journal of Orthopsychiatry, 57,* 316–331.

Sameroff, J. A., & Seifer, R. (1989). Early contributions to development risk. In J. Rolf, A. S. Masten, D. Cicchetti, K. H. Nuechterlein, & S. Weintraub (Eds.), *Risk and protective factors in the development of psychopathology* (pp. 52–66). Cambridge: Cambridge University Press.

Scales, P. (1997). The role of family support programs in building developmental assets among young adolescents: A national survey of services and staff training needs. *Child Welfare, 76,* 611–635.

Scheier, L., Botvin, G., & Baker, L. (1997). Risk and protective factors as predictors of adolescent alcohol involvement and transitions in alcohol use: A prospective analysis. *Journal of Studies on Alcohol, 58,* 652–667.

Schorr, L. (1997). *Common purpose: Strengthening families and neighborhoods to rebuild America.* New York: Anchor Books.

Schorr, L., & Schorr, D. (1988). *Within our reach: Breaking the cycle of disadvantage.* Doubleday: New York.

Sieving, R. E., Beuhring, T., Resnick, M., Bearinger, L. H., Shew, M. L., Ireland, M., et al. (2001). Development of adolescent self-report measures from the National Longitudinal Study of Adolescent Health. *Journal of Adolescent Health, 28,* 73–81.

Sieving, R., Hellerstedt, W., McNeely, C., Fee, R., Snyder, J., & Resnick, M. (2006). Reliability of self-reported contraceptive use and sexual behaviors among adolescent girls. *Journal of Sex Research, 42,* 159–167.

Turner, S., Norman, E., & Zunz, S. (1995). Enhancing resiliency in girls and boys: A case for gender specific adolescent prevention programming. *Journal of Primary Prevention, 16,* 25–38.

U.S. Congress. (1988). *Healthy children: Investing in the future.* Washington, DC: Office of Technology Assessment.

U.S. Congress. (1991a). *Adolescent health: Volume 1. Summary and policy options.* Washington, DC: Office of Technology Assessment.

U.S. Congress. (1991b). *Adolescent health: Volume II. Background and the effectiveness of selected prevention and treatment services.* Washington, DC: Office of Technology Assessment.

Vakalahi, H. (2001). Adolescent substance use and family-based risk and protective factors: A literature review. *Journal of Drug Education, 31*(1), 29–46.

Vance, J. E., Bowen, N. K., Fernandez, G., & Thompson, S. (2002). Risk and protective factors as predictors of outcome in adolescents with psychiatric disorder and aggression. *Journal of the American Academy of Child & Adolescent Psychiatry, 41*(1), 36–43.

Weist, M., Freedman, A., & Paskewitz, D. (1995). Urban youth under stress: Empirical identification of protective factors. *Journal of Youth and Adolescence, 24*, 705–721.

Werner, E. (1989). High-risk children in young adulthood: A longitudinal study from birth to 32 years. *American Journal of Orthopsychiatry, 59*, 72–81.

Werner, E. E., & Smith, R. S. (1992). *Overcoming the odds: High risk children from birth to adulthood.* Cornell University Press: Ithaca, NY: Cornell University Press.

Wilson, D. (2001). Protective factors associated with American Indian adolescents' safer sexual patterns. *Maternal and Child Health Journal, 5*(4), 273–280.

Wolkow, K. E., & Ferguson, H. B. (2001). Community factors in the development of resiliency: Considerations and future directions. *Community Mental Health Journal, 37*(6), 489–498.

World Health Organization. (2002). *Broadening the horizon: Balancing protection and risk for adolescents.* Geneva: Author.

Yates, A. (1987). Current status and future directions of research on the American Indian child. *American Journal of Psychiatry, 144*, 1135–1142.

7 Moral and Spiritual Dimensions of the Healthy Person: Notes from the Founders of Modern Psychology and Psychiatry

Paul C. Vitz

Institute for the Psychological Sciences
New York University, Emeritus

In this chapter, I will present a summary of the characteristics of the healthy or ideal person as described or clearly implied by the important modern theorists of psychology and psychiatry. This is a large task and could easily take a book-length treatment. Instead, I will highlight what these thinkers have emphasized about the nature of human flourishing. After presenting this material, we will then evaluate and reflect on it.

For present purposes, modern psychology—and from now on I will include much of psychiatry within this general term—is taken to begin with Sigmund Freud. No doubt, if medical and biological psychiatry had been our topic, our starting point would have been different, but our interest is with that general field of psychology that has had a major impact on our society, especially on how the educated public thinks about the mind today. Hence we start with Freud.

Sigmund Freud's theoretical writings are rich and varied, and he was an extraordinarily complex and often contradictory person. (There are many good summaries of Freud's work, for example, Monte, 1999, Chapter 2; as well as critical evaluations such as Macmillan, 1997.) But we will focus on his relatively straightforward major contributions to our special topic. First and foremost was Freud's emphasis on increasing knowledge about our own mind, especially our unconscious mind. Behind this search was the moral assumption that such understanding was good, both in the sense of being therapeutic for the patient and as a contribution to the general growth of human knowledge. Freud was just as interested in the development of psychological knowledge as a field as he was in the welfare of the individual patient. Freud is therefore a part of the Enlightenment project, and psychoanalysis was the procedure for increasing our conscious psychological self-understanding. Often, this involved uncovering early childhood traumas and lifting repressions. The psychoanalytic mantra "where id was, ego will be" summarizes this approach well. In short, the "talking cure," with its free association, emotional catharsis, and psychological insight, was Freud's major contribution to how we could become healthier.

In his personal comments—as distinct from his psychoanalytic theories— Freud was also known for his remark that the basis of the good life is "love and work." However, neither love, in the usual sense of the term, nor work is directly emphasized in psychoanalytic writings. Indeed, both were often interpreted as sublimated—that is, disguised and transformed—sexuality, within Freud's theoretical framework.

As for spirituality and similar higher goals, Freud explicitly rejected them by saying that he was there to guide the patient in his analysis but that the synthesis was up to the patient and was not a proper part of psychoanalysis or even, in his judgment, of science. Indeed, Freud scathingly rejected the move to higher, more purposive psychology as expressed in the writings of Carl Jung and Alfred Adler (Roazen, 1975, pp. 204, 229). There are several reasons to see some of this rejection as rooted in Freud's personal motivations and anxieties. Freud also had important rational reasons, however, as he was attempting to make psychoanalysis a new natural science (he failed; see Macmillan, 1999). Freud clearly recognized that once psychology moved from determinism and the person's past to teleology and the person's future—to the goals of life— then it was leaving modern natural science behind. He was correct in this assessment. After all, science is not about the purposes or ideals of life. These topics are proper to philosophy and theology.

Hence, in this discussion of the present theories, the difference between the scientific and clinical evidence from which they are derived and the meaning of this difference for the good of human life should be kept in mind. Many of the theories treated here are, because of their explicit goals and purposes, better understood as applied philosophies of life, not as scientific theories.

In spite of this criticism, all of these approaches should be evaluated seriously. In part, their importance comes from the new clinical material they present, but even the philosophical, moral, and theological aspects are often explained and argued in significant ways. In many respects, these psychologies represent the best modern secular thought about what it means to be human.

Perhaps in time, we will think these theorists simply reinvented the wheel. That is, they may help us understand the good and healthy life in ways similar to previously existing philosophical and religious traditions. Even if this should be so, I think we will understand our older traditions in a much more thorough and detailed way. Modern scientific evidence, and thoughtful psychological/psychiatric response to it, is giving us something new, namely, a knowledge about the person that is deeper, richer, and more convincing than that which existed prior to it.

We turn now to Carl Jung, a former student of Freud's. (For Jung, too, there are many good summaries; for example, Monte, 1999, Chapter 7.) Jung, of course, had a very different notion of the unconscious, one filled with universal and inherited archetypes rather than sexuality and aggression, as was the case with Freud. Nevertheless, very much like Freud, it was the conscious understanding of this unconscious that was seen as a prerequisite to psychological health. But Jung went much further than Freud in the direction of spirituality and in describing the goal of the positive life. Besides understanding one's unconscious, one was also to integrate previously denied or unknown aspects of our personality (e.g., archetypes) with the rest of one's personality. This process of integration, which Jung called *individuation*, was a difficult and time-consuming activity but presumably well worth it. According to Jung, this process constituted *self-realization* and was an ongoing one, to be pursued throughout life, even after Jungian psychotherapy was over.

Besides self-realization, Jung explicitly addressed spirituality as a desirable goal of life. That is, Jung and his followers interpreted self-realization as a kind of spiritual journey, in part because it involved dealing with archetypes such as the archetype of God and the Earth Mother, and in part because the experience of contact with one's archetypes was often of a religious nature. (For some of the spiritual emphasis of Jung, see Jacobi, 1973, especially pp. 60–61.) Although Jung began his life as a traditional scientific rejecter of religion, he ended as a believer in religion and advocate of spirituality, which he proposed as an important part of genuine human flourishing. One support for his spiritual emphasis is the recent claim by his biographer Richard Noll (1997) that Jung was in many ways trying to found a kind of neognostic religion. Another piece of evidence for this Jungian concern with the spiritual is the frequent use of Jung in the publications of many writers on New Age spirituality.

Next we take up the other of the three major founders of modern psychology, also a former student of Freud: Alfred Adler (1929, 1964; see also Ansbacher & Ansbacher, 1956). Like Freud and Jung, Adler, too, was a physician, and like them he turned away from biological science to a more psychological approach to human well-being. Like Freud and Jung, Adler believed that there was an unconscious, knowledge of which was a good and useful thing. But this unconscious was a much smaller part of Adlerian psychology than it was for Freud and Jung. Adler understood human mental health as involving the development of the conscious ego or self, which increasingly was able to free itself from past psychological pathologies and barriers. His emphasis on overcoming inferiority and on the ego and its conscious choices was a radical break from Freud. Adler developed the idea of the creative self and saw one purpose of psychotherapy as the development of the healthy self. By contrast, Freud's emphasis was on relieving unconscious conflicts of an especially crippling kind. As mentioned, Freud was very skeptical about ideas, such as Adler's, that a conscious self, with its growth and development, was possible especially within a scientific framework. As Freud reportedly once put it, "The best that psychoanalysis can do is to return the patient to the normal level of human misery." But Adler, like Jung, went further than this. He not only worked to help patients overcome their inferiority complexes; he went on to claim that the creative self was an important goal of psychotherapy. In doing this, Adler was emphasizing something similar to Jung's notion of self-realization.

In addition to his preoccupation with the conscious self and its healthy growth, Adler, unlike either Freud or Jung, strongly emphasized the interpersonal life of the patient. Quite explicitly, Adler proposed that a genuine interest in the well-being of others was necessary for the well-being of the individual. For Adler, the obvious fact that we are social creatures was not ignored. He called this concern for others *Gemeinschaftsgefühl*—a term translated into English as "social interest." Adler went so far as to say that the absence of social interest in a person's life was the *primary cause* of his or her mental pathologies (Ansbacher & Ansbacher, 1956, p. 91). This concern for the welfare of others was in marked contrast with the thinking of Freud and Jung, both of whom ignored social and adult interpersonal life in their theoretical positions. It is somewhat ironic that in Freud's personal comment on love and work as the meaning of life, he was implicitly supporting Adler's emphasis on positive concern for others and on the creative self.

Adler, however, unlike Jung, had no specific emphasis on anything that might be called "spirituality."

A group of neo-psychoanalytic theorists known as *ego psychologists* developed many of Freud's ideas, especially in the years after his death. Among these theorists I include Anna Freud (1936, 1952), and particularly Heinz Hartmann (1939/1958, 1964), but also others. Although they maintained a strong commitment to Freud's unconscious, and to many other of his ideas, they did develop a much more comprehensive understanding of the Freudian ego. In the process, they inevitably gave an emphasis and importance to the ego and some of its conscious life that were new. Hartmann, in particular, proposed that the ego had its own energy, independent of the id, and that there were many ego functions that took place free of id or superego pressures. One of the things that these theorists set the stage for was the notion of the ego as having its own capacities or ego strengths. These ego strengths were separate from and more positive than the more neurotic ego defense mechanisms. Many later psychoanalysts have continued to focus on ego strengths and their importance for psychological health.

We now turn to another group of post-Freudian psychoanalysts generally called object relations theorists. This category includes Melanie Klein (1932, 1957/1975), as well as Greenberg and Mitchell (1983), D. W. Winnicott (1958), and W. R. D. Fairbairn (1952). These thinkers focused on early childhood and how experiences in the first year or two of life set up later pathologies. They had almost nothing to say about spirituality or about such notions as self-actualization or other expressions of adult psychological health, but they made one major contribution to our concerns: All of them, in various ways, strongly emphasized early interpersonal relationships, normally between the child and mother or mother figure. Klein believed that the infant was born with an innate internal representation of the mother and even the father, and of relationships between itself and them, and between the mother and father. We are not going into the theoretical issues about how innate and specific these early internalized representations of others are. Our interest is in the fact that all of these theorists, even Winnicott and Fairbairn, who emphasized experience rather than "innateness," focused on the enormous importance of these early relationships. All of the object relations theorists thought that humans were born at least with a strong predisposition to early bonding, to intense early relationships that were then internalized and, if pathologic in nature, harmed the person throughout his or her life. In short, these theorists agreed that we are "hardwired," either for actual relationships (e.g., Klein) or at any rate for strong predispositions to early relationships.

With John Bowlby (1958, 1969, 1973, 1980) and Mary Ainsworth (1963, 1982), we see another very strong emphasis on early interpersonal relations, but from quite a different perspective compared with that of the object relations theorists. Bowlby and Ainsworth conceptualized the bond between mother and child under the general term of *attachment theory*. Their approach saw the human mother-and-infant bond as another example of the general primate mother-and-infant bond. Thus, this attachment was seen as intrinsic to our animal nature. Although it has specific human components, this bond was viewed as essential for survival of the infant because without close attachment, all infant primates are extraordinarily vulnerable to premature death. In particular, these theorists looked at the ways in which this bond could be disrupted or broken—the results being something known as separation anxiety. In a positive mother–child bond, the mother becomes a secure base for the child, from which the child can then explore the environment. But when the attachment bonding has been damaged by the mother's absence or by other maternal failures of a significant kind, the child is plagued by long-term anxiety and ambivalence about attachment. Such negative responses fall into two major types: the first consists of those who withdraw from relationships or avoid them because of their fear of future abandonment; the other type becomes excessively clinging and clutching in relationships, again out of fear—but in this case the strategy is to try to control and hold on to the other.

Recent research has begun exploring how adult romantic relationships are often strongly affected by early attachment problems. (On this topic of early attachment relations as affecting adult lives, see Collins and Read, 1990; Feeney and Noller, 1991; Hazen and Shaver, 1987; Kilpatrick and Davis, 1994; Simpson, 1990; Solomon and George, 1999.)

But for present purposes, we need only note the following about this important research and underlying theory: First, early human attachment is foundational for all primates and can be presumed to be biologically predetermined, or hardwired, if you wish. Second, reliable and positive attachment in early life predisposes one to a positive and psychologically healthy adulthood, including lower levels of hostility and greater ego resilience. Disrupted attachment has the opposite effects; for example, more depression, anxiety, and psychosomatic illness (see Eagle, 1995, pp. 142–143). Such positive attachments, both in childhood and later, seem to be at the core of what one means by the experience of love.

Yet another major theorist, one of the most popular and widely quoted today, is Erik Erikson (1950/1963, 1959, 1982; for a good summary, see Monte, 1999, Chapter 6). Erikson took Freud's five psychosexual stages—oral, anal, phallic, latency, and genital—and added to them three new stages relating to adulthood. Moreover, at all stages, he added to Freud's sexual emphasis an important social component. For example, in the first stage, the infant, centered on the mother, is not only involved in orality, the infant is developing either trust or mistrust as basic attitudes toward life—a psychosocial phenomenon. At the fifth stage—adolescence, ages 12 to 20—the teenager is not only experiencing the beginnings of adult sexuality and revisiting the Oedipal motives of Stage 3, he is also preoccupied with identity that is psychosocial in that identity involves one's relations with others. For example, to what group? what tribe? what people do I belong? Such questions are central to the identity crisis of this stage. At the sixth stage—early adulthood, from about age 20 to 30 (one of Erikson's new stages)—the psychosocial crisis is one of intimacy or love, versus isolation or loneliness. Here Erikson brings in aspects of love—including sexuality—as a necessary component of human happiness. The seventh stage—mature adulthood, roughly ages 30 to 65—is focused on what Erikson calls *generativity*. Here he identifies such activities as being concerned with raising children, with the community, with building a business or career that helps others and the society, as a necessary and major expression of our health. The virtue or ego strength at this stage is called *care*. To fail at this stage is to fall into stagnation. Stages 6 and 7 can be seen as much more developed expressions of Adler's social interest and of Freud's original comment about love and work.

The final stage of adult life, from 65 on, for Erikson involves the virtue of wisdom. It is based on a realistic retrospective integration of one's life—a certain distancing from personal goals in their narrow sense, and a peaceful and wise understanding of life in general that can be passed on to others. Failure at this stage leads to despair—and to bitterness about how one has lived, or not lived.

Unlike other psychoanalysts, Erikson also focused on the positive outcome of successfully dealing with each psychosocial stage. The positive outcome was called an *ego strength* or *virtue*, and in introducing the time-honored term of *virtue* into psychology, Erikson was identifying characteristics necessary for psychological health and, I believe, preparing the way for very recent work by Seligman and other "positive" psychologists (Seligman & Csikszentmihalyi, 2002). One of these virtues was hope derived from basic trust developed in the first year of life (many have seen this basic trust as necessary for religious faith). Other Eriksonian virtues include purpose, competence, fidelity, and, as noted, love; the capacity for caring; and wisdom. Erikson, by expanding the focus of psychology to the adult years and to positive dimensions of character, has done more perhaps than any other psychologist to identify or lay the groundwork for our topic today.

Another group of important psychologists includes Erich Fromm (1941, 1947, 1956) and the related existential psychologists. Fromm was concerned with identifying unhealthy ways in which large social and economic factors gave rise to mental problems, proposing, in a sense, that there are cultural neuroses. He stressed the need to separate oneself from social influences that might create sadistic or masochistic character types, or even strongly conformist types. To counter these effects, Fromm proposed the importance of human freedom and the need to overcome our fear of freedom in order to live an authentic and independent life. He argued that people who remained free in their psychological choices became *productive types*, and closely related to this concept was his development of the *biophiliac type*—a person who loved life and growth. Fromm saw such people as the most psychologically healthy. He contrasted them with the necrophilous personality, who desired death, decay, and destruction. In addition, Fromm strongly emphasized the importance of love and loving relationships for the healthy person.

The more typical existential psychologists, such as Rollo May (1953, 1969, 1981) and Viktor Frankl (1959, 1963), like Fromm, also emphasized the importance of freedom and free will in the development of personality. May claimed that courage and creativity were important properties of the positive existential person. Frankl is well-known for his position that people need a higher sense of meaning in order to function well. He put the search for such transcendent and higher meaning at the center of his notion of the ideal person, and his therapy was devoted to helping people find such higher meaning, whether this was religious or spiritual or philosophical or political.

Two other important theorists are Abraham Maslow (1961, 1964, 1970) and Carl Rogers (1942, 1961). These familiar psychologists proposed that self-actualization was the primary positive goal of psychotherapy and of life in general. Maslow was best known for his clear emphasis on self-actualization. One of his contributions was to focus on the psychology of what he called healthy and relatively normal people. He was concerned that too much psychological theory was derived from people with pathologies. It was time, he thought, to look to healthier people as positive models. After satisfying the lower, deficiency needs for biological survival, and for love, belonging, and esteem, the healthy person went on to higher needs and in the process actualized the self. Some of these higher needs included the motivation for truth, beauty, justice, goodness, simplicity, and meaning. Self-actualized people expressed their healthiness in pursuing these higher needs. One other important aspect of Maslow's psychology was his concept of the peak experience, which only occurred in the lives of self-actualized people. The peak experience was described as a kind of mystical experience without any specific religious content—a kind of oneness with all of life and the cosmos. This was proposed as an explicitly secular religious experience available to all as a consequence of having reached the level of self-actualization. Later in his life, shortly before he died, Maslow contributed to the founding of transpersonal psychology—a psychology that emphasized spirituality and related states. Along with his peak experience, Maslow was proposing a sort of spirituality open to everyone as the highest level for human psychology. After Carl Jung, Maslow is the most frequently cited psychologist in the New Age spirituality literature. What we need to keep in mind for our purposes is that Maslow proposed his kind of contentless spirituality as a mark of the highest and healthiest person.

Carl Rogers was similar in his emphasis on self-actualization, although Rogers's ideal was often termed the *fully functioning person*. For Rogers, the actualization of the self was a process representing the ideal person, a process that was defined by constantly changing and being in touch with one's feelings in a way that lasted throughout life. He did not, however, address any form of spirituality per se.

One of the grave criticisms of both Rogers and Maslow, and Jung as well, is that by ignoring interpersonal relations in adult life as important to personality formation and happiness, they contributed greatly to America's love affair with the autonomous isolated individual. This neglect of the importance of relationships has done much in the past few decades to contribute to our prevalent culture of narcissism and self-indulgence (see Vitz, 1977/1994).

The major approach coming after the humanistic or self psychologies of Maslow and Rogers is called cognitive and behavioral psychology. Theorists in this area include William Glasser, Albert Ellis, and Aaron Beck. Glasser (1965), a psychiatrist, is well-known for his *reality therapy*, with its central focus on the patient consciously taking responsibility for his or her behavior. Ellis (1962) and Beck (1976) identify irrational thought processes commonly found in people suffering from depression and anxiety. They both develop similar approaches to helping patients change their thinking patterns and engage in daily behaviors that reinforce new, healthier thoughts and self-understanding. All these theorists criticized patients who saw themselves as victims; they developed strategies for leaving such a self-representation behind.

As a result, despite the rigid determinism of the theoretical founders of behaviorism (e.g., B. F. Skinner), all of today's cognitive and behavioral theorists help the patient make conscious decisions to change, to take responsibility, and to construct a better life.

The final theorists under consideration here are Martin Seligman and associates, whose recent contributions (e.g., Seligman & Csikszentmihalyi, 2002) are known to many, but let us briefly refresh our memories. Seligman has proposed what is called a *positive psychology*. He contrasts this with most of the previous psychology, which concentrated on people's problems and pathologies. This *negative psychology*, to which he himself made important contributions with his concept of *learned helplessness*, he believes was a necessary early preoccupation of psychology. Seligman argues, however, that it is now time to focus much more on the ways in which positive human traits are learned and developed. It is not only that such positive aspects of the person are intrinsically good and rewarding, they also *protect* a person from psychological harm. For example, positive psychologists have begun to study how such human ego strengths or virtues as hope and optimism are developed. Seligman calls for research on such traits as happiness, responsibility, wisdom, creativity, courage, and spirituality. Positive psychologists have also begun to look at the development of human resilience. Even gratitude has received major attention (McCullough, Kilpatrick, Emmons, & Larson, 2001). I would also include in positive psychology the recent interesting work on the psychology of forgiveness (Enright & Fitzgibbons, 2000). Today's growing psychological interest in religion as a source of well-being can also be seen as part of this general phenomenon (see Johnson, Chapter 10, this volume).

Conclusions

I would now like to summarize and integrate some of the implications of the preceding large number of theorists for our understanding of the psychologically (or psychiatrically) healthy person.

First, we see an initial focus on becoming knowledgeable—gaining insight—about one's unconscious. Later, whether this was called the unconscious or just neglected past experience, this continued self-knowledge was a common psychological virtue in all the theorists. Implicit in this is the idea that the unexamined life is not worth living. And so self-understanding, then, is seen as an extremely important and universal aspect of the positive life.

Second, we see in a very general sense that over time psychology shifted from an emphasis on the unconscious and on the past to an emphasis on the conscious mind. In particular, psychological theorists propose that conscious choice—free will—is a central positive quality for the healthy life. Even classical psychoanalysis, which in theory denied free will and claimed that our mental life was completely determined, operated in fact under the assumption of free will; how else account for "where id was, ego will be"? Likewise, cognitive and behavioral psychologists rejected theoretical determinism for a big emphasis on freedom, choice, and responsibility.

Third, we see a general move from concern with pathologies and problems to more emphasis, in recent years, on higher and positive aspects of the person. Adler started with his concept of social interest and the creative self; Jung had self-realization; Erikson's adult psychological stages made specific positive contributions; similar concepts also show up in Maslow (with his characteristics of the self-actualized person), many of the existentialists, and, of course, more recently in Seligman. This general trend means that over the century psychologists began to agree on various familiar positive traits as central to human psychological health. These include such general traits as self-fulfillment and ego strength, as well as particular characteristics like hopefulness, caring, responsibility, resilience, creativity, and wisdom.

Fourth, quite recently, we have seen the concern with psychological well-being move beyond ego strengths or virtues to the spiritual life itself. Jung pioneered this general thrust, Maslow came in with the *peak experience* and *transpersonal psychology* in the 1960s, and today we see a widespread cultural interest in the transcendent. Emerging in contemporary psychology is a general belief that the good life involves a significant spiritual component.

Finally, a fifth important point about psychological health can be extracted from our historical summary. At the beginning, psychology heavily stressed the mental health of the individual, often considered as independent of other people; the individual was a kind of autonomous system. In part, this was an outcome of the early, almost universal one-on-one model of psychotherapy. And no doubt this individual and his or her psychological self-fulfillment is an extremely important part of well-being. But coming somewhat later, beginning with Adler and moving up through object relations and especially Bowlby and Ainsworth, and including today's many interpersonal psychologists and psychoanalysts, we have a different emphasis. These theorists underline the extent to which healthy interpersonal relations, beginning in infancy, are central to our psychological health. Increasingly, we understand the person as intrinsically related to others. That is, the process of becoming a person is in many ways dependent upon others and our relationships with them. Throughout our life, it is in the development of our interpersonal relationships that we become a well-functioning person. In some ways, this process is in serious conflict with the far more familiar idea proposed by many ego and self psychologists—and supported by our political and economic culture—that it is in separation from others and in individuation that we find identity and personal fulfillment.

No doubt, part of genuinely healthy maturation is learning to separate and individuate—to become independent and free of others—even though in fact we are never totally free. After all, we always carry our early relationships inside us. But given our growth in freedom, the question remains, what is "freedom for"? Is it "just another word for nothing left to lose," as the song goes? It seems to me that the purpose of freedom is not to be hoarded for its own sake, but to be spent—as we spend money. That is, yes, we choose individual fulfillment but we also increasingly understand that we choose relationships with others. In all serious choices we spend—we lose—some freedom; but the cost is worth it, for without commitment to particular goals and particular people, life would be empty indeed.

References

Adler, A. (1929). *The problems of neurosis* (P. Mairet, Ed.). New York: Harper.

Adler, A. (1964). *Social interest: A challenge to mankind*. New York: Putnam.

Ainsworth, M. (1963). The development of infant-mother interaction among the Ganda. In B. M. Foss (Ed.), *Determinants of infant behavior* (pp. 67–104). New York: Wiley.

Ainsworth, M. (1982). Attachment: Retrospect and prospect. In C. Parkes & J. Stevenson-Hinde (Eds.), *The place of attachment in human behavior* (pp. 3–30). New York: Basic Books.

Ansbacher, H., & Ansbacher, R. (1956). *The individual psychology of Alfred Adler: A systematic presentation in selections from his writings*. New York: Harper.

Beck, A. (1976). *Cognitive therapy and emotional disorders*. New York: International Universities Press.

Bowlby, J. (1958). The nature of a child's tie to his mother. *International Journal of Psychoanalysis*, 39, 350–373.

Bowlby, J. (1969). *Attachment and loss: Vol. I. Attachment*. New York: Basic Books.

Bowlby, J. (1973). *Attachment and loss: Vol. II. Separation*. New York: Basic Books.

Bowlby, J. (1980). *Attachment and loss: Vol. III. Loss.* New York: Basic Books.

Collins, N., & Read, A. (1990). Adult attachment, working models, and relationship quality in dating couples. *Journal of Personality and Social Psychology, 58,* 644–663.

Eagle, M. (1995). The developmental perspectives of attachment and psychoanalytic theory. In S. Greenberg, R. Muir, & J. Kerr (Eds.), *Attachment theory: Social, developmental and clinical perspectives* (pp. 123–150). Hillsdale, NJ: Analytic Press.

Ellis, A. (1962). *Reason and emotion in psychotherapy.* New York: Lyle Stuart.

Enright, R. D., & Fitzgibbons, R. P. (2000). *Helping clients forgive: An empirical guide for resolving anger and restoring hope.* Washington, DC: American Psychological Association.

Erikson, E. (1959). *Identity and the life cycle: Selected papers.* Psychological issues, Monograph No. 1, Vol. 1. New York: International Universities Press.

Erikson, E. (1963). *Childhood and society* (2nd ed.). New York: Norton. [Original work published 1950]

Erikson, E. (1982). *The life cycle completed.* New York: Norton.

Fairbairn, W. R. D. (1952). *An object-relations theory of the personality* . New York: Basic Books.

Feeney, J., & Noller, P. (1991). Attachment style and verbal descriptions of romantic partners. *Journal of Personal and Social Relationships, 8,* 87–215.

Frankl, V. (1959). The spiritual dimension in existential analysis and logotherapy. *Journal of Individual Psychology, 15,* 157–165.

Frankl, V. (1963). *Man's search for meaning.* New York: Simon & Schuster.

Freud, A. (1936). The ego and the mechanisms of defense (rev. ed.). Vol. 2 of *The writings of Anna Freud.* New York: International Universities Press.

Freud, A. (1952). The mutual influences in the development of ego and id. In *The writings of Anna Freud: Vol. 4. Indications for child analysis and other papers* (pp. 30–44). New York: International Universities Press.

Fromm, E. (1941). *Escape from freedom.* New York: Avon.

Fromm, E. (1947). *Man for himself.* Greenwich, CT: Fawcett

Fromm, E. (1956). *The art of loving.* New York: Harper

Glasser, W. (1965). *Reality therapy: A new approach to psychiatry.* New York: Harper & Row.

Greenberg, J., & Mitchell, S. (1983). *Object relations in psychoanalytic theory.* Cambridge, MA: Harvard University Press.

Hartmann, H. (1958). *Ego psychology and the problem of adaptation* (D. Rapaport, Trans.). New York: International Universities Press. [Original work published 1939]

Hartmann, H. (1964). *Papers on psychoanalytic psychology: Psychological issues.* Monograph No. 14. New York: International Universities Press.

Hazen, C., & Shaver, P. (1987). Attachment as an organizational framework for research for close relationships. *Psychological Inquiry, 5,* 1–22.

Jacobi, J. (1973). *The psychology of C. G. Jung* (8th ed.). New Haven, CT: Yale University Press.

Kilpatrick, L., & Davis, K. (1994). Attachment style, gender, and relationship stability: A longitudinal analysis. *Journal of Personality and Social Psychology, 66,* 502–512.

Klein, M. (1932). *The psycho-analysis of children.* London: Hogarth Press.

Klein, M. (1975). Envy and gratitude. In *Envy and gratitude and other works, 1946–1964.* New York: Delacorte Press, 1975. [Original work published 1957]

Macmillan, M. (1997). *Freud evaluated: The completed arc.* Cambridge, MA: MIT Press.

Maslow, A. (1961). *Toward a psychology of being.* New York: Van Nostrand.

Maslow, A. (1964). *Religions, values and peak-experiences.* New York: Viking.

Maslow, A. (1970). *Motivation and personality* (2nd ed.). New York: Harper & Row.

May, R. (1953). *Man's search for himself.* New York: Norton.

May, R. (1969). *Love and will.* New York: Norton.

May, R. (1981). *Freedom and destiny.* New York: Norton.

McCullough, M. E., Kilpatrick. S. D., Emmons, R. A., & Larson, D. B. (2001). Is gratitude a moral affect? *Psychological Bulletin, 127,* 249–266.

Monte, C. F. (1999). *Beneath the mask: An introduction to theories of personality* (6th ed.). Fort Worth, TX: Harcourt Brace.

Noll, R. (1997). *The Aryan Christ: The secret life of Carl Jung.* New York: Random House.

Roazen, P. (1975). *Freud and his followers*. New York: Knopf.

Rogers, C. (1942). *Counseling and psychotherapy*. Boston: Houghton Mifflin.

Rogers, C. (1961). *On becoming a person*. Boston: Houghton Mifflin.

Seligman, M., & Csikszentmihalyi, M. (2002). Positive psychology: An introduction. *American Psychologist, 55*, 5–14.

Simpson, J. (1990). Influence of attachment styles on romantic relationships. *Journal of Personality and Social Psychology, 59*, 571–580.

Solomon, J., & George, C. (1999). *Attachment disorganization*. New York: Guilford.

Vitz, P. C. (1994). *Psychology as religion: The cult of self-worship* (2nd ed.). Grand Rapids, MI: Eerdmans. [Original work published 1977]

Winnicott, D. W. (1958). *Through paediatrics to psycho-analysis*. London: Hogarth Press.

IV
Connecting to the Transcendent

8 Hardwired for God: A Neuropsychological Model for Developmental Spirituality

Andrew B. Newberg

University of Pennsylvania

Stephanie K. Newberg

Council for Relationships

The study of religious and spiritual phenomena from a neuropsychological and developmental perspective presents a number of complex issues, the most important of which is to determine whether such an approach may open a window to understanding how religion and spirituality are intimately linked with human biology and psychology throughout the life cycle. This can ultimately help in the understanding of how human beings are "hardwired" for God. The implication here is not necessarily one of design; that is, that the brain was specifically created to accommodate a concept and experience of God. Rather, being hardwired implies that the brain functions underlying religious and spiritual experiences are built into the brain's structures over the life span of the person. (How and why these mechanisms are "built in" requires significant theological and philosophical debate that will not be addressed in this chapter.) The basic mechanisms associated with religious and spiritual experiences are correlated with essential brain functions, and the development of both mirrors each other. The notion that as the brain develops physiologically, the human concept of religion and spirituality also evolves accordingly supports the intimate link between human biology and spirituality. By exploring this link, we hope to elucidate how religion and spirituality become hardwired in the brain.

Neuropsychologically, religion and spirituality must be experienced by the human brain, which can then help to translate and interpret the experience and eventually modify outward behaviors accordingly. With this in mind, it is important to explore the wide variety of experiences that can be considered to be religious or spiritual and also to try to describe and identify these experiences. We can then explore these experiences in the context of human brain development and look for potential clues for understanding when such development may go awry. It is important to realize that it is difficult to examine religious and spiritual experiences such as meditation (d'Aquili & Newberg, 1993), near-death experiences (Newberg & d'Aquili, 1994), and other related phenomena in a manner comprehensive enough to accommodate multiple perspectives of the psychologist, neuroscientist, philosopher, and theologian. The study of religious and spiritual experiences, however, must begin with an understanding of these phenomena. These phenomena can then be superimposed upon a theoretical framework based on neurophysiology and developmental psychology.

Epidemiology and Description

Spirituality, religion, and faith are complex concepts that have been defined in many different ways. For this chapter, we define spirituality as distinct from religion or religiousness. Spirituality is usually regarded as less institutionally based and as more encompassing and inclusive of all groups and cultures than religiousness. Spirituality is also used to describe individual experiences such as those of transcendence and meaningfulness (Larson, Swyers, & McCullough, 1998; Spilka & McIntosh, 1996). According to a consensus conference report sponsored by the National Institute for Healthcare Research, the criteria for spirituality were described as "the feelings, thoughts, experiences, and behaviors that arise from a search for the sacred. The term 'search' refers to attempts to identify, articulate, maintain, or transform. The term 'sacred' refers to a divine being or Ultimate Reality or Ultimate Truth, as perceived by the individual" (Larson et al., 1998). This definition of spirituality was distinguished from the definition of religiousness. Religion and religiousness are not only contained in the above criteria but are also included in a "search for nonsacred goals (such as identity, belongingness, meaning, health, or wellness)." Religiousness also implies that the means and methods of the search "receive validation and support from within an identifiable group." It should be emphasized that these definitions were specifically intended to be operationalized approaches that would facilitate future scientific research.

The concept of faith is also extremely difficult to clearly characterize. Although the term *faith* has religious implications in terms of being a belief in a particular religious conceptualization, faith also can be considered from a neuropsychological perspective. As stated in the introduction, the neuropsychological perspective posits that all human experience is ultimately processed by the brain. The brain therefore can only provide a "secondhand rendition" of external reality. If this is the case, then human beings always have to have faith in their interpretation of that external reality as it is processed by the brain. Faith, in some sense, becomes absolutely essential for the human brain to function properly so that it assumes that the world as it is perceived and interpreted represents a reasonable one-to-one correlation with what is actually "out there." With this perspective in mind, faith clearly underlies the experiences and ideas associated with religion and spirituality. James Fowler (1981) has observed that faith is universal, recognizably similar regardless of one's specific beliefs or religion. In this regard, faith might be considered to refer to the quest for meaning and its relation to transcendence and how one uses the concept to derive purpose and set priorities within life. Thus, faith can evolve over the course of an individual's life span and will have mutual interactions with the person's sense of spirituality and religion.

To better understand spirituality and religion, scholars have attempted to identify the specific characteristics of experiences associated with these two concepts. A spiritual experience has been defined as a melting of boundaries and a merging with the surrounding environment (Rolbin, 1985) and as a unitary or *cosmic consciousness* (Bucke, 1961; Rowan, 1983). Spirituality has been discussed as a transcendence that occurs along a specified spiritual path that can be attained through practices such as meditation. "Through therapy or personal growth, we learn to open up to our own inner process, through mysticism we learn how to carry on with that same process into the deepest depths of all" (Rowan, 1983, p. 9). Maslow (1970) has described spirituality as a unity with all and the attainment of self-actualization. According to Rowan (1983), to attain a spiritual experience one must have discovered one's self through mindful awareness, therapy, personal growth, and/or meditation. However, there are clearly many examples of spontaneous spiritual experiences that include near-death experiences and religious conversions. It is also important to acknowledge that spiritual experiences likely reside along a continuum from relatively brief feelings of "awe" to profound unitary states, and we will consider this issue later (d'Aquili & Newberg, 1999).

With regard to the frequency of various spiritual experiences, it is likely that "lesser" spiritual experiences may occur in most people at least several times during their lives. Evidence for this prevalence can be found in the number of people who have stated that they believe in God (>90%) and that they have had some type of spiritual experience (>40%), including a sense of a presence, feelings of awe or peace during prayer or ritual, or even a perceived contact with angels or the deceased (Gallup, 1990). According to a survey of American Psychological Association members in full-time practice, 4.5% of patients reported spiritual experiences (Snedden, 1991). Most therapists did not view such experiences as necessarily pathologic, and 50% of the therapists themselves reported having spiritual experiences.

Recent studies indicate that psychiatric patients have spiritual needs that, if addressed appropriately, may aid in the process of psychological healing. In a survey of psychiatric and medical inpatients (20 to 89 years old), 80% considered themselves spiritual and 88% reported that they had spiritual needs (Fitchett, Burton, & Sivan, 1997). Koenig and Weaver (1997, p. 325) developed a chart that listed many examples of the psychological and spiritual needs of psychiatric patients. The three main categories were needs related to self, needs related to God, and needs related to others.

Despite the frequency of these various spiritual experiences, therapists typically do not ask patients about their religious beliefs and spiritual history (Neeleman & Persaud, 1995; Worthington, McCullough, & Sandage, 1995). This avoidance, however, might hinder proper diagnosis and management, as there is evidence that some psychopathologies may be directly related to problems associated with religion and spirituality. In addition, spirituality may be able to aid in the treatment of psychological disorders such as depression and anxiety. Thus, it seems necessary to consider spiritual experiences from a neuropsychological as well as a clinical perspective to provide some insight into the significance of such experiences and to begin to consider how to incorporate the exploration of these experiences into therapy.

The Neuropsychology of Spiritual Experiences

The study of spiritual experiences has important implications for a developmental spirituality, as it is frequently such experiences that can propel an individual along the developmental path. Furthermore, it may be that certain stages of spiritual development are associated with different types of spiritual experiences. There is clearly a wide variety of spiritual experiences that exist along a continuum ranging from mild feelings of "awe" to the sense of the "wholly other" of the divine being to what has been called *Absolute Unitary Being* (AUB) in many of the Eastern traditions such as Buddhism and Hinduism (Otto, 1970; Streng, 1978). Ninian Smart distinguishes between the experience of Otto's "wholly other" and the internal sense of ineffable unity defined as a mystical experience, predominately, although not exclusively, in Asian traditions. Smart (1967, 1969, 1978) has argued that certain strains of Hinduism, Buddhism, and Taoism differ markedly from prophetic religions such as Judaism and Islam and from religions related to the prophetic-like Christianity, in that the religious experience most characteristic of the former is *mystical* whereas that most characteristic of the latter is *numinous*. Of these two terms, it is the numinous that Smart seems to have an easier time explaining, as it obviously arises more spontaneously out of Western religious traditions. W. T. Stace (1961) goes further by distinguishing between what he calls extrovertive mystical experiences and introvertive mystical experiences. Extrovertive mystical experiences are differentiated by including a unifying vision in which all things are perceived as one and the more concrete apprehension of the One as an inner subjectivity, or life, in all things. Introvertive mystical experiences are distinguished by including a Unitary Consciousness that is nonspatial and nontemporal. Steven Katz (1978), in his critique of these typologies, maintains that not only do spiritual experiences differ in terms of the language of the culture in which they are embedded but also their very content is altered by the cultural experience the person brings to them.

A neurobiological analysis of spiritual experiences might clarify some of the issues regarding these experiences by allowing for a typology based on the underlying brain functions. With regard to the continuum of spiritual experiences, unitary states appear to play a crucial role. Although it is difficult to define what makes a given experience spiritual, the sense of having a union with some higher power or fundamental state of being seems a crucial part of spiritual experiences. To that end, this union helps reduce existential anxiety as well as provide a sense of control over the environment (d'Aquili, 1978; d'Aquili & Newberg, 1998; Smart, 1967, 1969).

The bottom line in understanding the phenomenology of subjective spiritual experience is to understand that every experience involves a sense of the unity of reality at least somewhat greater than the baseline perception of unity in day-to-day life (d'Aquili, 1986). This may be related to altered functioning of the brain structures typically involved in helping to construct the self/other dichotomy. Usually the self/other dichotomy functions to help us distinguish our self from the rest of the external world. It has been suggested that the left posterior superior parietal lobe may be responsible for this function because it is involved in differentiating graspable from nongraspable objects (Van Heertum & Tikofsky, 1995). In human beings, it has been suggested that the functions of this structure have been elaborated to allow for the self/other dichotomy (Joseph, 1996). This dichotomy is normally based on input from all of the sensory systems.

In cases of meditation, it has been suggested that there is a differential blocking or *deafferentation* of input into the posterior superior parietal lobe, which progressively diminishes the strength of the self/other dichotomy (d'Aquili & Newberg, 1993). Thus, if the continuum of spiritual experience relies heavily on the progressive sense of unity, this should be associated with progressive blocking of input into the posterior superior parietal lobe. This creates a sense of increased unity over multiplicity. It should also be mentioned that the right posterior superior parietal lobe is involved in orienting ourselves within three-dimensional space (Joseph, 1996). We have proposed that the blocking of input into this structure may result in the alterations in the sense of space and time that are often described during spiritual experiences. Thus, both the left and right posterior superior parietal lobe are likely involved in spiritual experiences. Brain imaging studies of meditative experiences have supported the notion that the superior parietal lobe is affected. In particular, studies have reported a relative decrease in activity in the superior parietal lobes during meditation and related spiritual practices (see Figures. 1 and 2; Newberg, Alavi, Baime, Mozley, & d'Aquili, 2001; Newberg, Pourdehnad, Alavi, & d'Aquili, 2003).

At the extreme end of the continuum of spiritual experiences is the state of Absolute Unitary Being, which is described in the mystical literature of all the world's great religions. When a person is in that state, he or she loses all sense of discrete being. Even the difference between self and other is obliterated. There is no sense of the passing of time, and all that remains is a perfect, timeless, undifferentiated consciousness. When such a state is suffused with positive affect, there is a tendency to describe the experience, after the fact, as personal. Such experiences are often described as a perfect union with God (the *Unio Mystica* of the Christian tradition) or the perfect manifestation of God in the Hindu tradition. When such experiences are accompanied by neutral

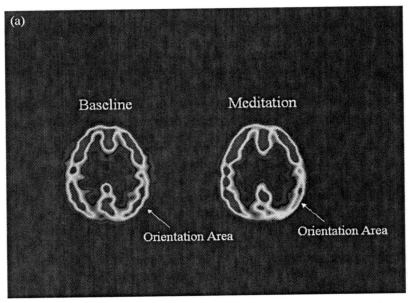

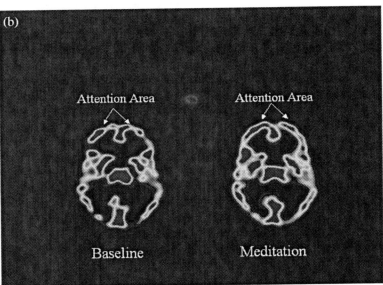

Figure 1. The figures were obtained during an ongoing study of the neurophysiologic correlates of meditation. Briefly, we have been studying highly experienced Tibetan Buddhist meditators using a brain imaging technology called single-photon emission computed tomography (SPECT). SPECT imaging allows us to image the brain and determine which areas are active by measuring blood flow. The more blood flow an area has, the more active it is. The images show the results from a baseline scan on the left (i.e., at rest) and during a "peak" of meditation shown on the right. Two sets of images were taken, showing slightly different parts of the brain. Part (a) shows that there is decreased activity in the parietal lobe (lower right portion of the brain image

affect, they tend to be described, after the fact, as impersonal. These states are described in concepts such as the abyss of Jacob Boeme, the Void or Nirvana of Buddhism, or the Absolute of a number of philosophical or mystical traditions. Whether the experience is interpreted personally as God or impersonally as the Absolute, it nevertheless possesses a quality of transcendent wholeness without any temporal or spatial division whatsoever. We have postulated that these rare states of AUB are associated with the total blocking of input into the posterior superior parietal lobe (d'Aquili, 1982; d'Aquili & Newberg, 1993).

We propose that even in more ordinary perceptions, whenever the sense of wholeness exceeds the sense of multiplicity of parts or of discrete elements in the sensorium, there is an affective discharge via the right brain–limbic connections that Schwartz, Davidson, and Maer (1975) have shown to be of such importance. This tilting of the balance toward an increased perception of wholeness, depending on its intensity, can be experienced as beauty, romantic love, numinosity, or the religious awe described by Smart; religious exaltation in the perception of unity in multiplicity (described by Stace as extrovertive mystical experience); and, eventually, various trance states culminating in AUB.

As there is an increasing sense of unity, there is the perception of ever greater approximations of some more fundamental reality (d'Aquili, 1986). Furthermore, the more the blocking of input into the right posterior superior parietal lobe in excess of a state of balance with the analytic functions of the left hemisphere, the stronger will be the associated emotional charge. Thus, in any perception such as of a piece of music, a painting, a sculpture, or a sunset, there is a sense of meaning and wholeness that transcends the constituent parts. In aesthetic experiences such as those just described, this transcendence is mild to moderate. We would locate the overarching sense of unity between two persons in romantic love as the next stage in this continuum. Feelings of numinosity or religious awe occur when there is a very marked sense of meaning and wholeness extending well beyond the parts perceived or well beyond the image generated but in a "wholly other" context. Both Otto (1970) and Smart (1969) have described this experience in detail. It is often considered (rather incorrectly, we feel) to be the dominant Western mystical experience. It is experienced when an archetypal symbol is perceived or when certain archetypal elements are externally constellated in a myth. As we move from numinosity along the continuum, we reach the state of religious exaltation that Bucke (1961) has called *cosmic consciousness*. This state is characterized by

Figure 1. shows up as lighter rather than the darker on the left image) during meditation. This area of the brain is responsible for giving us a sense of our orientation in space and time. We hypothesized that blocking all sensory and cognitive input into this area during meditation is associated with the sense of "no space and no time," which is so often described in meditation. Part (b) shows that the front part of the brain, which is usually involved in focusing attention and concentration, is more active during meditation (increased dark activity). This makes sense, because meditation requires a high degree of concentration. We also found that the more activity increased in the frontal lobe, the more activity decreased in the parietal lobe. (Continued)

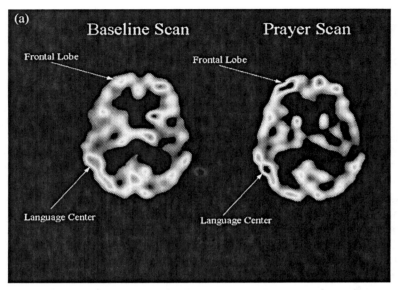

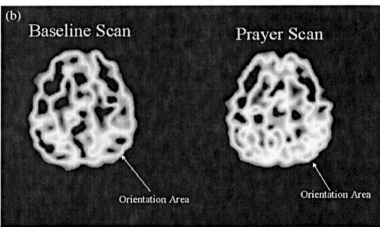

Figure 2. This set of images resulted from a study of Christian nuns during meditative prayer. The first set of images (a) demonstrates increased activity in the frontal lobes (same as Buddhists) but increased activity in the inferior parietal lobe (the language center). This latter finding makes sense in relation to the nuns doing a verbally based practice (prayer) rather than visualization (Buddhists). The second set of images (b) shows that the nuns, like the Buddhists, also decreased the activity in the orientation area (superior parietal lobes)

a sense of meaning and wholeness extending to all discrete being, whether subjective or objective. The essential unity and purposefulness of the universe are perceived as a primary datum despite the perception and knowledge of evil in the world. During this state, nothing whatsoever escapes the mantle of wholeness and purposefulness. But this state does not obliterate discrete being, and it certainly exists within a temporal context. This roughly corresponds with Stace's extrovertive mystical experience.

Several other brain structures are likely to be important with regard to spiritual experiences. It is likely that there is increased activity in two structures of the limbic system, the amygdala and the hippocampus, resulting in the strong affective component described as part of spiritual experiences (Saver & Rabin, 1997). Electrical stimulation of these two structures has also resulted in various sensory experiences, visions, and emotional discharges similar to some of those that occur during spiritual experiences (Penfield & Perot, 1963; Valenstein, 1973). Limbic stimulation during spiritual experiences may be modulated by activity in the posterior superior parietal lobes as well as the frontal lobes, as these structures are all intimately interconnected (Joseph, 1996). During practices such as meditation, stimulation of the limbic system may result from activity in the frontal cortex, which is known to modulate emotional responses via its connections with two limbic structures, the amygdala and the hippocampus. Increased frontal lobe activity has been shown to occur during meditation and likely occurs during other types of spiritual practices (Herzog et al., 1990–1991; Lazar et al., 1999; Newberg et al., 2001). This frontal lobe activity is also likely associated with the concomitant experience of intense awareness and alertness reported during such experiences. See Figures 1 and 2 for examples of changes in the frontal lobes and other regions associated with spiritual practices such as prayer or meditation (Newberg et al., 2001; Newberg et al., 2003). Mention should also be made of the connections between the limbic system and autonomic nervous system with regard to spiritual experiences. Alterations in autonomic activity during various spiritual practices have been demonstrated in a number of studies (Corby, Roth, Zarcone, & Kopell, 1978; Jevning, Wallace, & Beidebach, 1992; Kesterson, 1989; Sudsuang, Chentanez, & Veluvan, 1991). It seems likely that the feelings of the heart racing or of extreme calmness that may occur during different spiritual practices may be associated with alterations in the functioning of the autonomic nervous system. Such alterations may also help to explain other physiologic changes, including those in heart rate, blood pressure, and respiratory rate.

Although spiritual experiences and the unitary continuum are crucial, it is also important to realize how they are elaborated into myth formation. A myth presents a problem of ultimate concern to a society. We have typically considered myth formation based on several prominent cognitive functions. These cognitive functions include those of causality, binary operations, affect value response, and holistic perceptions. These basic brain functions are also subserved by specific brain structures and their interactions within the brain's neural network. The ability to observe causality and to relate one event to another in a sequential ordering appears to be located in the superior temporal lobe in conjunction with the inferior parietal region (Mills & Rollman, 1980; Pribram & Luria, 1973; Swisher & Hirsch, 1971). The ability to generate a sense of binary opposites, so that we can compare concepts such as good and evil or right and wrong, is also likely associated with the inferior parietal regions (Gardner, Silverman, Wapner, & Surif, 1978; Gazzaniga & Miller, 1989). This binary function has particular relevance to religious experiences and especially myth formation. Religious myths tend to involve opposites that are in some form of conflict and are then resolved through the myth process (d'Aquili, 1978). When we initially observe a pair of opposites, we encounter a sense of arousal because of the incongruity between the opposites. We desire a resolution and revised understanding because of the holistic abilities of the brain, most likely associated with the superior parietal region (Nebes & Sperry, 1971; Schiavetto, Cortese, & Alain, 1999; Sperry, Gazzaniga, & Bogen, 1969). The initial binary tension enhances activity in the autonomic nervous system, particularly in the sympathetic system that subserves the sense of arousal and the "fight or flight" response. The parasympathetic system, which underlies quiescent functions, may be stimulated upon resolution of the opposites within a myth. Thus, the existential problem that is presented in the myth is solved by some resolution or unification of the seemingly irreconcilable opposites that constitute the problem, and such a resolution is associated with strong emotional and visceral experiences. The ability to assign emotional valence to various thoughts and stimuli involved in the myth is associated with the connections between the limbic system and the other cognitive processes. Clearly, this emotional response is crucial for religious myth as well as spiritual experiences.

Developmental Spirituality

Given the preceding description of the neuropsychological correlates of religious and spiritual experiences, as well as their elaboration in myth, it is now possible to consider a developmental spirituality. This developmental spirituality considers how spiritual perspectives and concepts evolve over the course of the human life span and how they parallel human brain development. It is well-known that the human brain is not static in its structures or functions throughout life. It is this ability to change and adapt that gives the brain its power to enable human beings to survive, grow, and learn new things to ever enhance and modify thoughts and behaviors and experiences. Enough studies of brain function and structure have been performed to yield an overall model of human brain development from infancy, through adolescence, and into adulthood and old age. The brain changes that occur should have a direct impact upon human thoughts and behaviors and consequently on religious and spiritual experiences. In this section, we will outline a neuropsychologically based developmental spirituality in which we consider the developmental stages of brain function and compare them with the stages of spiritual development. We will use James Fowler's (1981) conception of structural faith development in his book, *Stages of Faith*, as a framework for this analysis. However, it should be stated clearly that spiritual development is likely to be more complex (Oser, 1991; Tamminen, 1994) and involve more subtle changes than will be elaborated here. Furthermore, this chapter represents an initial attempt to intimately link brain development with spiritual development. Some of the speculative concepts considered will hopefully lay the foundation for future analyses and studies in order to more clearly establish and substantiate this link.

Infancy

Fowler described the stage that precedes the first structural, developmental faith stage as *Undifferentiated Faith*. Because there is little in the way of higher cognitive functions, especially with regard to integrating sensory phenomena, there can be no identifiable or differentiated faith or belief system. The infant operates almost exclusively in a stimulus-response mode. This implies that at this level, there can be no conception of a well-defined religion or spiritual viewpoint. Even if the person is raised in a highly devoted religious family, the infant cannot cognitively absorb this information in order to derive an understanding of any particular religious perspective. In spite of the lack of higher cognitive processing, this is the stage at which the seeds of trust, hope, and love are developed through the infant's caregivers. It is imperative at this stage that the environment in which an infant is raised provides enough consistency and nurturance and is not one in which there is deprivation. Such deprivation, at least in animal models, results in a significant lack of neuronal complexity and interconnectedness, which ultimately lays the foundation for future brain development (Black, 1998; Kuhn & Schanberg, 1998). This pre-stage is therefore critical for overall development, both psychologically and spiritually, for the individual. Even though there are no higher processing steps, this pre-stage helps to lay the foundation for future development and benefits from an environment that provides the basis for courage, autonomy, hope, trust, and strength to prepare for faith and spiritual development and subsequent stages. If there are neglect or inconsistencies in care, the infant may lock into patterns of isolation and despair and not integrate the concept of mutuality. Such isolation is arguably associated with an overall lack of connection, not only between the neurons in the individual's brain, but also between the individual and the rest of his or her environment. If such a lack of connection persists beyond this stage, then the individual's association areas may not form adequately, thus preventing the person from being able to explore spirituality and meaning in the first place. Such a phenomenon is known to occur with specific sensory systems in which an inability to make the appropriate neuronal connections early in life causes a reorganization of the brain's structure and function. This reorganization typically prevents these brain structures from functioning in their "normal" capacity, even though they might be able to acquire new functions (Gazzaniga, 2000).

From the physiologic developmental perspective, the undifferentiated stage is associated with the state of brain function during this infancy period. It has been shown that the brain function pattern changes throughout the first year of life with initial increases in the sensorimotor cortex, thalami, brain stem, and cerebellar vermis (Chugani & Phelps, 1986; Chugani, Phelps,

& Mazziotta, 1987). These are central systems that subserve brain-stem reflexes and visuomotor integrative performance that are typically displayed in infant behavior (Chugani, 1992). However, there are no significant higher cortical functions and, subsequently, no strong evidence of well-integrated cognitive functioning. As visuospatial and visuo-sensorimotor integrative functions are acquired and primitive reflexes are reorganized, there is increasing activity in the primary visual cortex, parietal and temporal regions, basal ganglia, and cerebellar hemispheres (Andre-Thomas & Saint Anne Dargassies, 1960; Parmelee & Sigman, 1983). This also coincides with maturation of the EEG at around 2 to 3 months of age (Kellaway, 1979). At this time, there is still relatively decreased activity in the association areas that are necessary for higher cognitive processing. At 8 to 9 months, there is increasing activity in the frontal lobes and association areas coinciding with the advent of cognitive thinking and hypothesis forming, social interaction, and higher-order thinking. This also correlates with the time that a child begins to develop the concept of object permanence and understands that things that are removed from immediate sensory perception can still exist. This is likely associated with the ability for neurons representing sensory information to connect with memory functions and association areas that are becoming activated.

We would argue that the initial pre-stage lasts up to approximately 1 year, at which time the metabolic pattern observed on brain scans *qualitatively* resembles that of the adult brain (Chugani, 1992). However, this stage may extend up to 2 years until verbal skills are more highly developed (as suggested by Fowler). From the spiritual development perspective, an undifferentiated state is likely associated with the structures that are functioning during the first year with no clear evidence of higher cognitive processing, no clearly defined sense of self, and a strong reliance on visual and motor responses. Because the association areas are not mature, any information coming into the infant is essentially unprocessed and, in that respect, is viewed by the infant in an undifferentiated manner. For example, faces generally appear the same or at least cannot readily be differentiated until several months of age, a skill that progressively develops as the higher-order processing brain structures mature (Gauthier & Nelson, 2001; Morton & Johnson, 1991). The inability to process sensory information is somewhat similar to the notion of *deafferentation*, which refers to the ability to block or prevent incoming sensory or neuronal input from reaching a structure (d'Aquili & Newberg, 1993). Because sensory input arriving at the association areas cannot be further processed, the result would be a state similar to a deafferented association area observed during spiritual experiences. However, because there is no higher cognitive processing, even the association areas cannot respond normally owing to an immature functional status. Thus, this state is not the same as absolute unitary states that are attributed to high spiritual experiences. Specifically, there is an absence of any notion of self, either in an ego context or a universal context. On the other hand, there should theoretically be some remarkable similarities, and it has been remarked by a number of mystical traditions that the ultimate goal of spiritual pursuits is to return to a time in which the mind was at its beginning. For example, the ancient Taoist text, the *Lao Tzu*, contains the following passages (Chan, 1963):

Chapter 10
Can you keep the spirit and embrace the One without departing from them?
Can you concentrate your vital force (ch'i) and achieve the highest degree of weakness like an infant?
Chapter 55
He who possesses virtue in abundance
May be compared to an infant.

Childhood: Stages 1 and 2

Fowler refers to the first stage of faith as the *Intuitive-Projective* stage, and he describes this to occur between the ages of 2 and 6 years. A child in this stage is beginning to develop the ability to use speech to organize his sensory experience into meaning. A child is able to sort out and gain some control over the world through her use of language and symbolic representations. At this point, children's thought processes are not reversible, and the concept of causality is poorly understood. Children at this stage assume that their perspective is the only perspective, and their thinking is magical, episodic, and not constrained by stable logical operations. Their conversations can be described as dual monologues in which they have their own train of thought and cannot respond to another in a reciprocal manner. In general, during this stage a child has integrated and conceptualized God in the way in which society has ingrained it into her through fantasy, stories, and dramatic representations. This stage is largely characterized by fantasy-filled, imaginative processes that are unconstrained by logical thought processes.

It is interesting that during this stage, neurophysiologic development is associated with a progressive increase in overall brain metabolism. In absolute brain metabolism, the neonate's brain, which is typically 30% lower than that of adults, continually increases until it reaches the adult level at about age 2 (Chugani, 1992; Kennedy & Sokoloff, 1957). It continues to increase until about age 4, at which point there is a plateau. We would suggest that because of this aspect of neurophysiologic development, this Intuitive-Projective stage of spiritual development actually lasts until the age of 4 with an overlap with the next stage up to approximately age 6. The initial increase in metabolism is primarily in the neocortex, which attains almost twice the metabolic activity as in adults (Kennedy & Sokoloff, 1957). Central structures such as the brain stem and cerebellum do not demonstrate an increase. Intermediate increases occur in the basal ganglia and thalamus. The initial increased metabolism is likely associated with the overproduction of neurons and their connections (Huttenlocher, 1979; Huttenlocher & deCourten, 1987).

We would suggest that this might explain the increase in fantasy and imaginative powers of children at this age. Their brain is establishing so many different connections all of the time that there is tremendous expansion and overconnectedness between neurons that are not typically related in the adult brain. The result is that there are few clearly defined rules, and there is a sense of blending many different experiences and ideas. The child would therefore perceive the world as comprising many overlapping ideas, experiences, and feelings, and would likely see things in ways that appear to be a fantasy to older individuals who have already reduced their neural interconnections and developed more concrete rules associated with their better defined neural connections.

Children in this first stage will likely not see any problem blending ideas about God with very mundane issues. They may not form clear senses of opposites such as right and wrong or justice and injustice, which will come when the overconnectedness is cut back during the developmental process. Children during this stage begin to form their first sense of self-awareness, which is most likely associated with a greater maturity of the association areas, particularly the superior parietal region in which the sense of self, in conjunction with the other association areas, is ultimately formed. Due to the overconnectedness of sensory neurons with the association areas, however, the developing self is seen as highly interwoven with the external world. Thus, the self may participate in various fantasies and dream states. On the other hand, with this developing sense of self comes the beginning of an ability to experience concepts of death, sex, strong taboos within society, and the ultimate conditions of existence. However, young children will not likely be able to make sense of these complex issues in the same way a mature adult would, as they might not be able to clearly distinguish death from life and wrong from right until their association areas are fully able to process such ideas.

This stage of development can be influenced by the external environment. Problems can arise during this time if a child develops images of terror and destructiveness in the reinforcement of societal taboos. For example, primary caretakers who are very critical, rigid, and use violent and destructive images can cause a child to internalize these negative concepts. Similarly, young children may be taught to associate negative images with religion and spirituality rather than more positive conceptions of something greater than themselves. Children may also develop mood disorders that may delay their ability to incorporate religious and spiritual ideals, symbols, and rituals into their lives. Consequently, the child may not be able to develop strong senses of self, independence, or autonomy—which are crucial to progress to future stages. From a neurophysiologic perspective, the neuronal connections associated with negative fantasies may become stronger, making such a negative perspective more pervasive during subsequent stages of development.

The initiating factor that propels a child to the next stage is the capacity for concrete operational thinking (Piaget, 1932), at which point a child begins to discern and become curious about what is and is not "real." Fowler refers to the second stage as the *Mythic-Literal* stage, which he describes as occurring during the school-age years (6 to 10 years of age). During this stage, a child begins to internalize stories, beliefs, and observances that symbolize belonging to a community or group, enabling the composition of a worldview and ideology. Beliefs are related to literal interpretations of religions or doctrines and are usually composed of moral rules and attitudes.

From the neurologic development perspective, this stage appears to coincide with a plateau phase in brain metabolism such that the overall activity throughout the brain remains higher than in the adult, but there is no longer an increase in activity (Chugani et al., 1987). It is believed that during this time, from the age of 4 to 9, there continues to be a slower overproduction of neuronal connections, and there is a very active cutting back of connections (Chugani, Phelps, & Mazziotta, 1989). The removal of inappropriate connections is likely associated with the establishment of specific rules by which neural connections are allowed to continue. If the connection that $1 + 2 = 3$ is correct, then the other connections that might lead to $1 + 2 = 2$ and $1 + 2 = 4$ will be pruned away. In this manner, very specific and possibly literal rules of behavior, language, emotion, and thought are established. Although there is still some overproduction of neuronal connections during this stage, the emphasis on the cutting back of these connections may account for the transition from a very imagination- and fantasy-oriented stage to a very literal- and rule-based stage.

As we have described in previous work, these rules are likely associated with the elaboration of myth in order to provide information and understanding of the world around us (d'Aquili & Newberg, 1999). These myths are also based on a number of specific cognitive functions, including those that subserve the ability to view things in a binary, quantitative, linguistic, holistic, and abstract manner. Thus, in this stage of development, stories, drama, and myth are the primary venues in which ideas are experienced. This is particularly relevant to the development of the sense of self and the connection of this self to the world. In terms of establishing the sense of self, this stage also begins to provide very concrete rules for determining what is and what is not the self and what is and not "real" (Fowler, 1981). These rules guide the orientation function of the brain to provide a definitive sense of self that is now more clearly separated from the fantasies and holistic world experience. However, this sense of self is still not fully matured.

All of these developments, if they become too rigidly determined, can lead the child's cognitive and emotional perspectives, as well as faith-based concepts, to become trapped in the "narrative." Thus, if a child's environment is constantly controlling and judging, she ultimately will have difficulty formulating her own spiritual concepts and reflecting on the value of those concepts. Although there is increased accuracy in taking the perspective of other people into consideration, there is also an excessive sense of reliance on reciprocity with the sacred (Fowler, 1981). This can even lead to the distortion of the individual's sense of self or possibly to becoming self-destructive if the child feels he deserves punishment on the basis of his relationship with the sacred.

Adolescence to Early Adulthood: Stage 3

The factor initiating transition to the third stage is the implicit contradiction within authoritative stories that leads to reflection on meanings and conflicts. In this regard, the concrete thinking that establishes myths is confronted by new information, exposure to other perspectives, and higher cognitive processes that result in a reconsideration of the literal aspect of Stage 2. Fowler refers to the third stage, which usually takes place during adolescence and into early adulthood, as the *Synthetic-Conventional* stage. Formal operational thinking and mutual perspective taking characterize it. Neurophysiologically, this corresponds with a time in which the overall metabolism in the brain begins to decrease (probably from the age of 11 to 20). This is associated with the pruning of neuronal connections in order to establish the primary connections that will take the person into adulthood. Plasticity of the brain decreases notably during the decreasing metabolism phase of brain development (Chugani et al., 1989).

There is still significant room, however, for developing and learning new ideas and concepts. It is simply that these new ideas are not as likely to be foundational concepts so much as they are building upon the connections made during the previous stages of development. Thus, new concepts of mathematics might continue to be learned, but they are built upon the fundamental laws of quantitation that have become engrained in the person's brain structures. Likewise, a person's sense of spirituality is more likely to be built upon previously established notions of religion and spirituality. During this time there is significant elaboration of basic ideas and deeper incorporation into the person's overall world perspective. Because the connections that are established and lost during this time will likely become the individual's neurophysiologic "setup" throughout the rest of her life, this is a crucial period of development. This is the period in which the person's basic approach to life, relationships, self, and spirituality is galvanized and fully elaborated.

This is also a complex stage owing to a variety of factors, including biological ones associated with various hormonal states associated with puberty and sexual maturation as well as the time in which the individual's world begins to extend beyond the family into peer and other cohort groups. The individual begins to develop a more coherent orientation within the world in the midst of more complex and diverse involvements and understandings. In this stage, values and information become synthesized, which provides for a sense of identity and outlook. Conversely, this stage can also be characterized as a conformist stage because one is attuned to the expectations and judgments of significant others that can actually prevent the development of independent perspectives and provide less opportunity to examine individual beliefs and doctrines systematically. All of these factors affect the pruning process of the neuronal connections, establishing which will survive and which will fall away.

As a result, the person's individual approach to life and various ideologies is beginning to be solidified. Such a process also can result in defining differences among ideologies and the individuals who adhere to discrepant ideologies. This can lead to alienation and possible violence toward others if the environment in which the person lives is depriving and prone to scapegoating. This is where hatred and intergroup rivalries can occur and where cults and powerful leaders can provide a safe and important context to nurture vulnerabilities relating to the need to conform. In particular, rituals that can activate the same biological mechanisms described earlier for spiritual experiences also can enhance a sense of unity among individuals adhering to the same ideology or myth (d'Aquili & Newberg, 1999). Thus, if the myth is embodied within a ritual, then the participants experience a sense of unity and a decrease in intragroup aggression. However, there is a subsequent increase in intergroup aggression toward those individuals and groups that are not participating in the same myth or ritual.

The initiating factor to the next stage is frequently the experience of leaving home or receiving more education, which precipitates the examination of self, values, and background. In addition to the establishment of the basic functionality of the brain as determined by the neuronal connections, this is also the stage in which the cognitive functions described in the previous section become fully established. The binary and causal functions, for example, are now able to function fully and base that function, in part, on the connections established between and within the brain structures subserving these functions. Thus, for a given individual, the basic cognitive functions achieve a fully operational state. These functions, however, have not yet been used to their fullest extent to help the person examine beliefs and doctrines systematically. This appears to occur in the fourth stage.

Adulthood: Stage 4

Fowler refers to the fourth stage as the *Individuative-Reflective* stage. This stage occurs when there is an interruption of reliance on external sources of authority. In addition, there is critical distancing from one's assumptive value system, which Fowler believes leads to the emergence of the executive ego. Fowler defines the executive ego as the internal process by which a person chooses his beliefs and a relocation of authority within himself and is prepared to take full responsibility for his choices. A new identity begins to be formed with new personal affiliations and lifestyle choices. This stage usually occurs during young adulthood but can happen as late as ages 30 to 40. It is a time when one begins to take responsibility for one's own choices irrespective of what others in one's former or present community feel.

Neurophysiologically, this stage is associated with the full development of the cognitive and emotional processes that are now significantly more stable than in all of the previous stages. A limited number of new connections are made, and limited pruning occurs (at least they are in balance). Thus, the cognitive functions of the individual are operating for the first time in their full manner and can be brought to bear on all types of experiences and ideas (both internally and externally generated). This is likely associated with the ability to establish a well-defined identity and to imbue that self with a set of cognitive, affective, and behavioral processes that together help to define the self. The overall brain metabolism is highly stable as well, reflecting this overall mature stage of the human brain. In fact, the metabolism remains at this level until the end of the fourth decade of life.

There is an ability at this stage to critically and objectively reflect on identity and outlook and translate symbols into concepts with deeper meanings. This may be based on the person's fully functioning orientation mechanism as well as on other cognitive functions that can analyze and reflect on all aspects of the person's life. There is also the struggle for self-fulfillment as a primary concern versus service to and being for others and the question of being committed to the relative versus the possibility of an absolute. The initiating factor that propels a person to Stage 5 is disillusionment with one's compromises and recognition that life is more complex than one's ability to use logic and abstract thinking, which leads to the search for a more multileveled approach to life truth through other traditions.

Fowler refers to the fifth stage as *Conjunctive Faith*. This stage generally occurs at midlife. At this stage, the individual is ready for significant encounters with other traditions in a quest for meaning and value in life. As the individual gains access to various perspectives, each one will augment and correct aspects that will eventually enable him to sort out the most real and true ones. There is now an integration of the self that was previously unrecognized or suppressed. The end result is a reclaiming and reworking of one's identity and faith through understanding one's life and how it relates to humanity.

Neurophysiologically, this stage is associated with a decrease in overall brain metabolic activity (Newberg & Alavi, 1997). This decrease begins around the age of 40 and slowly progresses throughout the remainder of the individual's life. This decrease, while unknown to the person, may reflect or at least contribute to the notion of disillusionment, as the brain no longer appears to be able to find the answers it was striving so hard to find with its full complement of functions. As connections are lost, there may be a sense that the answers are slipping away and that it is unlikely they will be obtained on the current path. The self may also be perceived to be somewhat slipping away, as the connections between the neurons subserving the self and the sensory and cognitive input become diminished. The result may be a concern that the self can no longer face the struggle to know and understand.

The last stage Fowler refers to as *Universalizing Faith*. The transition to this stage "involves an overcoming of a paradox through a moral and ascetic actualization of the universalizing apprehensions" (p. 200). In universalizing faith, there is a sense of unity between the self and the tenets of the individual's religious tradition. This may represent a sense of union of the self with God or ultimate reality. This union may result from various spiritual practices or experiences such as those described earlier in this chapter. In fact, this type of experience likely arises from the deafferentation of sensory and cognitive inputs into the association areas that subserve the orientation abilities of the brain. That there is already a concomitant decrease in overall neuronal function and interconnectedness may actually contribute to this type of experience typically occurring in older individuals. There may also be a conception of various faiths having similar characteristics. As such, there is not only a sense of union within a given tradition but also a notion of universalization across traditions, that is, that all faiths have similar perspectives and derive from a similar root. Depending on the depth and extension of the universalizing sense, there is partly a recapitulation of the undifferentiated faith stage in which all things are considered to be part of a greater, integrated whole.

It is interesting to note that physiologically, the brain of an older individual begins to decrease activity in the association areas similar to what is found in the infant brain. It is not a coincidence that individuals suffering from disorders such as Alzheimer disease can actually have brain metabolic patterns that appear almost identical to that of an infant (Newberg & Alavi, 1996). The difference here is that such an experience is built upon the entire developmental basis of the individual as they progress through the various stages.

Conclusions

In outlining a neuropsychological developmental spirituality, we have combined the phenomenological aspects of spiritual development with observed changes in brain function over the life span of the human being, providing a hypothetical framework upon which to base future studies of normal and abnormal development. The ability to observe potential physiologic and clinical sources of "abnormal" spiritual development may prove to be a valuable interface from which to design interventions that may help prevent such problems from arising. It appears that there is a strong correlation between a number of the characteristics of spiritual development and the changing function of specific brain structures from infancy through adulthood. This developmental approach suggests a deep interconnection between neurophysiology and spirituality and supports the notion that spirituality is "hardwired" into the brain.

References

Andre-Thomas, C. Y., & Saint Anne Dargassies, S. (1960). The neurological examination of the infant. London: Medical Advisory Committee of the National Spastics Society.
Black, J. E. (1998). How a child builds its brain: Some lessons from animal studies of neural plasticity. Preventive Medicine, 27, 168–171.
Bryant, P. E. (1992). Arithmetic in the cradle. Nature, 358, 712–713.
Bucke, R. M. (1961). Cosmic consciousness. Secaucus, NJ: Citadel Press.
Chan, W. T. (1963). The source book in Chinese philosophy. Princeton, NJ: Princeton University Press.
Chugani, H. T. (1992). Functional brain imaging in pediatrics. Pediatric Clinics of North America, 39, 777–799.
Chugani, H. T., & Phelps, M. E. (1986). Maturational changes in cerebral function in infants determined by [18]FDG positron emission tomography. Science, 231, 840–843.

Chugani, H. T., Phelps, M. E., & Mazziotta, J. C. (1987). Positron emission tomography study of human brain functional development. *Annals of Neurology, 22,* 487–497.

Chugani, H. T., Phelps, M. E., & Mazziotta, J. C. (1989). Metabolic assessment of functional maturation and neuronal plasticity in the human brain. In C. von Euler, H. Forssberg, & H. Lagercrantz (Eds.), *Neurobiology of early infant behavior* (pp. 323–330). New York: Stockton Press.

Corby, J. C., Roth, W. T., Zarcone, V. P., & Kopell, B. S. (1978). Psychophysiological correlates of the practice of tantric yoga meditation. *Archives of General Psychiatry, 35,* 571–577.

d'Aquili, E. G. (1978). The neurobiological bases of myth and concepts of deity. *Zygon, 13,* 257–275.

d'Aquili, E. G. (1982). Senses of reality in science and religion. *Zygon, 17,* 361–384.

d'Aquili, E. G. (1986). Myth, ritual, and the archetypal hypothesis: Does the dance generate the word? *Zygon, 21,* 141–160.

d'Aquili, E. G., & Newberg, A. B. (1993). Religious and mystical states: A neuropsychological substrate. *Zygon, 28,* 177–200.

d'Aquili, E. G., & Newberg, A. B. (1998). The neuropsychological basis of religion: Or why God won't go away. *Zygon, 33,* 187–201.

d'Aquili, E. G., & Newberg, A. B. (1999). *The mystical mind: Probing the biology of religious experience.* Minneapolis: Fortress Press.

Fitchett, G., Burton, L. A., & Sivan, A. B. (1997). The religious needs and resources of psychiatric patients. *Journal of Nervous and Mental Disorders, 185,* 320–326.

Fowler, J. W. (1981). *Stages of faith.* San Francisco: HarperCollins.

Gallup, G. (1990). *Religion in America: 1990.* Princeton, NJ: Princeton Religion and Research Center.

Gardner, H., Silverman, J., Wapner, W., & Surif, E. (1978). The appreciation of antonymic contrasts in aphasia. *Brain and Language, 6,* 301–317.

Gauthier, I., & Nelson, C. A. (2001). The development of face expertise. *Current Opinion in Neurobiology, 11,* 219–224.

Gazzaniga, M. S. (2000). *The new cognitive neurosciences.* Cambridge, MA: MIT Press.

Gazzaniga, M. S., & Miller, G. A. (1989). The recognition of antonymy by a language-enriched right hemisphere. *Journal of Cognitive Neuroscience, 1,* 187–193.

Herzog, H., Lele, V. R., Kuwert, T., Langen, K.-J., Kops, E. R., & Feinendegen, L. E. (1990–1991). Changed pattern of regional glucose metabolism during yoga meditative relaxation. *Neuropsychobiology, 23,* 182–187.

Huttenlocher, P. R. (1979). Synaptic density in human frontal cortex: Developmental changes and effects of aging. *Brain Research, 163,* 195–205.

Huttenlocher, P. R., & deCourten, C. (1987). The development of synapses in striate cortex of man. *Human Neurobiology, 6,* 1–9.

Jevning, R., Wallace, R. K., & Beidebach, M. (1992). The physiology of meditation: A review. A wakeful hypometabolic integrated response. *Neuroscience and Biobehavioral Reviews, 16,* 415–424.

Joseph, R. (1996). *Neuropsychology, neuropsychiatry, and behavioral neurology.* Baltimore: Williams & Wilkins.

Katz, S. (1978). Language, epistemology, and mysticism. In S. Katz (Ed.), *Mysticism and philosophical analysis* (pp. 22–74). New York: Oxford University Press.

Kellaway, P. (1979). An orderly approach to visual analysis: Parameters of the normal EEG in adults and children. In D. W. Klass & D. D. Daly (Eds.), *Current practice of clinical electroencephalography* (pp. 69–147). New York: Raven Press.

Kennedy, C., & Sokoloff, L. (1957). An adaptation of the nitrous oxide method to the study of the cerebral circulation in children: Normal values for cerebral blood flow and cerebral metabolic rate in childhood. *Journal of Clinical Investigation, 36,* 1130.

Kesterson, J. (1989). Metabolic rate, respiratory exchange ratio and apnea during meditation. *American Journal of Physiology, R256,* 632–638.

Koenig, H. G., & Weaver, A. J. (1997). *Counseling troubled older adults: A handbook for pastors and religious caregivers.* Nashville, TN: Abingdon Press.

Kuhn, C. M., & Schanberg, S. M. (1998). Responses to maternal separation: Mechanisms and mediators. *International Journal of Developmental Neuroscience, 16,* 261–270.

Larson, D. B., Swyers, J. P., & McCullough, M. E. (1998). *Scientific research on spirituality and health: A consensus report* . Rockville, MD: National Institute of Healthcare Research.

Lazar, S. W., Bush, G., Gollub, R. L., Fricchione, G. L., Khalsa, G., & Benson, H. (2000). Functional brain mapping of the relaxation response and meditation. *NeuroReport, 11*, 1581–1585.

Maslow, A. H. (1970). *Religions, values, and peak experiences.* New York: Viking Press.

Mills, L., & Rollman, G. B. (1980). Hemispheric asymmetry for auditory perception of temporal order. *Neuropsychologia, 18*, 41–47.

Morton, J., & Johnson, M. H. (1991). CONSPEC and CONLERN: A two-process theory of infant face recognition. *Psychological Review, 98*, 164–181.

Nebes, R. D., & Sperry, R. W. (1971). Hemispheric disconnection syndrome with cerebral birth injury in the dominant arm area. *Neuropsychologia, 9*, 249–259.

Neeleman, J., & Persaud, R. (1995). Why do psychiatrists neglect religion? *British Journal of Medical Psychology, 68*, 169–178.

Newberg, A. B., & Alavi, A. (1996). The study of the neurological disorders using positron emission tomography and single photon emission computed tomography. *Journal of the Neurological Sciences, 135*, 91–108.

Newberg, A. B., & Alavi, A. (1997). Neuroimaging in the in vivo measurement of regional function in the aging brain. In S. U. Dani, A. Hori, & G. F. Walter (Eds.), *Principles of neural aging* (pp. 397–408). Amsterdam: Elsevier Science.

Newberg, A., Alavi, A., Baime, M., Mozley, P. D., & d'Aquili, E. (2001). The measurement of regional cerebral blood flow during the complex cognitive task of meditation: A preliminary SPECT study. *Psychiatry Research: Neuroimaging, 106*, 113–122.

Newberg, A. B., & d'Aquili, E. G. (1994). The near death experience as archetype: A model for "prepared" neurocognitive processes. *Anthropology of Consciousness, 5*, 1–15.

Newberg, A., Pourdehnad, M., Alavi, A., & d'Aquili, E. (2003). Cerebral blood flow during meditative prayer: Preliminary findings and methodological issues. *Perceptual and Motor Skills, 97*, 625–630.

Oser, F. K. (1991). The development of religious judgment. *New Directions for Child Development, 52*, 5–25.

Otto, R. (1970). *The idea of the holy.* New York: Oxford University Press.

Parmelee, A. H., & Sigman, M. D. (1983). Perinatal brain development and behavior. In M. Haith & J. Campos (Eds.), *Biology and infancy* (Vol. 2, pp. 95–155). New York: Wiley.

Penfield, W., & Perot, P. (1963). The brain's record of auditory and visual experience. *Brain, 86*, 595–695.

Piaget, J. (1932). *The moral judgment of the child.* London: Routledge & Kegan Paul.

Pribram, K. H., & Luria, A. R. (1973). *Psychophysiology of the frontal lobes.* New York: Academic Press.

Rolbin, S. B. (1985). The mystical quest: Experiences, goals, changes, and problems. *Dissertation Abstracts International, 47*, 940A–941A.

Rowan, J. (1983). The real self and mystical experiences. *Journal of Humanistic Psychology, 23*, 9–27.

Saver, J. L., & Rabin, J. (1997). The neural substrates of religious experience. *Journal of Neuropsychiatry and Clinical Neurosciences, 9*, 498–510.

Schiavetto, A., Cortese, F., & Alain, C. (1999). Global and local processing of musical sequences: An event-related brain potential study. *NeuroReport, 10*, 2467–2472.

Schwartz, G. E., Davidson, R. J., & Maer, F. (1975). Right hemisphere lateralization for emotion in the human brain: Interactions with cognitions. *Science, 190*, 286–288.

Smart, N. (1967). History of mysticism. In P. Edwards (Ed.), *Encyclopedia of philosophy* (pp. 419–428). London: Macmillan.

Smart, N. (1969). *The religious experience of mankind.* London: Macmillan.

Smart, N. (1978). Understanding religious experience. In S. Katz (Ed.), *Mysticism and philosophical analysis* (pp. 10–21). New York: Oxford University Press.

Snedden, L. (1991). Mystical experience as a clinical issue in psychology. *Dissertation Abstracts International, 51*, 4589B.

Sperry, R. W., Gazzaniga, M. S., & Bogen, J. E. (1969). Interhemispheric relationships: The neocortical commissures; syndromes of hemisphere disconnection. In P. J. Vinken & C. W. Bruyn (Eds.), *Handbook of clinical neurology* (Vol. 4., pp. 273–290). Amsterdam: North Holland.

Spilka, B., & McIntosh, D. N. (1996, August). *Religion and spirituality: The known and the unknown.* Paper presented at the annual meeting of the American Psychological Association. Toronto, Canada.

Stace, W. T. (1961). *Mysticism and philosophy.* London: Macmillan.

Streng, F. (1978). Language and mystical awareness. In S. Katz (Ed.), *Mysticism and philosophical analysis* (pp. 141–169). New York: Oxford University Press.

Sudsuang, R., Chentanez, V., & Veluvan, K. (1991). Effects of Buddhist meditation on serum cortisol and total protein levels, blood pressure, pulse rate, lung volume and reaction time. *Physiology and Behavior, 50,* 543–548.

Swisher, L., & Hirsch, I. (1971). Brain damage and the ordering of two temporally successive stimuli. *Neuropsychologia, 10,* 137–152.

Tamminen, K. (1994). Religious experiences in childhood and adolescence: A viewpoint of religious development between the ages of 7 and 20. *International Journal for the Psychology of Religion, 4,* 61–85.

Valenstein, E. S. (1973). *Brain control: A critical examination of brain stimulation and psychosurgery.* New York: John Wiley & Sons.

Van Heertum, R. L., & Tikofsky, R. S. (Eds.). (1995). *Cerebral SPECT imaging.* New York: Raven Press.

Worthington, E. L., McCullough, M. E., & Sandage, S. J. (1995). Empirical research on religion and psychotherapeutic processes and outcomes: A 10 year review and research prospectus. *Psychological Bulletin, 119,* 448–487.

9 A Tale of Two Religious Effects: Evidence for the Protective and Prosocial Impact of Organic Religion

Byron R. Johnson

Baylor University

Surveys continue to reveal that a majority of Americans are highly religious. Therefore, it is not surprising that many with an interest in civil society have been particularly intrigued by the questions of what role religion and religious practices and beliefs, or what has been termed *organic religion* (Johnson, 2004; Johnson, Thompkins, & Webb, 2002), may play in contributing to wide-ranging outcomes relevant in contemporary society. As a social scientist, I am intrigued not only with these questions but also with empirical answers as to how religion affects the way people actually live.

Over the past two decades, scientists have carried out a good deal of such empirical work, and we are now able to objectively discuss, if not answer, many of these questions. In fields ranging from medicine and public health to the social and behavioral sciences, scholars have studied the general influence of religion and religious practices on a wide range of health and social outcomes for adults. In an effort to organize this research systematically and bring clarity to this area, I reviewed and assessed, in summary fashion, more than 600 studies of organic religion and a wide array of health-related outcomes for children, youth, and families.

What do we know about the influence of religious practices on health and various social outcomes for youth and adolescents? The short answer is that we know much less about religious influences on youth, as research on adolescent samples remains a grossly understudied area. Having acknowledged this considerable gap in knowledge, a key question to answer is whether the influence of religion or religious practices on adolescents and youth is markedly different or similar to the influence on adults. Are findings from studies examining the linkages between youth and adolescent religiosity and health outcomes relevant for adults, and vice versa? Many empirical studies from diverse fields of scientific inquiry document that behavior patterns initiated during adolescence are directly related to future adult behavior and outcomes; for example, there is compelling empirical evidence that many causes of adult illness and even death are linked to adolescent behavior patterns (see McGinnis & Foege, 1993). Conversely, both common sense and volumes of research show that families and parenting are directly related to diverse adolescent and youth outcomes. Survey data suggest that both youth and adult samples reveal similar response patterns when religion and religious practices are examined.

Religion and Youth

Survey work confirms that as a group, American youth, like adults, are quite religious and that they exhibit high levels of proreligious beliefs, attitudes, and behaviors (Gallup & Bezilla, 1992). For example, 95% of American teens aged 13 to 17 believe in God, 76% believe that God observes their actions and rewards or punishes them, and 93% believe that God loves them (Thornton & Camburn, 1989).

In addition to reporting relatively high levels of religious belief and affiliation, significant portions of the American youth population indicate that they regularly engage in religious practices. For example, 42% of teenagers report that they frequently pray alone, 36% report that they read the Bible weekly or more often, 41% report that they are currently involved in Sunday school, and 36% say they are involved with a church youth group (Gallup & Bezilla, 1992). How important is religion in the lives of high school seniors? Approximately two thirds of high school seniors indicate that religion is either a *very* important or *pretty* important part of their life. In addition to importance, attendance at religious services is another potentially relevant indicator of the role of religion in the lives of young people and their families (Monitoring the Future, 1998).

Parents and other family members are typically children's primary sources of socialization and thus pass on to children the norms and values that will shape the way they behave in society. For many, then, religion often represents a key secondary socialization influence that is integral to parents' belief systems and is instrumental as they attempt to instill in their children beliefs and values that are consistent with their own.

We know that behaviors initiated in children and adolescents are clearly linked to future adult behavior and outcomes. We also know that parents and the family represent the primary socializing agents for children. Further, we know that the influence of religion is broad and not relegated to any one segment of the population. The parallels and common linkages between research on religion in both adult and youth samples warrant a review that integrates rather than segregates these important bodies of knowledge.

Organic Religion

I use the term *organic religion* to represent the influence of religion practiced over time, such as with children who were raised and nurtured in religious homes. Religious activities, involvements, practices, and beliefs, therefore, tend to be very much part of everyday life for many people throughout the life course. Although organic religion is still understudied, empirical research on its impact on various outcome factors has resulted in a substantial and mounting body of scientific.

Protective and Prosocial Influences

There are two separate but related literatures to review. First, I will examine studies documenting the role of organic religion in protecting or shielding individuals from deleterious outcomes. Then, I will review research that examines the role of organic religion in promoting an array of prosocial or beneficial outcomes. This examination of organic religion is based on both methodological and theoretical considerations. Methodologically, the study of organic religion is interesting because the literature offers diverse methodological approaches across various disciplines from which to draw a number of substantive conclusions about the influence of religion or religious commitment. Theoretically, organic religion is interesting because of the complex relationships, both indirect and direct, that may exist not only between religious practice and overall health and well-being but also with a host of other key independent and dependent variables. For example, if (organic) religion tends to reduce one's likelihood for hypertension, depression, suicide, and alcoholism, is it reasonable to hypothesize that faith-based programs or intentional religion[1] may be viewed as interventions that effectively treat hypertension, depression, suicide, and alcoholism (Johnson et al., 2000)?[2]

Religious Practice as a Protective Factor

Over the past several decades, a notable body of empirical evidence has emerged that examines the relationship between religion or religious practices

---

[1]Intentional religion is the exposure to religion one receives at a particular time in life for a particular purpose. Here religion, in an intentional way, "enters the system," if you will, in order to meet a particular need at a particular time in a person's life. For example, a child from a rundown neighborhood is actively matched with a volunteer mentor from a religious organization. A drug addict enrolls in a faith-based/conversion-oriented drug rehabilitation program after several unsuccessful attempts at sobriety in secular treatment programs.
[2]In a systematic review of research on faith-based organizations, Johnson and colleagues (2002) find that research on faith-based organizations has been largely overlooked by researchers and often relies on weak research designs but is nonetheless almost uniformly positive.

and a host of social and health-related outcomes (see, e.g., Levin, 1994; Levin & Vanderpool, 1987, 1992). In an important publication, Duke University researcher Harold Koenig and colleagues systematically reviewed much of this work (Koenig, McCullough, & Larson, 2001). This lengthy and detailed review of hundreds of studies focuses on scholarship appearing in refereed journals and, in sum, demonstrates that the majority of published research is consistent with the notion that religious practices or religious involvement are associated with beneficial outcomes in mental and physical health. These outcome categories include mortality, hypertension, depression, alcohol use or abuse and drug use or abuse, and suicide. Social science research also confirms that religious commitment and involvement in religious practices are significantly linked to reductions not only in delinquency among youth and adolescent populations but also in criminality in adult populations. As can be seen in Appendix A, in summary fashion, I review approximately 500 research studies on eight important health-related outcomes where religion variables have not been excluded in the analyses.

Mortality

A substantial body of research reveals an association between intensity of participation in religious activities and greater longevity. I reviewed studies that examined the association between degree of religious involvement and survival. The systematic review of this literature revealed that 75% (46 of 61) of these published studies conclude that higher levels of religious involvement have a sizable and consistent relationship with greater longevity (Figure 1). This association is found independent of the effect of confounders such as age, sex, race, education, and health. McCullough and colleagues conducted a meta-analytic review that incorporated data from more than 125,000 subjects and similarly concluded that religious involvement had a significant and substantial association with increased length of life (McCullough, Hoyt, Larson, Koenig, & Thoresen, 2000). In fact, longitudinal research in a variety of different cohorts has also documented that frequent religious attendance is associated with a significant reduction in the risk of dying during study follow-up periods ranging from 5 to 28 years (Koenig et al., 1999; Musick, Koenig, Hays, & Cohen, 1999; Strawbridge, Cohen, Shema, & Kaplan, 1997).

It is well documented that the negative health consequences many Americans experience in adulthood (e.g., lung cancer) are the result of behaviors (such as smoking) initiated during adolescence. Research similarly confirms that other adolescent behaviors, such as alcohol and illicit drug use, sexual activity, dietary patterns, and physical inactivity, are linked to adult health outcomes (Centers for Disease Control and Prevention, 1997, pp. 1–2; McGinnis & Foege, 1993). Unintentional injuries from motor vehicle accidents, drowning, and firearms account for more than 60% of all injury deaths among American teenagers (Sells & Blum, 1996). Intentional injuries, specifically homicide and suicide, are the second and third leading causes

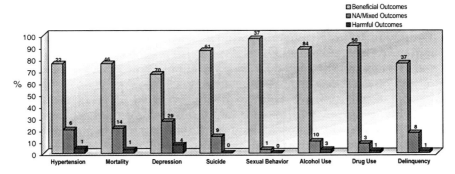

Figure 1. Research examining the relationship between religion and health outcomes (8 fields of study; total of 498 studies reviewed)

of death among adolescents (DiClemente, Hansen, & Ponton, 1996). Using data from the Monitoring the Future project, sociologist John Wallace has documented that religious commitment is significantly associated with a lower likelihood of adolescent unintentional and intentional injury (Wallace, 2002).

Hypertension

Hypertension is defined as a sustained or chronic elevation in blood pressure. The most common of cardiovascular disorders, hypertension affects about 20% of the adult population and is one the major risk factors in 20% to 50% of all deaths in the United States (National Heart, Lung, and Blood Institute, 1997). Although there is strong evidence that pharmacological treatment can lower blood pressure, there remains concern about the adverse side effects of such treatments. For this reason, social epidemiologists are interested in the effects of socioenvironmental determinants of blood pressure. Among the factors shown to correlate with hypertension is religion. Indeed, epidemiologic studies have found that individuals who report higher levels of religious activities tend to have lower blood pressure (Graham et al., 1978; Larson et al., 1989; Scotch, 1963). As can be seen in Figure 1, the current review indicates that 76% (22 of 29) of these studies found that religious activities or involvement tend to be linked with reduced levels of hypertension. Only one of the studies reviewed found that increasing religiosity was linked to a harmful outcome. As 50 million Americans suffer from high blood pressure, it would be prudent to conduct additional research to determine whether and how religious communities may play an intentional role in contributing to hypertension control and prevention.

Depression

Depression is the most common of all mental disorders, and approximately 330 million people around the world suffer from it. People with depression are also at increased risk for use of hospital and medical services and for early death from physical causes (Covinsky et al., 1999; Koenig, Shelp, Goli, Cohen, & Blazer, 1989). People who are frequently involved in religious activities and who highly value their religious faith are at reduced risk for depression. Religious involvement seems to play an important role in helping people cope with the effects of stressful life circumstances. Prospective cohort studies and quasi-experimental and experimental research all suggest that religious or spiritual activities may lead to a reduction in depressive symptoms. These findings have been replicated across a number of large, well-designed studies and are consistent with much of the cross-sectional and prospective cohort research that has found less depression among the more religious. A total of 103 studies examining the religion-depression relationship were reviewed for this essay (Appendix A). As illustrated in Figure 1, religious involvement tends to be associated with less depression in 68% (70 of 103) of these studies.

Suicide

Suicide now ranks as the ninth leading cause of death in the United States. This is particularly alarming when one considers that suicides tend to be underestimated, as many of these deaths are coded as accidental. The problem of suicide is particularly problematic among adolescent males (Ghosh & Victor, 1994). A substantial literature documents that religious involvement (as measured, for example, by frequency of religious attendance, frequency of prayer, and degree of religious salience) is associated with less suicide, suicidal behavior, suicidal ideation, as well as less tolerant attitudes toward suicide across a variety of samples from many nations. This consistent inverse association is found in studies using both group and individual-level data. In total, as can be seen in Figure 1, 87% (61 of 70) of the studies reviewed on suicide found these beneficial outcomes. Although several studies had mixed results, none of the studies found religiosity to be associated with increasing suicidal tendencies.

Promiscuous Sexual Behaviors

Out-of-wedlock pregnancy, often a result of sexual activity among adolescents, is largely responsible for the nearly 25% of children age 6 or younger who are below the federal poverty line. About half of 9th to 12th graders report that they have had sexual intercourse at least once, and 36% report that they have had sexual intercourse during the past 3 months (Centers for Disease Control and Prevention, 1997). According to the CDC, unmarried motherhood is also associated with significantly higher infant mortality rates. Further, sexual promiscuity increases significantly the risk of teen pregnancy and of contracting sexually transmitted diseases (Kann et al., 1991). Studies in this review generally show that those who are religious are less likely to engage in premarital sex or extramarital affairs or to have multiple sexual partners. In fact, approximately 97% of those studies reviewed reported significant correlations between increased religious involvement and lower likelihood of promiscuous sexual behaviors (Figure 1). None of the studies found that increased religious participation or commitment was linked to increases in promiscuous behavior.

Drug and Alcohol Use

The abuse of alcohol and illicit drugs ranks among the leading health and social concerns in the United States today. According to the National Institute on Drug Abuse, approximately 111 million persons are current alcohol users in the United States. About 32 million of these engage in binge drinking, and another 11 million Americans are heavy drinkers. Additionally, some 14 million Americans are current users of illicit drugs (National Institute on Drug Abuse, 1997). Both chronic alcohol consumption and abuse of drugs are associated with increased risks of morbidity and mortality (Bravender & Knight, 1998; Chick & Erickson, 1996). I reviewed more than 150 studies that examined the relationship between religiosity and drug use (n = 54) or alcohol use (n = 97) and abuse. As can be seen in Figure 1, the vast majority of these studies demonstrate that participation in religious activities is associated with less of a tendency to use or *abuse* alcohol (87%) or drugs (92%). These findings hold regardless of the population under study (i.e., children, adolescents, and adult populations), or whether the research was conducted prospectively or retrospectively (Appendix A). The greater a person's religious involvement, the less likely it is that he or she will initiate alcohol or drug use or have problems with these substances if they are used (Wallace, 2002; in addition to alcohol and drug use, Wallace found that frequent religious attendance is inversely related to cigarette smoking among high school seniors). Only four of the studies reviewed reported a positive correlation between religious involvement and increased alcohol or drug use. Interestingly, these four tend to be some of the weaker with regard to methodological design and statistical analyses (one of the four studies does not have any statistical analysis, and none of the four has multiples of even some controls).

Delinquency

There is growing evidence that religious commitment and involvement help protect youth from delinquent behavior and deviant activities (for systematic reviews of this literature, see Baier & Wright, 2001; Johnson, Li, Larson, & McCullough, 2000). Recent evidence suggests that such effects persist even if there is not a strong prevailing social control against delinquent behavior in the surrounding community (Johnson, Larson, Li, & Jang, 2000). There is mounting evidence that religious involvement may lower the risks of a broad range of delinquent behaviors, including both minor and serious forms of criminal behavior (Evans et al., 1996). There is also preliminary evidence that religious involvement may have a cumulative effect throughout adolescence and thus may significantly lessen the risk of later adult criminality (Jang & Johnson, 2001). Additionally, there is growing evidence that religion can be used as a tool to help prevent high-risk urban youth from engaging in delinquent behavior (Johnson, Jang, Larson, & Li, 2001; Johnson, Larson, Jang, & Li, 2000). For example, youth living in poverty tracts in urban environments, or what criminologists call disorganized communities, are at particular risk for a number of problem behaviors, including poor school performance, drug use and other delinquent activities, and more (Johnson, 2000; Johnson, Larson, Li, et al., 2000). However, youth from these same disorganized communities who participate in religious activities are significantly less likely to be involved in the deviant activities described earlier. In this way, religiously committed youth are "resilient" to the negative consequences of living in rundown communities.

Religious involvement may provide networks of support that help adolescents internalize values conducive to behavior that emphasizes concern for others' welfare. Such processes may contribute to the acquisition of positive attributes that give adolescents a greater sense of empathy toward others, which in turn makes them less likely to commit acts that harm others. Similarly, once individuals become involved in deviant behavior, it is possible that participation in specific kinds of religious activity can help steer them back to a course of less deviant behavior and, more important, away from potential career criminal paths. Such recent research confirms that religiosity helps youth to be resilient even in the midst of poverty, crime, and other social ills commonly linked to deleterious outcomes.

Research on adult samples is less common but tends to represent the same general pattern—that religion reduces criminal activity by adults. An important study by T. David Evans and colleagues found that religion, indicated by religious activities, reduced the likelihood of adult criminality as measured by a broad range of criminal acts. The relationship persisted even after secular controls were added to the model. Further, the finding did not depend on social or religious contexts (Evans, Cullen, Dunaway, Burton, 1995; Johnson, Larson & Pitts, 1997). A small but growing literature focuses on the links between religion and family violence. Several recent studies find that regular religious attendance is inversely related to abuse among both men and women (Ellison & Anderson, 2000; Ellison, Bartkowski & Anderson, 1999). Looking at Figure 1, we can see that 80% (37 of 46) of these studies show that reductions in delinquency and criminal acts are associated with higher levels of religious activity and involvements.

In sum, a review of the research on religious practices and health-related outcomes indicates that, in general, higher levels of religious involvement are associated with reduced hypertension, longer survival, less depression, lower levels of drug and alcohol use and abuse, less promiscuous sexual behaviors, reduced likelihood of suicide, lower rates of delinquency among youth, and reduced criminal activity among adults. As can be seen in Figure 1, this substantial body of empirical evidence demonstrates a very clear picture: Those who are most involved in religious activities tend to fare better with respect to important and yet diverse outcome factors. Thus, aided by appropriate documentation, religiosity is now beginning to be acknowledged as a key protective factor that buffers or shields youth from harmful outcomes.

Religious Practice as a Prosocial Factor

In the first section of this chapter, I addressed the role of religion as a protective factor against diverse harmful outcomes. A number of researchers have documented the protective effect of religiosity. Less commonly acknowledged by researchers, however, is the contribution of organic religion in enhancing appropriate behavior. In this section, I examine the effect of religious involvement and practices in promoting positive outcomes, or what sociologists refer to as prosocial behavior. I reviewed four separate literatures that encompass the study of organic religion and prosocial behavior (Appendix B).

Well-Being

Well-being has been referred to as the positive side of mental health. Symptoms for well-being include happiness, joy, satisfaction, fulfillment, pleasure, contentment, and other indicators of a life that is full and complete (Koenig et al., 2001, p. 97). Many studies have examined the relationship between religion and the promotion of beneficial outcomes. Although a number of these studies tend to be cross-sectional, a significant number are prospective cohort studies (Blazer & Palmore, 1976; Graney, 1975; Markides, 1983; Musick, 1996; Tix & Frazier, 1997; Willits & Crider, 1998). As indicated in Figure 2, the vast majority of these studies (some 80% of the 99 studies reviewed) reported some positive association between religious involvement and greater happiness, life satisfaction, morale, positive affect, or some other measure of well-being. The large number of studies on religion and well-being included younger and older populations as well as African Americans and Caucasians from various denominational affiliations. Only one study found a negative correlation between religiosity and well-being, and this study was conducted in a small, nonrandom sample of college students (Appendix B).

Hope, Purpose, and Meaning in Life

Many religious traditions and beliefs have long promoted positive thinking and an optimistic outlook on life. Not surprisingly, researchers have

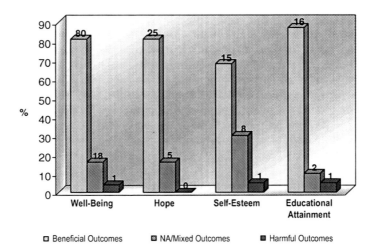

Figure 2. Research examining the relationship between religion and well-being outcomes (4 fields of study; total of 171 studies reviewed).

examined the role religion may or may not play in instilling hope and meaning, or a sense of purpose in life for adherents. Researchers have found, on the whole, a positive relationship between measures of religiosity and hope (Sethi & Seligman, 1993), in both clinical and nonclinical settings (Herth, 1989; Raleigh, 1992; Ringdal, 1996). All told, 25 of the 30 studies reviewed (83%) document that increases in religious involvement or commitment are associated with having hope or a sense of purpose or meaning in life (Figure 2). Similarly, studies show that increasing religiousness is also associated with optimism (Sethi & Seligman, 1993), as well as larger support networks, more social contacts, and greater satisfaction with support (Bradley, 1995; Ellison & George, 1994; Koenig et al., 1999). In fact, 19 of the 23 studies reviewed conclude that increases in religious involvement and commitment are associated with increased social support.

Self-Esteem

Most people would agree that contemporary American culture places too much significance on physical appearance and the idea that one's esteem is bolstered by one's looks. Conversely, a common theme of various religious teachings would be that physical appearance, for example, should not be the basis of self-esteem. Religion provides a basis for self-esteem that is not dependent upon individual accomplishments, relationships with others (e.g., "who you know"), or talent. In other words, a person's self-esteem is rooted in the individual's religious faith as well as the faith community as a whole. Of the studies reviewed, 65% (15 of 23) conclude that religious commitment and activities are related to increases in self-esteem (Figure 2).

Educational Attainment

The literature on the role of religious practices or religiosity on educational attainment represents a relatively recent development in the research literature (Jeynes, 2003, 2004; Regnerus, 2000, 2001). In the past decade or so, a number of researchers have sought to determine whether religion hampers or enhances educational attainment. Even though the development of a body of evidence is just beginning to emerge, some 84% (16 of 19) of the studies reviewed find that religiosity or religious activities are positively correlated with improved educational attainment (Figure 2).

To summarize, a review of the research on religious practices and various measures of well-being reveals that, in general, higher levels of religious involvement are associated with increased levels of well-being, hope, purpose, meaning in life, and educational attainment. As can be seen in Figure 2, this substantial body of evidence shows quite clearly that those who are most involved in religious activities tend to be better off on critical indicators of well-being. Just as the studies reviewed earlier document that religious commitment is a protective factor that buffers individuals from various harmful outcomes (e.g., hypertension, depression, suicide, and delinquency), there is mounting empirical evidence to suggest that religious commitment is also a source for promoting or enhancing beneficial outcomes (e.g., well-being, purpose or meaning in life). This systematic review of a large number of diverse studies concludes that, in general, the effect of religion on physical and mental health outcomes is remarkably positive. These findings have led some religious health care practitioners to conclude that further collaboration between religious organizations and health services may be desirable (Levin, 1984; Miller, 1987; Olson, 1988). According to Peterson (1983), "These phenomena combined point to the church as having powerful potential to affect the health of half the population.... We are convinced that a church with a vigorous life of worship, education, and personal support together with the promotion of wellness has more of an impact on the health of a community than an addition to the hospital or another doctor in town. Right now this is a hunch; in five years, we'll have the data to prove it" (p. 17). This enthusiasm notwithstanding, more research using longitudinal and experimental designs is needed to further address important causal linkages between organic religion and myriad social and behavioral outcomes.

In a previous systematic review of research examining the role of religiosity in crime and delinquency, I found not only that the literature documents that religious commitment is generally linked to reductions in delinquent behavior, but also that this finding was most pronounced in those studies utilizing more rigorous research methods (Johnson, Li, et al., 2000). The scientific study of organic religion has grown in impressive ways over the past several decades. Researchers are now in a position to cite many quality studies in peer-reviewed journals that indicate a striking correspondence between religiosity and general health and well-being for children, youth, and families.

Conclusions

This review confirms that religious influences do affect the behavior of many adolescents in multiple settings such as family, peers, and school. The vast majority of studies document the importance of religious influences in protecting youth from harmful outcomes as well as promoting beneficial and prosocial outcomes. The beneficial relationship between religion and health behaviors and outcomes is not simply a result of religion's constraining function or what it discourages—drug use, suicide, or delinquent behavior—but also of what it encourages, namely, behaviors that can enhance hope, well-being, or educational attainment.

Although some researchers have identified low religiosity as a risk factor for adolescent health risk behaviors, religion measures are not routinely included in adolescent research, and research that explicitly examines religion and health among young people remains rare. Future research on adolescent health and social outcomes should include multiple measures of religious practices and beliefs. It is time for researchers and federal funding agencies to discontinue the pattern of overlooking this important line of policy-relevant research. New research will allow us to more fully understand the ways in which religion directly and indirectly affects health and social outcomes. Churches, synagogues, mosques, inner-city blessing stations, and other houses of worship represent some of the few institutions that remain within close proximity of most adolescents, their families, and their peers. Research now confirms that they can play an important role in promoting the health and well-being of those they serve.

References

Baier, C. J., & Wright, B. E. (2001). If you love me, keep my commandments: A meta-analysis of the effect of religion on crime. *Journal of Research in Crime and Delinquency, 38*, 3–21.

Blazer, D. G., & Palmore, E. (1976). Religion and aging in a longitudinal panel. *Gerontologist, 16*, 82–85.

Bradley, D. E. (1995). Religious involvement and social resources: Evidence from the data set Americans' Changing Lives. *Journal for the Scientific Study of Religion, 34*, 259–267.

Bravender. T., & Knight, J. R. (1998). Recent patterns of use and associated risks of illicit drug use in adolescents. *Current Opinions in Pediatrics, 10*, 344–349.

Centers for Disease Control and Prevention. (1997). Leading causes of mortality and morbidity and contributing behaviors in the United States. Available at http://www.cdc.gov/nccdphp/dash/ahsumm/ussumm.htm.

Chick, J., & Erickson, C. K. (1996). Conference summary: Consensus conference on alcohol dependence and the role of pharmacotherapy in its treatment. *Alcohol Clinical and Experimental Research, 20*, 391–402.

Covinsky, K. E., Kahana, E., Chin, M. H., Palmer, R., Fortinsky, R. H., & Landefield, C. S. (1999). Depressive symptoms and three-year mortality in older hospitalized medical patients. *Annals of Internal Medicine, 130*, 563–569.

DiClemente, R. J., Hansen, W. B., & Ponton, L. E. (1996). Adolescents at risk: A generation in jeopardy. In R. J. DiClemente, W. B. Hansen, & L. E. Ponton (Eds.), *Handbook of adolescent health risk behavior* (pp. 1–4). New York: Plenum Press.

Ellison, C. G., & Anderson, K. L. (2001). Religious involvement and domestic violence among U. S. couples. *Journal for the Scientific Study of Religion, 40,* 269–286.

Ellison, C. G., Bartkowski, J. P., & Anderson, K. L. (1999). Are there religious variations in domestic violence? *Journal of Family Issues, 20,* 87–113.

Ellison, C. G., & George, L. K. (1994). Religious involvement, social ties, and social support in a southeastern community. *Journal for the Scientific Study of Religion, 33,* 46–61.

Evans, T. D., Cullen, F., Burton, V., Dunaway, R. G., Payne, G., & Kethineni, S. (1996). Religion, social bonds, and delinquency. *Deviant Behavior, 17,* 43–70.

Evans, T. D., Cullen, F. T., Dunaway, R. G., & Burton, V. S. (1995). Religion and crime reexamined: The impact of religion, secular controls, and social ecology on adult criminality. *Criminology, 33,* 195–224.

Gallup, G. H., Jr., & Bezilla, R. (1992). *The religious life of young Americans.* Princeton, NJ: George H. Gallup International Institute.

Ghosh, T. B., & Victor, B. S. (1994). Suicide. In R. E. Hales, S. C. Yudofsky, and J. A. Talbott (eds.), *Textbook of Psychiatry* (pp. 1251–1271). Washington, DC: American Psychiatric Association.

Graham, T. W., Kaplan, B. H., Cornono-Huntley, J. C., James, S. A., Becker, C., Hames, C. G., et al. (1978). Frequency of church attendance and blood pressure evaluation. *Journal of Behavioral Medicine, 1,* 37–43.

Graney, M. J. (1975). Happiness and social participation in aging. *Journal of Gerontology, 30,* 701–706.

Herth, K. (1989). The relationship between level of hope and level of coping response and other variables in patients with cancer. *Oncology Nursing Forum, 16,* 67–72.

Jang, S. J., & Johnson, B. R. (2001). Neighborhood disorder, individual religiosity, and adolescent use of illicit drugs: A test of multilevel hypotheses. *Criminology, 39,* 109–144.

Jeynes, W. (2003). The effects of the religious commitment of twelfth graders living in non- intact families on their academic achievement. *Marriage and Family Review, 35*(1/2), 77–97.

Jeynes, W. (2004). Comparing the influence of religion on education in the United States and overseas: A meta-analysis. *Religion & Education, 31*(2), 1–15.

Johnson, B. R. (2000). *A better kind of high: How religious commitment reduces drug use* (CRRUCS Report 2000-2). Philadelphia: University of Pennsylvania, Center for Research on Religion and Urban Civil Society.

Johnson, B. R. (2004). Religious programs and recidivism among former inmates in Prison Fellowship programs: A long-term follow-up study. *Justice Quarterly, 21*(2), 329–354.

Johnson, B. R., Jang, S. J., Larson, D. B., & Li, S. D. (2001). Does adolescent religious commitment matter? A reexamination of the effects of religiosity on delinquency. *Journal of Research in Crime and Delinquency, 38,* 22–44.

Johnson, B. R., Larson, D. B., Jang, S. J., & Li, S. D. (2000). The "invisible institution" and Black youth crime: The church as an agency of local social control. *Journal of Youth and Adolescence, 29,* 479–498.

Johnson, B. R., Larson, D. B., Li, S. D., & S. J. Jang. (2000). Escaping from the crime of inner cities: Church attendance and religious salience among disadvantaged youth. *Justice Quarterly, 17,* 377–391.

Johnson, B. R., Larson, D. B., & Pitts, T. G. (1997). Religious programming, institutional adjustment and recidivism among former inmates in Prison Fellowship programs. *Justice Quarterly, 14,* 145–166.

Johnson, B. R., Li, S. D., Larson, D. B., & McCullough, M. (2000). Religion and delinquency: A systematic review of the literature. *Journal of Contemporary Criminal Justice, 16,* 32–52.

Johnson, B. R., Thompkins, R. B., & Webb, D. (2002). *Objective hope—Assessing the effectiveness of faith-based organizations: A review of the literature* (CRRUCS Report 2002-1). Philadelphia: University of Pennsylvania, Center for Research on Religion and Urban Civil Society.

Kann, L., Anderson, J. E., Holtzman, D., Ross, J., Truman, B. I., Collins, J. J., et al. (1991). HIV-related knowledge, beliefs, and behaviors among high school students in the United States: Results from a national survey. *Journal of School Health, 61,* 397–401.

Koenig, H. G., Hays, J. C., Larson, D. B., George, L. K., Cohen, H. J., McCullough, J. E., et al. (1999). Does religious attendance prolong survival? A six year follow-up study of 3,968 older adults. *Journal of Gerontology, 54A,* M370–M377.

Koenig, H. G., McCullough, M. E., & Larson, D. B. (2001). *Handbook of religion and health.* New York: Oxford University Press.

Koenig, H. G., Shelp, F., Goli, V., Cohen, H. J., & Blazer, D. G. (1989). Survival and health care utilization in elderly medical inpatients with major depression. *Journal of the American Geriatrics Society, 37,* 599–606.

Larson, D. B., Koenig, H. G., Kaplan, B. H., Greenberg, R. S., Logue, E., & Tyroler, H. A. (1989). The impact of religion on men's blood pressure. *Journal of Religion and Health, 28* , 265–278.

Levin, J. S. (1984). The role of the Black church in community medicine. *Journal of the National Medical Association, 76,* 477–483.

Levin, J. S. (1994). Religion and health: Is there an association, is it valid, and is it causal? *Social Science Medicine, 38,* 1475–1482.

Levin, J. S., & Vanderpool, H. Y. (1987). Is frequent religious attendance really conducive to better health? Toward an epidemiology of religion. *Social Science Medicine, 24,* 589–600.

Levin, J. S., & Vanderpool, H. Y. (1992). Religious factors in physical health and the prevention of illness. In K. I. Pargament, K. I. Maton, & R. E. Hess (Eds.), *Religion and prevention in mental health: Research, vision, and action* (pp. 83–104). Binghamton, NY: Haworth Press.

Markides, K. S. (1983). Aging, religiosity, and adjustment: A longitudinal analysis. *Journal of Gerontology, 38,* 621–625.

McCullough, M. E., Hoyt, W. T., Larson, D. B., Koenig, H. G., & Thoresen, C. E. (2000). Religious involvement and mortality: A meta-analytic review. *Health Psychology, 19,* 211–222.

McGinnis, J. M., & Foege, W. H. (1993). Actual causes of death in the United States. *Journal of the American Medical Association, 270,* 55–60.

Miller, J. (1987). Wellness programs through the church. *Health Values, 11,* 3–6.

Monitoring the Future: A Continuing Study of American Youth 12th-Grade Survey. (1998). L. D. Johnston, J. G. Bachman, and P. M. O'Malley (principal investigators). Ann Arbor: University of Michigan, Institute for Social Research.

Musick, M. A. (1996). Religion and subjective health among Black and White elders. *Journal of Health and Social Behavior, 37,* 221–237.

Musick, M. A., Koenig, H. G., Hays, J. C., & Cohen, H. J. (1999). Religious activity and depression among community-dwelling elderly persons with cancer: The moderating effect of race. *Journal of Gerontology, 53B,* S218–S227.

National Heart, Lung, and Blood Institute. (1997). *Sixth report of the Joint National Committee on Prevention, Detection, Evaluation, and Treatment of High Blood Pressure.* Bethesda, MD: National Institutes of Health.

National Institute on Drug Abuse. (1997). *National Household Survey on Drug Abuse, 1997.* Bethesda, MD: Author.

Olson, L. (1988). The religious community as a partner in health care. *Journal of Community Health, 13,* 249–257.

Peterson, B. (1983). Renewing the church's health ministries: Reflections on ten years' experience. *Journal of Religion and the Applied Behavioral Sciences, 4,* 16–22.

Raleigh, E. D. H. (1992). Sources of hope in chronic illness. *Oncology Nursing Forum, 19,* 443–448.

Regnerus, M. D. (2000). Shaping schooling success: Religious socialization and educational outcomes in metropolitan public schools. *Journal for the Scientific Study of Religion, 39,* 363–370.

Regnerus, M. D. (2001). *Making the grade: The influence of religion upon the academic performance of youth in disadvantaged communities* (CRRUCS Report 2001-3). Philadelphia: University of Pennsylvania, Center for Research on Religion and Urban Civil Society.

Ringdal, G. I. (1996). Religiosity, quality of life, and survival in cancer patients. *Social Indicators Research, 38,* 193–211.

Scotch, N. (1963). Sociocultural factors in the epidemiology of Zulu hypertension. *American Journal of Public Health, 53,* 1205–1213.

Sells, C. W., & Blum, R. W. (1996). Current trends in adolescent health. In R. J. DiClemente, W. B. Hansen, & L. E. Ponton (Eds.), *Handbook of adolescent health risk behavior* (pp. 5–34). New York: Plenum.

Sethi, S., & Seligman, M. (1993). The hope of fundamentalists. *Psychological Science, 5,* 58.

Strawbridge, W. J., Cohen, R. D., Shema, S. J., & Kaplan, G. A. (1997). Frequent attendance at religious services and mortality over 28 years. *American Journal of Public Health, 87*, 957–961.

Thornton, A., & Camburn, D. (1989). Religious participation and adolescent sexual behavior and attitudes. *Journal of Marriage and the Family, 51*, 641–653.

Tix, A. P., & Frazier, P. A. (1997). The use of religious coping during stressful life events: Main effects, moderation, and medication. *Journal of Consulting and Clinical Psychology, 66*, 411–422.

Wallace, J. M. (2002). *Is religion good for adolescent health?* (CRRUCS Report 2002-2). Philadelphia: University of Pennsylvania, Center for Research on Religion and Urban Civil Society.

Willits, F. K., & Crider, D. M. (1998). Religion and well-being: Men and women in the middle years. *Review of Religious Research, 29*, 281–294.

TABLE 9.1.Appendix A: Review of Research Examining the Relationship Between Religion and Health Outcomes

Outcome/investigators	Type	Method	N	Population	Location	Religious variable	Controls	Findings
HYPERTENSION								
Armstrong (1977)	CC	C	418 vs. Cs	CDA	Australia	D (SDA vs. n-SDA)	MC	NA
Beutler (1988)	CT	C	120	CDA	Netherlands	Laying on of hands	N	NA
Blackwell (1976)	CT	C	7	MP	—	Transcendental Med	N	B
Brown D (1994)	CS	S	537	CDA, B, M	Norfolk, VA	Religious scale, ORA, D	MC	NA
Graham (1978)	CS	R	355	CDA, W, M	Georgia	ORA	MC	B
Hafner (1982)	CT	C	21	MP	—	Meditation	N	NA
Hixson (1998)	CS	C	112	CDA, F	North Carolina	RC, RE, IR	SC	B
Hutchinson (1986)	CS	R	357	CDA	West Indies	ORA	SC	B
Koenig (1988)	CS	S	106	MP, E	Illinois	ORA, NORA, IR	SC	B
Koenig (1998a)	PC	R	4,000	CDA, E	North Carolina	D, ORA, NORA	MC	B
Lapane (1997)	CS	R	5,145	CDA	Rhode Island	Church membership	MC	B
Larson (1989)	CS	S	401	CDA, M	Georgia	ORA, SR	MC	B
Leserman (1989)	CT	C	27	MP	Boston	Relaxation response	N	NA
Levin (1985)	CS	R	1,125	CDA-Mex-Am	Texas	ORA, SR	N	H
Livingston (1991)	CS	R	1,420	CDA, B	Maryland	Church affiliation	MC	B
Merritt (2000)	Exp	C	74	CDA, B, young	Durham, NC	ORA, NORA, IR	SC	B
Miller (1982)	CT	C	96	MP	—	Healing prayers	N	B
Patel (1975)	CT	C	34	MP	England	Yoga	N	B
Patel (1976)	CT	C	27	MP	England	Yoga	N	B
Pollack (1977)	CT	C	20	MP	New York City	Trans Meditation	N	NA
Schneider (1995)	CT	C	111	CDA, B, E	Oakland, CA	Trans Meditation	N	B
Scotch (1963)	CS	R	1,053	CDA	South Africa	ORA, CM	SC	B
Stavig (1984)	CS	R	1,757	CDA-Asians	California	(Affiliation vs. N)	MC	B
Steffen (2000)	CS	—	—	CDA	North Carolina	RC (from COPE)	MC	B
Sudstuang (1991)	CT	C	52	M (ages 20–25)	Thailand	Buddhist meditation	N	B
Timio (1988)	PC	S	144 vs. Cs	R (Ca nuns)	Italy	Ca nuns vs. other	MC	B
Walsh (1980)	CS	C	75	Immigrants	Ohio	ORA	MC	B
Walsh (1998)	CS	C	137	Immigrants	Toledo, OH	ORA, SR	MC	B
Wenneberg (1997)	CT	C	39	CDA, M	Iowa City, IA	Trans Meditation	N	B

MORTALITY

Study						"Religiosity"		
Abramson (1982)	PC	S	387	E, 100%M	Israel	Trans Meditation	MC	NA
Alexander (1989)	CT	C	73	E	Massachusetts	Trans Meditation	N	B
Berkel (1983)	CC	R	522 deaths	CDA	Netherlands	D (SDA vs. N-SDA)	SC	NA
Berkman (1979)	PC	R	6,928	CDA	Alameda, CA	CM	MC	B
Bolduan (1933)	CC	R	14,047 +Cs	CDA	New York City	D (Jewish vs. non-J)	SC	M
Bryant (1992)	PC	R	473	CDA, E, B	National US	ORA	MC	B
Comstock (1967)	CC	R	234	Stillborn babies	Maryland	ORA	SC	B
Comstock (1971)	CC	R	189	ASCVD deaths + CS	Maryland	ORA	SC	B
Comstock (1972)	CC	R	54,848	CDA	Maryland	ORA	SC	B
Comstock (1977)	CC	R	47,423	CDA	Maryland	ORA	SC	NA
De Gouw (1995)	RS	S	1,523	R (monks)	Netherlands	Monks vs. others	SC	B
Dwyer (1990)	CS	R	3,063 counties	CDA	National US	D, CM	MC	B
Enstrom (1989)	CC	R	9,844 vs. 3,199	CDA-Mormons	California	ORA (Mor vs. n-M)	SC	B
Gardner (1982a)	CC	S	1,819 deaths	M, Mormons	Utah	Lay-priesthood level	SC	B
Gardner (1982b)	CC	S	1,354 deaths	F, Mormons	Utah	ORA	SC	B
Glass (1999)	PC	R	2,761	CDA, E	New Haven, CT	ORA	MC	B
Goldbourt (1993)	PC	R	10,059	CDA, M	Israel	Orthodox vs. secular Jews	MC	B
Goldman (1995)	PC	R	7,500	CDA, E	National US	ORA	MC	B
Goldstein (1996)	CC	R	15,520 + Cs	CDA	Rhode Island	D (Jewish vs. non-Jewish)	SC	NA
Hamman (1981)	CC	R	25,822 (1,226)	CDA (Amish)	Indiana, OH, PA	D (Amish vs. non-Amish)	SC	M
Harding le Riche (1985)	CS	C	289	R (clergy)	Canada	Clergy vs. MDs	N	B
Helm (2000)	PC	R	3,851	CDA, E	North Carolina	NORA	MC	B
Hogstel (1989)	CS	C	302	CDA, E (>85)	Texas	RB, Christian living	NS	B
House (1982)	PC	R	2,754	CDA	Tecumseh	ORA	MC	B
Hummer (1999)	PC	R	21,204	CDA	National US	ORA	N	B
Idler (1991)	PC	R	2,812	CDA, E	New Haven, CT	ORA, NORA	MC	NA
Kastenbaum (1990)	CC	S	487	Saints	World	Sainthood vs. others	SC	B
King H (1968)	CC	S	609 deaths	R (Lutheran)	US & Canada	Clergy vs. others	SC	B
King H (1970)	CC	S	4,106 deaths	R (clergy)	US, England	Clergy vs. others	SC	B
King H (1971)	CC	S	1,387 deaths	R (Anglican)	US	Clergy vs. others	SC	B
King H (1980)	CC	S	5,207 deaths	R (Prot, W, M)	US	Clergy vs. others	SC	B
Locke (1980)	CC	R	3,446 deaths	R (Baptist)	National US	Clergy vs. others	SC	B

(Continued)

Appendix A (*Continued*)

Outcome/investigators	Type	Method	N	Population	Location	Religious variable	Controls	Findings
Janoff-Bulman (1982)	PC	C	30	NH, E	Massachusetts	SR	SC	H
Jarvis (1977)	CC	R	1,169 deaths	CDA, Mormons	Canada	D (Mormon vs. non-m)	SC	NA
Kark (1996b)	PC	S	3,900	Kibbutz members	Israel	Relig vs. secular kibbutz	MC	B
Koenig (1995b)	PC	S	262	MP	Durham, NC	RC	MC	NA
Koenig(1998)	PC	S	1,000	MP	Durham, NC	RC	MC	NA
Koenig (1999a)	PC	R	3,968	CDA, E	North Carolina	D (Jew vs. non-J)	MC	B
Krause (1998a)	PC	R	819	CDA, E	National US	ORA, NORA, RC	MC	B
Lemon (1964)	PC	R	10,059	CDA, M	Israel	Orthodox vs. secular Jews	MC	B
LoPrinzi (1994)	PC	S	1,115	MP (advanced CA)	United States	"Feelings re: religiosity"	MC	NA
Madigan (1957)	CC	R	6,932 deaths	R (Catholic)	National US	Clergy vs. others	SC	B
Madigan (1961)	CC	S	1,247 deaths	R (Catholic Priests)	National US	Priests vs. others	SC	B
Musick (1999)	PC	R	3,617	CDA	National US	ORA	MC	B
Needleman (1988)	CC	R	1920–1971	CDA	Montreal, Can	D (Jew vs. non-Jews)	SC	NA
Ogata (1984)	CC	S	1,396 deaths	R (Zen Priests)	Japan	Priests vs. others	SC	B
Oxman 1995	PC	S	232	MP (open heart surgery)	New Hampshire	ORA, SR, RC	MC	B
Oman (1998)	PC	S	1931	CDA, E	Marin, CA	ORA	MC	B
Oman (1999)	PC	S	1931	CDA, E	Marin, CA	ORA	MC	B
Oxman (1995)	PC	S	232	MP (open-heart surgery)	New Hampshire	ORA, SR, RC	MC	B
Palmore (1982)	PC	C	252	CDA, E	North Carolina	SR	MC	NA
Reynolds (1981)	PC	R	193	NH, E	Los Angeles	RC	NS	B
Ringdal (1995)	PC	S	253	MP (cancer)	Norway	RB	SC	B
Ringdal (1996)	PC	S	253	MP (cancer)	Norway	RB	SC	B
Rogers (1996)	PC	R	15,938	CDA, E	National US	ORA	MC	B
Schoenbach (1986)	PC	R	2,059	CDA	Georgia	ORA	MC	B
Seeman (1987)	PC	R	4,175	CDA	Alameda, CA	CM	MC	B
Strawbridge (1997)	CC	R	5,286	CDA	Alameda, CA	ORA	MC	B
Taylor RS (1959)	CC	C	2,657 deaths	R (Catholic nuns)	MA, NY	Nuns vs. others	SC	B
Yates (1981)	CS	C	71	MP (adv CA)	Michigan	RB, RE, SR, ORA	N	NA
Zuckerman (1984)	PC	S	225	CDA, E	New Haven, CT	D, ORA, SR, RC	SC	B

DEPRESSION

Study								
Ai (1998)	CS	S	151	MP (with CABG)	Michigan	SR, ORA, NORA	MC	M
Alvarado (1995)	CS	C	200	CS, CDA	Fresno, CA	D, ORA, RB, SR	SC	B
Azhar (1995b)	CT	C	32 vs. 32 Cs	PP	Malaysia	Religious psychotherapy	N	B
Ball (1990)	CS	S	51	PP	London, England	ORA	N	NA
Belavich (1995)	CS	C	222	CS	Ohio	RC scales	SC	M
Bickel (1998)	CS	C	245	CM (Presbyterians)	—	RC scales	N	B
Bienenfeld (1997)	CS	C	89	R, E, 100%F	Ohio	RC m	MC	B
Blaine (1995)	CS	C	144	CS	Buffalo, NY	SR, ORA, miscellaneous	N	B
Blalock (1995)	PC	C	300	MP (arthritis), E	North Carolina	RC	MC	B
Blaney (1997)	PC	C	40	HIV+	Miami, FL	RC	MC	B
Braam (1997)	CS	R	2,817	CDA, E	Netherlands	ORA	MC	B
Braam (1997)	PC	S	177	CDA, E	Netherlands	SR	N	B
Braam (1998)	CS	R	3,020	CDA, E	Netherlands	D, giving up ORA	MC	B
Braam (1999)	CS	R	3,051	CDA, E	Netherlands	"Religious climate"	MC	M
Braam (1999)	CS	S	13 nations	CDA, E	Europe	D, ORA, SR, O	MC	B
Brant (1995)	CS	—	179	CDA, 100% B	—	RC scale	N	M
Brown D (1987)	CS	R	451	CDA, B	Richmond, VA	Scale	SC	NA
Brown D (1990)	CS	R	451	CDA, 100% B	Richmond, VA	D, ORA, RCm	MC	B
Brown D (1992)	CS	R	927	CDA, 100% B	Norfolk, VA	RCm	MC	NA
Brown D (1994)	CS	R	527	CDA, 100% BM	Southeast US	D, ORA, RCm	MC	B
Brown GW (1981)	CS	S	355	CDA, 100% F	Scotland	ORA	N	B
Idler (1992)	PC	R	2,812	CDA, E	New Haven, CT	ORA, SR, RC	MC	B
Ellison (1995)	CS	R	2,956	CDA	North Carolina	D, ORA, NORA	MC	B
Ellison (1997)	PC	—	—	CDA, B	National US	ORA, RB	N	B
Ellison (1997)	PC	—	—	CDA, B	National US ?	"Religious guidance"	N	B
Fehring (1987)	CS	C	170	CS	Wisconsin	RWB, RCm	N	NA
Fernando (1975,1978)	CC	C	117 vs. Cs	PP	London, England	D, ORA	N	B
Ferraro (1998)	CS	R	3,497	CDA	National US	D, ORA, NORA, SR, RC	MC	M
Gallemore (1969)	CC	C	62 vs. Cs	PP	Durham, NC	D, RE, Relig history	N	M
Genia (1991)	CS	C	309	CDA	Washington, DC	D, IR, ER	N	B
Genia (1993)	CS	C	309	CDA	Washington, DC	D, IR, ER	N	B
Griffith (1984)	PC	C	16	CM	Barbados	"Mourning"	N	B

(Continued)

Appendix A (*Continued*)

Outcome/investigators	Type	Method	N	Population	Location	Religious variable	Controls	Findings
Grosse-Holtforth (1996)	CS	C	97	NHP	Durham NC	IR, RC	SC	NA
Hallstrom (1984)	CS	S	800	CDA, 100% F	Sweden	ORA, NORA, RB	MC	B
Hertsgaard (1984)	CS	R	760	CDA, F, farms	North Dakota	ORA, D	MC	B
Husaini (1999)	CS	R	995	E, CDA	Nashville	ORA, NORA	MC	NA
Idler (1987)	CS	R	2,811	CDA, E	New Haven, CT	ORA, SR, RC	MC	B
Jensen L (1993)	CS		3,835	CS	UT, TX, WI, ID	D, "religiosity"	SC	B
Johnson W (1992)	CT	C	10	Christians	Indiana	Christian vs. non-Chr	N	NA
Johnson W (1994)	CT	C	32	Christians	Hawaii	Christian vs. non-Chr	N	NA
Jones-Webb (1993)	CS	R	3,724	CDA	National US	D (agnostic/N)	MC	B
Kendler (1997)	CS	C	1,902	CDA, twins	Virginia	RB, ORA, NORA, SR	MC	B
Kennedy (1996)	PC	R	1,855	CDA, E	Bronx, NY	ORA, D	MC	B
Koenig (1988)	CS	S	106	MP, E	Illinois	ORA, NORA, IR	SC	B
Koenig (1992)	PC	S	850	MP, E	Durham, NC	D, RC	MC	B
Koenig (1994)	CS	R	853 vs. 1,826	Baby boomers	Durham, NC	D, ORA, SR, NORA	MC	B
Koenig (1995a)	CS	R	96	Prisoners	Butner, NC	RB, ORA, RC	N	B
Koenig (1995)	CS	S	850	MP, E	Durham, NC	D, RC	MC	B
Koenig (1997)	CS	R	4,000	CDA, E	North Carolina	D, ORA, NORA	MC	NA
Koenig (1998)	CS	C	115	NH, E	Durham, NC	RC	MC	B
Koenig (1998)	PC	S	87	MP, E	Durham, NC	IR, ORA, NORA	MC	B
Koenig (1998)	CS	S	577	MP, E	Durham, NC	RC, ORA, NORA, SR	MC	M
Kroll (1989)	CS	1/M	52	PP	Minnesota	RB, RE, ORA	N	NA
Levin (1985)	CS	R	1,125	CDA-Mex-Am	Texas	ORA, SR	N	NA
Lubin (1988)	CS	R	1,543	CDA	National US	D (affil vs. N)	N	B
Malzberg (1973)	CC	S	40,000+	PP	New York	Jewish vs. non-Jewish	N	NA
Maton (1989)	CS	C	81/68	Bereaved parents/HS	Maryland	Spiritual support	MC	B
McIntosh (1995)	CS	R	1,644	CDA, E	National US	Religious volunteering	MC	B
Meador (1992)	CS	C	2,850	CDA	Durham, NC	D (Pentecostal vs. other)	MC	NA
Miller L (1997)	PC	—	60/151	Mothers, children	New York	D, SR	MC	B
Mitchell (1993)	CS	R	868	CDA, E	North Carolina	RB religious intervention	MC	M
Morris P (1982)	PC	C	24	Chronically ill	United Kingdom	Pilgrimage to Lourdes	N	B
Morse (1987)	CS	C	156	E, CDA	Massachusetts	CM, ORA, RC	SC	B

(Continued)

Mosher (1997)	CS	C	461	HS (Catholic)	St. Louis	Scale	N	B
Musick (1998a)	CS	R	586	CDA, B	Detroit	ORA, RC (prayer)	MC	B
Musick (2000)	PC	R	10,008	CDA	National US	ORA, RB	MC	M
Musick (1998b)	PC	R	3,007	CDA, E	North Carolina	ORA, NORA	MC	B
Neeleman (1994)	CC	S	73 vs. 25 Cs	PP	London England	ORA, NORA, RB, SR	SC	H
Nelson (1990)	CS	C	68	E, CDA	Texas	IR-ER scale	N	B
Nelson (1989)	CS	C	26	E, NH	Texas	"Religious activity"	N	B
O'Connor (1990)	CS	C	176	E, NH	Quebec, Can	IR scale (French)	N	B
O'Laoire (1997)	CT	C	96/406	CDA	San Francisco	Prayer for others	N	B
Park (1990)	PC	C	83/83	CS (religious)	Delaware	IR, ER, O	SC	M
Pecheur (1984)	CT	C	21	Depressed Christians	—	Religious CBT	N	NA
Plante (1992)	CS	C	86	CS	Santa Clara, CA	SR, D	N	NA
Plante (1997)	CS	C	102	CS	California	SR, NORA, ORA, RC	N	B
Pressman (1990)	CS	C	30	MP, E, F	Chicago	ORA, SR, RC	SC	B
Propst (1980)	CT	C	44	Mildly depressed Christians	Oregon	Religious imagery	N	B
Propst (1992)	CT	C	59	Depressed Christians	Oregon	Religious CBT	N	B
Rabins (1990)	CS	C	62	Caregivers of Alz D&CA pts	Baltimore	RC	MC	B
Rabins (1990b)	PC	C	62	Caregivers of Alz D&CA pts	Baltimore	RC	MC	B
Razali (1998)	CT	C	203	PP	Malaysia	Religious psychotherapy	N	B
Ross (1990)	CS	R	401	CDA	Illinois	D, SR	MC	B
Ryan (1993)	CS	C	105/151/342	CS, CM	—	IR, ER, O, Q, misc.	N	B
Schafer (1997)	CS	C	282	CS	Chico, CA	RB, RC, ORA, NORA	MC	H
Sherkat (1992)	CS	C	156	CDA bereaved	Southeast US	D, ORA, NORA	MC	NA
Siegel (1990)	CS	C	825	CDA,E	Southern CA	D, ORA, NORA	MC	B
Smith B (1996)	PC	—	131	CDA	Missouri, Illinois	CM	N	B
Sorenson (1995)	PC	S	261	Teenage mothers	S.W. Ontario	RC, ORA, SR	SC	H
Spendlove (1984)	CS	R	179	CDA, W, F	Salt Lake City	D, ORA, SR	MC	NA
Spiegel (1983)	PC	S	58	MP (breast CA)	California	IR, ORA, CM, D	MC	H
Strayhorn (1990)	CS	S	201	Parents of Head Start kids	Pittsburgh	Family ORA, NORA	MC	H
Strawbridge (1998)	CS	R	2,537	E, CDA	Alameda, CA	ORA, NORA	N	B
Tamburrino (1990)	CS	C	71	F post-abortion dysphoria	Ohio	ORA, NORA, SR	MC	M
Toh (1997)	CT	C	46	CDA, religious	Pasadena, CA	Conversion	N	B
VandeCreek (1995)	CS	C	150	CDA (relatives)	Ohio	Lay counselors in church	N	B
Veach (1992)	CS	C	148	CS & health pros	Nevada	Spiritual experience	SC	B

Appendix A (Continued)

Outcome/investigators	Type	Method	N	Population	Location	Religious variable	Controls	Findings
Watson P (1988)	CS	C	314/181	CS	Tennessee	IR, ER	SC	B
Watson P (1989)	CS	C	1,397	CS	Tennessee	IR, ER	N	B
Watson P (1990)	CS	C	2,435	CS	Tennessee	IR, ER, miscellaneous	N	B
Williams D (1991)	PC	R	720	CDA	New Haven, CT	D, ORA	MC	B
Wright (1993)	CS	C	451	HS, Ad	Texas	IR, ORA	SC	B
Zhang (1996)	CS	C	320/452	CS	China & US	ORA, NORA,	MC	B
SUICIDE								
Bagley (1989)	CS	R	679	CDA	W.Canada	D, RC	N	M
Bainbridge (1981)	RS	S	78 large cities	Suicide rates (1926)	National US	D, CM	SC	B
Bainbridge (1989)	RS	S	75 large cities	Suicide rates (1980)	National US	CM	SC	B
Beehr (1995)	CS	S	177 police	Suicidal thoughts	Eastern US	RC	MC	NA
Breault (1982)	RS	S	42 countries	Suicide rates	United Nations	Religious books/papers	MC	B
Breault (1986)	RS	S	State/county	Suicide rates	National US	D (Ca vs other) CM	MC	B
Burr (1994)	RS	S	294	SMSAs Suicide rates	National US	D (Ca vs other) CM	MC	B
Cameron (1973)	CS	C	144	Handicapped	Michigan	SR (value of religion)	N	B
DeMan (1987)	CS	C	150	CDA	Quebec, Can	SR	MC	B
Ellis J (1991)	CS	C	100	CS	Tennessee	RWB	N	B
Ellison CG (1997)	RS	R	296 SMSAs	Suicide rates	National US	D homogeneity	MC	B
Feifel (1980)	CS	C	616	PP, prison, other	Los Angeles	SR	MC	B
Fernquist (1995–96)	RS	S	9 countries	Suicide rates	Europe	Religious books	SC	B
Hasselback (1991)	RS	S	261 c. tracts	Suicide rates	Canada	D (% N)	MC	B
Hoelter (1979)	CS	C	205	CS	Indiana	ORA, RB, SR, O	N	B
Horton (1973)	CS	C	3 cases	Ad (schizophrenic)	New Haven, CT	"Mystical experi"	N	B
Johnson D (1980)	CS	R	1,530	CDA	National US	D, ORA, SR	N	B
Kandel D (1991)	CS	R	593	Ad	New York	ORA	N	B
Kaplan K (1995)	CS	C	117	Cs	Detroit, MI	IR, ER, Q, Misc	SC	B
King S (1996)	CS	C	511	CS	Connecticut	D, ORA	N	B
Kirk (1979)	CC	C	20 vs. 20 Cs	PP	Detroit, MI	D, ORA	N	NA
Kranitz (1968)	CC	C	20 vs. 20 Cs	PP	Los Angeles	Misc	N	NA
Krull (1994)	RS	S	—	Suicide rates	Quebec, Can	D (% N)	MC	B
Lee D (1987)	CS	C	317	CS	Illinois	SR	N	B

Study								
Lester (1987)	RS	S	49 states	Suicide rates	United States	ORA	SC	B
Lester (1988)	RS	R	49 states	Suicide rates	United States	ORA	SC	B
Lester (1992)	RS	R	13 nations	Suicide rates	Cross-national	RB	N	B
Lester (1993)	CS	C	103	CS	—	"Religiosity"	SC	B
Levav (1988)	CS	R	1,200	CDA	Israel	"Religiosity"	SC	NA
Long D (1991)	CS	C	147	Members of MS society	Cincinnati, OH	RB, SR, O	SC	B
LoPresto (1995)	CS	C	282	CS	Baltimore, MD	SR	SC	B
Marks (1977)	CS	S	98/29 vs. Cs	Ad suicide attempt	National US	ORA	N	B
Martin WT (1984)	RS	R	—	Suicide rates	National US	ORA	N	B
Minear (1981)	CS	C	394	CS	New England	D, ORA, SR, RB	N	B
Mireault (1996)	CS	C	104	E	Quebec, Can	SR	MC	NA
Neeleman (1997)	CS	R	23,085	CDA (attitude)	Europe, US,CAN	D, ORA, RB	MC	B
Neeleman (1998)	CS	R	1,729	CDA	National US	ORA, NORA, SR, RB	MC	B
Neeleman (1998)	RS	S	11 provinces	Suicide rates	Netherlands	Religiousness	MC	B
Neeleman (1999)	RS	S	26 countries	Suicides rates	Europe & US	ORA, miscellaneous	MC	B
Nelson FL (1980)	CS	C	99	E, NH	Los Angeles	D, SR	N	B
Paykel (1974)	CS	R	720	CDA	Connecticut	ORA, NORA, CM	MC	B
Pescosolido (1989)	RS	S	404 counties	Suicides	National US	D (J, Ca EP, MP,ORA)	MC	B
Resnick (1997)	CS	R	12,118	Ad	National US	SR	MC	NA
Salmons (1984)	D	S	294/149	Cs/MP	England	(Religious vs. non-R)	N	B
Schneider (1989)	Cs	C	108	Gay men	Los Angeles	D (no affiliation)	N	B
Schweitzer (1995)	CS	—	1,678	CS	Australia	D, SR	N	B
Shagle (1995)	CS	S	473	AD	Tennessee	ORA, SR	MC	B
Siegrist (1996)	CS	R	2,034	Ages 15–30 y.o.	Germany	D, ORA	MC	B
Simpson, M (1989)	RS	S	71 nations	Suicide rates	World	D (Ca, Prot, Islam)	SC	NA
Singh (1986)	CS	R	6,521	CDA (attitude)	National US	ORA, miscellaneous	MC	B
Stack (1983a)	RS	S	25 nations	Suicide rates	World	Produce religious book	MC	B
Stack (1983b)	RS	S	—	Suicide rates	National US	ORA	SC	B
Stack (1983c)	RS	S	Nations	Suicide rates	World	Produce religious book	SC	B
Stack (1985)	RS	S	—	Suicide rate	National US	ORA	SC	NA
Stack (1991a)	RS	S	National	Suicide rate	Sweden	Produce religious book	SC	B
Stack (1991b)	CS	R	1,687	CDA	National US	D, ORA	SC	B

(Continued)

Appendix A (*Continued*)

Outcome/investigators	Type	Method	N	Population	Location	Religious variable	Controls	Findings
Stack (1992a)	RS	S	—	Suicide rates	Finland	Produce religious book	MC	B
Stack (1992b)	CS	R	5,726	CDA	National US	D, ORA	MC	B
Stack (1994)	CS	R	4,946f, 4,475m	CDA	National US	ORA	MC	B
Stack (1995)	CS	R	1,197b, 8,204w	CDA	National US	ORA	MC	B
Stack (1998)	CS	R	1,500+	CDA	National US	Religiosity	MC	B
Stark (1983)	RS	S	214 SMSAs	Suicide rates	United States	CM, D	MC	B
Stein (1989)	CS	S	525	Ad	Israel	SR	MC	B
Stein (1992)	CS	S	525	Ad	Israel	SR	MC	B
Steininger (1978)	CS	C	732	HS, CS	New Jersey	"Religion a waste"	N	B
Stillion (1984)	CS	C	198	HS	Southern US	SR	N	B
Trovato (1992)	RS	S	9 provinces	Suicide (young)	Canada	D (N)	SC	B
Truett (1992)	CS	C	7,620 twins	CDA	Australia	D, ORA	SC	B
Wandrei (1985)	PC	S	706	F, attempts	San Francisco	D, miscellaneous	SC	B
Zhang (1996)	CS	C	320/452	CS	China & US	ORA, NORA, SR, RB	MC	B
SEXUAL BEHAVIOR								
Beck (1991)	PC	R	2,000+	Youth 14-22	National US	D, DORA	MC	B
Billy (1993)	CS	R	3,321	CDA, M, 20-39	National US	D (vs. N)	MC	B
Brown S (1985)	CS	R	702	Ad, B, F	National US	ORA	MC	B
Cardwell (1969)	CS	C	187	CS	New England	(5 dimensions)	N	B
Clayton (1969)	CS	S	887	CS	Florida	RB	N	B
Cochran (1991)	CS	R	14,979	CDA	National US	ORA, SR, RB, CM, D	MC	B
Cullari (1990)	CS	C	208	HS	Pennsylvania	Ca vs. public school	N	B
Davids (1982)	CS	C	208	CS, Jewish	Ontario, Can	D, SR	N	B
DuRant (1990)	CS	R	202	Ad, F, Hispanic	National US	D, DORA	MC	B
Forliti (1986)	CS	C	8,165/10,467	Ad/parents, CM	United States	RB, ORA, SR	N	B
Fox (1989)	CS	C	196	CS	Southern US	ORA, NORA, RB, RB,RE	N	B
Goldscheider (1991)	CS	R	8,450	CDA, F	National US	ORA, D	SC	B
Gunderson (1979)	CS	C	327	CS	Houston	ORA, D, SR	MC	B
Haerich (1992)	CS	C	204	CS	Riverside, CA	ORA, SR, IR, ER	N	B
Heltsley (1969)	CS	C	1,435	CS	United States	D, religion scale	SC	B
Hendricks (1984)	CC	C	48 vs. 50 Cs	Ad, B fathers	Columbus, OH	ORA, NORA	DF	B

Study			N	Sample	Location	Measures		
Herold (1981)	CS	C	514	CS, HS	Ontario, Can	ORA	SC	B
Jensen L (1990)	CS	C	423	CS, ages 17-25	Oklahoma & WI	ORA	N	B
Kandel D (1990)	CS	R	2,711	Young adults	National US	ORA, D	MC	B
Kinsey (1953)	CS	R/S	5,940	CDA, F, W	National US	ORA, SR	N	B
Mahoney (1980)	CS	C	441	CS	Washington	SR	N	B
Miller PY (1974)	CS	R	2,064	Ad, W	Illinois	SR	SC	B
Mol (1970)	CS	R	1,825	CDA	Australia	RB, ORA	N	B
Naguib (1966)	CS	R	5,896	CDA, F	Maryland	ORA, D (any vs. N)	N	B
Nicholas (1995)	CS	S	1,817	CS	South Africa	Scale	N	M
Parfrey (1976)	CS	R	444	CS	Ireland	ORA, RB	N	B
Poulson (1998)	CS	C	210	CS	Greenville, NC	SR	SC	B
Resnick (1997)	CS	R	12,118	Ad	National US	SR	MC	B
Rohrbaugh (1975)	CS	C	475/221	HS/CS	Colorado	ORA, RB, RE	N	B
Rosenbaum (1990)	CS	R	2711	CDA 19-20	National US	ORA	MC	B
Ruppel (1970)	CS	R	437	CS	N. Illinois	RB, miscellaneous	MC	B
Seidman (1992)	CS	R	7,011	CDA, F	National US	ORA, D	MC	B
Sheeran (1996)	CS	C	682	HS	Scotland	SR	N	B
Studer (1987)	CS	C	224	Ad-18	Detroit	ORA	SC	B
Thornton (1989)	PC	R	888	Ad-18	Detroit	D, ORA, SR	MC	B
Werebe (1983)	CS	C	386	Ad	France	D, ORA	N	B
Woodroof (1985)	CS	C	477	CS (Christian)	United States	IR ER, miscellaneous	SC	B
Wright (1971)	CS	C	3,850	CS	England	RB, ORA, miscellaneous	N	B
ALCOHOL/USE ABUSE								
Adelekan (1993)	CS	S/R	636	CS	Nigeria	SR,D Muslim vs Chr	N	B
Adlaf (1985)	CS	R	2,066	Ad	Ontario, Can	D, ORA, SR	SC	B
Alexander F (1991)	CS	R	156	CDA, retired	Southern CA	Religious vs. secular	N	B
Alford (1991)	PC	C	157	AD, PP	Nebraska	AA participation	N	B
Amoateng (1986)	CS	R	17,000	HS seniors	National US	ORA, SR	MC	B
Beeghley (1990)	CS	R	8,652	CDA	National US	ORA, SR, CM, RB	MC	B
Benson P (1989)	CS	R	12,000+	HS seniors	National US	ORA, SR	MC	B
Bliss (1994)	CS	C	143	CS (Catholic)	Ohio	ORA, SR	N	M
Bock (1987)	CS	R	4,289	CDA	National US	D, ORA, SR, CM	MC	B

(Continued)

Appendix A (Continued)

Outcome/investigators	Type	Method	N	Population	Location	Religious variable	Controls	Findings
Brizer (1993)	CC	C	65 vs. Cs	PP (alc/drg)	New York	ORA, NORA	N	B
Brown D (1994)	CS	S	537	CDA, B, M	Southeast US	Religious scale, ORA, D	MC	B
Brown H (1991)	PC	C	35 and 15	PP (alc)	—	12-step spiritual	N	B
Burkett (1974)	CS	C	855	HS	Pacific NW US	ORA	SC	B
Burkett (1977)	CS	S	837	HS	Pacific NW US	ORA, RB	SC	B
Burkett (1987)	PC	C	240	HS	Pacific NW US	ORA, SR, RB	MS	B
Cancellaro (1982)	CC	C	74 vs. Cs	Narcotic addicts	Kentucky	NORA, RE	N	B
Christo (1995)	PC	C	101	Poly-drug abuse	London	RB	N	B
Cochran (1989)	CS	R	3,065	Ad	Midwest US	ORA, SR, D	MC	B
Cochran (1991)	CS	R	3,065	Ad	Midwest US	ORA, SR, D	MC	B
Coleman (1986)	CC	S	50 vs. Cs	Opiate addicts	Philadelphia	ORA, SR	MC	M
Cook (1997)	CS	R/S	7,666	Youth (ages 12-30)	United Kingdom	RCm	N	B
Desmond (1981)	PC	C	248	PP (addicts)	San Antonio, TX	Religious rehab program	NS	B
Dudley R (1987)	CS	R	801	Youth (12–24)	North America	ORA, NORA, CM	SC	B
Engs (1980)	CS	S	1,691	CS	Australia	D, SR	N	B
Forliti (1986)	CS	C	8,165/10,467	Ad/parents, CM	United States	RB, ORA, SR	NS	B
Francis LJ (1993)	CS	S	4753	HS	England	ORA, RB	N	B
Guinn (1975)	CS	S/R	1,789	HS, Mex-Am	Texas	ORA	N	B
Hadaway (1984)	CS	R	600	Ad, public HS	Atlanta, GA	ORA,SR,NORA, O	SC	B
Hardert (1994)	CS	C	1,234	HS, CS	Arizona	"Religiosity"	MC	B
Hardesty (1995)	CS	C	475	HS, CS (16-19)	Midwest US	"Family religiousness"	N	B
Hater (1984)	CS	S	1,174	PP (opioid addicts)	National US	#4 ORA, SR	MC	NA
Hays (1986)	PC	R	1,121	Ad (13-18)	National US	#5 religiousness scale	MC	B
Hays (1990)	CS	—	415	HS	—	"Religious identification"	MC	B
Hundleby (1982)	CS	C	231	HS (Catholic)	Ontario, Can	ORA, NORA	N	NA
Hundleby (1987)	CS	S/R	2,048	HS (9th grade)	Ontario, Can	ORA	SC	B
Jang (2001)	PC	R	1,087	Youth (13–22)	National US	ORA, SR	MC	B
Jessor (1973)	PC	R	605/248	HS and CS	Colorado	ORA	N	B
Jessor (1977)	PC	R	432/205	HS and CS	Colorado	ORA, NORA, SR	N	B
Johnson B (2000) JQ	CS	R/R	2,358/4,961	Young BM/WM	Boston, Chi, Phil	ORA	MC	B
Johnson B (2001) RCD	PC	R	R	Youth	National US	ORA	MC	B

Kandel D (1984)	CS	R	1,325	CDA (24-25)	New York	ORA	MC	B
Khavari (1982)	CS	—	4,853	CDA	Milwaukee, WI	D, SR	N	B
Lorch (1985)	CS	S/R	13,878	HS	Colorado Springs	CM, ORA, SR	SC	B
McIntosh (1981)	CS	R	1,358	Ages 12-19	Texas	D, ORA, SR	MC	B
McLuckie (1975)	CS	R	27,175	Grades 7/12	Pennsylvania	D, ORA	MC	B
Mullen (1995)	CS	R	1,534	HS	Netherlands	D, ORA, RB	N	B
Ndom (1996)	CS	R	1,508	CS	Nigeria	D, SR	N	B
Newcomb (1986)	CS	S	791	Ad	Los Angeles	SR	N	B
Newcomb (1992)	PC	S	614	Ad	Los Angeles	SR	N	B
Oetting (1987)	CS	S	415	HS	Western US	SR, ORA	SC	B
Oleckno (1991)	CS	C	1,077	CS	Northern IL	ORA, SR	N	B
Parfrey (1976)	CS	R	444	CS	Ireland	ORA, RB	N	B
Resnick (1997)	CS	R	12,118	Ad	National US	SR	MC	B
Rohrbaugh (1975)	CS	C	475/221	HS/CS	Colorado	ORA, RB, RE	N	B
Tenant-Clark (1989)	CC	C	25 vs. 25 Cs	Ad, PP	Colorado	SR	N	B
Veach (1992)	CS	C	148	CS & health professionals	Nevada	Spiritual exp, etc.	N	H
Wallace, J (1998)	CS	R	5,000	HS	National US	D, ORA, SR	MC	B
Long K (1993)	PC	C	625	Grades 3-7	Montana	ORA, NORA	MC	B
Lorch (1985)	CS	S/R	13,878	HS	Colorado Springs	CM, ORA, SR	SC	B
Luna (1992)	CS	R	955	Medical, vet, law students	Spain	SR	N	B
Mathew (1995)	CC	C	62 vs. Cs	PP (alcoholics)	North Carolina	Mathew scale	N	B
Mathew (1996)	CC	C	62 vs. Cs	PP (alcoholics)	North Carolina	Mathew scale	N	B
McDowell (1996)	CS	S	101	PP (alcoholics)	New York	IR, ER, ORA, RB	N	NA
Midanik (1995)	CS	R	1,603	CDA drinkers	National U.S.	D, SR	MC	B
Mookherjee (1986)	CS	S	1,477	W, M (DWI rehab)	Tennessee	RB scale	N	NA
Moore (1995)	CS	C	2,366	Ad	Israel	D, SR	N	B
Moos (1979)	CS	C	122	Alcoholics	Palo Alto, CA	Moral-religion subscale	N	B
Mullen (1995)	CS	R	1,534	HS	Netherlands	D, ORA, RB	N	B
Mullen (1996)	CS	R	985	CDA> 35 yo	West Scotland	D	SC	B
Ndom (1996)	CS	R	1,508	CS	Nigeria	D, SR	N	B

(Continued)

Appendix A (*Continued*)

Outcome/investigators	Type	Method	N	Population	Location	Religious variable	Controls	Findings
Newcomb (1986)	CS	—	791	Ad	Los Angeles	SR	N	B
Oleckno (1991)	CS	—	1077	CS	Northern IL	ORA, SR	N	B
Parfrey (1976)	CS	R	444	CS	Ireland	ORA, RB	N	B
Park (1998)	CS	R	—	CDA	Korea	D, RCm	—	B
Patock-Peckham (1998)	CS	C	364	CS	Arizona	D, IR/ER	SC	M
Perkins (1987)	CS	S	860	CS	New York	SR, D, miscellaneous	MC	B
Poulson (1998)	CS	C	210	CS	Greenville, NC	SR	SC	B
Query (1985)	PC, D	S	96	PP ages 10–23	North Dakota	ORA, D	NS	B
Resnick (1997)	CS	R	12,118	Ad	National US	SR	MC	B
Richards D (1990)	CS	C	292	CDA	National US	"Universal force"	N	B
Schlegel (1979)	CS	R	842	HS	Ontario, Can	ORA, D (vs. N)	N	B
Strauss (1953)	CS	S	15,747	CS	National US	D, ORA	N	B
Taub (1994)	CT	C	118	Alcoholics	Washington, DC	TM	N	B
Taylor J (1990)	CS	R	289	CDA B, F	Pittsburgh	IR, NORA, RB	MC	B
Thorne (1996)	CS	R	990	CDA, E	Ohio	ORA, D	N	NA
Turner (1994)	CS	S	247	HS	Austin, TX	D (affil), ORA	MC	B
Waisberg (1994)	CT	C	131	PP	Ontario, Can	Spiritual program	N	H
Wallace (1972)	CS	R	4,000	CDA	Norway	ORA, NORA	MC	B
Wallace J (1998)	CS	R	5,000	HS	National US	D, ORA, SR	MC	B
Walters (1957)	CC	C	50 vs. Cs	Alcoholics	Topeka, KS	ORA, RE, NORA	NS	H
Wechsler (1979)	CS	R	7,170	CS	New England	D, ORA	N	B
Weill (1994)	PC	R	437	Ad (13–18)	France	ORA	N	B
Williams J (1986)	CS	C	36	Alcoholics	New York	Alcohol Anonymous	N	B
Zucker (1987)	PC	C	61	Alcoholics	Bronx, NY	D, SR ORA	N	H
DRUG USE/ABUSE								
Adelekan (1993)	CS	S/R	636	CS	Nigeria	SR, D	N	B
Adlaf (1985)	CS	R	2,066	Ad	Ontario, Can	D, ORA, SR	N	B
Amey (1996)	CS	R	11,728	HS	National US	OR, SR, D	MC	B
Amoateng (1986)	CS	R	17,000	HS seniors	National US	SR, ORA	MC	B
Bell (1997)	CS	R	17,952	CS (Catholic)	National US	SR	MC	B
Bliss (1994)	CS	C	143	CS	Ohio	ORA, SR	N	B

Study			N	Population	Location	Measures		
Bowker (1974)	CS	R	948	CS	Ivy College	ORA, D	N	B
Brownfield (1991)	CS	R	>800	Ad, W, M	Seattle, WA	D, ORA, SR	MC	B
Brunswick (1992)	PC	R	536	Ad B, (12–17)	Harlem, NY	ORA, SR	SC	B
Burkett (1974)	CS	C	855	HS	Pacific NW US	ORA	SC	B
Burkett (1977)	CS	S	837	HS	Pacific NW US	ORA, RB	SC	B
Burkett (1987)	PC	C	240	HS	Pacific NW US	ORA, SR, RB	MS	B
Cancellaro (1982)	CC	C	74 vs. Cs	Narcotic addicts	Kentucky	NORA, RE	N	B
Christo (1995)	PC	C	101	Polydrug abuse	London	RB	N	B
Cochran (1989)	CS	R	3,065	Ad	Midwest US	ORA, SR, D	MC	B
Cochran (1991)	CS	R	3,065	Ad	Midwest US	ORA, SR, D	MC	B
Coleman (1986)	CC	S	50 vs. Cs	Opiate addicts	Philadelphia	ORA, SR	MC	M
Cook (1997)	CS	R/S	7,666	Youth (ages 12–30)	United Kingdom	RCm	N	B
Desmond (1981)	PC	C	248	PP (addicts)	San Antonio, TX	Religious rehab program	NS	B
Dudley R (1987)	CS	R	801	Youth (12–24)	North America	ORA, NORA, CM	SC	B
Engs (1980)	CS	S	1,691	CS	Australia	D, SR	N	B
Forliti (1986)	CS	C	8,165/10,467	Ad/parents, CM	United States	RB, ORA, SR	NS	B
Francis LJ (1993)	CS	S	4753	HS	England	ORA, RB	N	B
Guinn (1975)	CS	S/R	1,789	HS, Mex-Am	Texas	ORA	N	B
Hadaway (1984)	CS	R	600	Ad, public HS	Atlanta, GA	ORA,SR,NORA, O	SC	B
Hardert (1994)	CS	C	1,234	HS, CS	Arizona	"Religiosity"	MC	B
Hardesty (1995)	CS	C	475	HS, CS (16-19)	Midwest US	"Family religiousness"	N	B
Hater (1984)	CS	S	1,174	PP (opioid addicts)	National US	#4 ORA, SR	MC	NA
Hays (1986)	CS	R	1,121	Ad (13–18)	National US	#5 religiousness scale	MC	B
Hays (1990)	CS	—	415	HS	—	"Religious identification"	MC	NA
Hundleby (1982)	CS	C	231	HS (Catholic)	Ontario, Can	ORA, NORA	N	B
Hundleby (1987)	CS	S/R	2,048	HS (9th grade)	Ontario, Can	ORA	SC	B
Jang (2001)	PC	R	1,087	Youth (13–22)	National US	ORA, SR	MC	B
Jessor (1973)	PC	R	605/248	HS and CS	Colorado	ORA	N	B
Jessor (1977)	PC	R	432/205	HS and CS	Colorado	ORA, NORA, SR	N	B
Johnson B (2000) JQ	CS	R/R	2,358/4,961	Young BM/WM	Boston, Chi, Phil	ORA	MC	B
Johnson B (2001) RCD	PC	R	—	Youth	National US	ORA	MC	B
Kandel D (1984)	CS	R	1,325	CDA (24–25)	New York	ORA	MC	B

(Continued)

Appendix A (*Continued*)

Outcome/investigators	Type	Method	N	Population	Location	Religious variable	Controls	Findings
Khavari (1982)	CS	—	4,853	CDA	Milwaukee, WI	D, SR	N	B
Lorch (1985)	CS	S/R	13,878	HS	Colorado Springs	CM, ORA, SR	SC	B
McIntosh (1981)	CS	R	1,358	Ages 12–19	Texas	D, ORA, SR	MC	B
McLuckie (1975)	CS	R	27,175	Grades 7/12	Pennsylvania	D, ORA	MC	B
Mullen (1995)	CS	R	1,534	HS	Netherlands	D, ORA, RB	N	B
Ndom (1996)	CS	R	1,508	CS	Nigeria	D, SR	N	B
Newcomb (1986)	CS	S	791	Ad	Los Angeles	SR	N	B
Newcomb (1992)	PC	S	614	Ad	Los Angeles	SR	N	B
Oetting (1987)	CS	S	415	HS	Western US	SR, ORA	SC	B
Oleckno (1991)	CS	C	1,077	CS	Northern IL	ORA, SR	N	B
Parfrey (1976)	CS	R	444	CS	Ireland	ORA, RB	N	B
Resnick (1997)	CS	R	12,118	Ad	National US	SR	MC	B
Rohrbaugh (1975)	CS	C	475/221	HS/CS	Colorado	ORA, RB, RE	N	B
Tenant-Clark (1989)	CC	C	25 vs. 25 Cs	Ad, PP	Colorado	SR	N	B
Veach (1992)	CS	C	148	CS & health professionals	Nevada	Spiritual exp, etc.	N	H
Wallace, J (1998)	CS	R	5,000	HS	National US	D, ORA, SR	MC	B
DELINQUENCY/CRIME								
Avtar (1979)	CS	C	54/59	CA/HS	Ottawa, Can	SR	N	B
Barrett (1988)	PC	S	326	Mex-Am clients	Texas	ORA	MC	B
Benda (1995)	CS	S	>1,000	HS	Arkansas & MD	ORA, SR	MC	B
Benda (1997)	CS	S	724	HS (9th–12th graders)	Arkansas & OK	ORA, SR	MC	B
Benson P (1989)	CS	R	>12,000	HS	National US	SR	MC	B
Burkett (1974)	CS	C	855	HS	Pacific NW US	ORA	SC	B
Carr-Saunders (1944)	CC	C	276 vs. 551	Delinquents	London, England	ORA	N	B
Chadwick (1993)	CS	R	2,143	Ad (Mormons)	Eastern US	ORA	MC	B
Cochran (1994)	CS	C	1,600	HS	Oklahoma	ORA, SR	MC	NA
Cohen (1987)	PC	S	976	Mothers/caretakers	New York	ORA	MC	B
Elifson (1983)	CS	R	600	Ad, public HS	Atlanta, GA	RB, SR, NORA	SC	NA
Evans (1995)	CS	S	477	CDA, 100% W	Midwest US	OR, SR, RB, D	MC	B
Fernquist (1995)	CS	—	180	CS	—	ORA, NORA	N	B

Forliti (1986)	CS	C	8,165/10,467	Ad/parents, CM	United States	RB, ORA, SR	NS	B
Freeman (1986)	CS	R/R	2,358/4,961	Young BM/WM	Boston, Chi, Phil	ORA	MC	B
Grasmick (1991)	CS	R	304	CDA	Oklahoma City	D ORA, SR	SC	B
Hater (1984)	CS	S	1,174	PP (opiate addicts)	National US	ORA, SR	MC	NA
Higgins (1977)	CS	R	1,410	HS (10th grade)	Atlanta, GA	ORA	SC	B
Hirschi (1969)	CS	R	4,077	HS	Northern CA	ORA	N	NA
Jang (2001)	PC	R	1,087	Youth (13-22)	National US	ORA, SR	MC	B
Johnson B (1987)	RS	S	782	Former prisoners	Florida	ORA, SR	MC	NA
Johnson B (1997)	CC	S	201 vs. 201	Prisoners - ex prisoners	New York	ORA, NORA	MC	B
Johnson B (2000)	CS	R/R	2,358/4,961	Young BM/WM	Boston, Chi, Phil	ORA	MC	B
Johnson B (2000b)	PC	R	226	Ad, B	National US	ORA	MC	B
Johnson B (2001)	PC	R	1,725	Youth	National US	ORA, SR	MC	B
Johnson B (2002)	CC	S	148 vs. 247	Former prisoners	Brazil	Religious program	SC	B
Kvaraceus (1944)	CS	S	700+	Ad	New Jersey	ORA	N	NA
Middleton (1962)	CS	—	554	CS	California, FL	RB, ORA, SR	N	B
Montgomery (1996)	CS	—	392	HS (Catholic), F	Great Britain	NORA	SC	B
Morris R (1981)	CS	C	134	CS	Tennessee	IR, ER	N	B
Parfrey (1976)	CS	R	444	CS	Ireland	ORA, RB	N	B
Peek (1985)	PC	—	817	HS, M	National US	Religiosity	MC	M
Pettersson (1991)	CS	R	118	Police districts	Sweden	ORA	SC	B
Powell (1997)	CS	S	521	HS high risk, B	Birmingham, AL	ORA, SR	MC	B
Resnick (1997)	CS	R	12,118	Ad	National US	SR	MC	NA

(Continued)

Appendix A (Continued)

Outcome/investigators	Type	Method	N	Population	Location	Religious variable	Controls	Findings
Rhodes (1970)	CS	R	21,720	HS	Tennessee	ORA, D, miscellaneous	MC	B
Rohrbaugh (1975)	CS	C	475/221	HS/CS	Colorado	ORA, RB, RE	N	B
Shcoll (1964)	CC	C	52 vs. 28 Cs	Ad delinquents	Illinois	RB, RE	N	H
Sloane (1986)	CS	R	1,121	HS	National US	ORA, SR	MC	B
Stark (1982)	CS	R	1,799	White boys	National US	RB, SR, ORA	N	B
Stark (1996)	CS	R	11,955	Ad	National US	D, ORA	SC	B
Wallace J (1998)	CS	R	5,000	HS	National US	D, ORA, SR	MC	B
Wattenburg (1950)	CS	S	2,137	Delinquent boys	Detroit, MI	ORA	N	B
Wickerstrom (1983)	CS	C	130	CS (Christian)	4 states	IR, ER	MC	B
Wright (1971)	CS	C	3,850/1,574	CS	England	RB, ORA, miscellaneous	N	B
Zhang (1994)	CS	C	1,026	CS	China,Taiwan,US	SR, NORA, ORA	MC	B

Type: CS, cross-sectional; PC, prospective cohort; RS, retrospective; CT, clinical trial; Exp, experimental; CC, case control; D, descriptive; CR, case report; Q, qualitative.

Method (sampling): R, random (probability or population-based sample); S, systematic sampling; C, convenience/purposive sample.

N: number of subjects in sample; Cs, controls.

Population: C, children; Ad, adolescents; HS, high school students; CS, college students; CDA, community dwelling adults; E, elderly; MP, medical patients; PP, psychiatric patients; NHP, nursing home patients; CM, church members; R, religious or clergy; F, female; M, male; B, black; W, white.

Location: city, state, or country.

Religious variables: ORA, organizational religious activities (religious attendance and related activities); NORA, (scripture study); SR, subjective religiosity; RCn, religious commitment; IR, intrinsic religiosity; ER, extrinsic religiosity; Q, quest; SWB, spiritual well-being; R, religious coping; M, mysticism; O, orthodoxy; RB, religious belief; RE, religious experience; CM, church membership; D, denomination; SDA, Seventh-Day Adventist.

Findings: NA, no association; M, mixed evidence; B, beneficial association with outcome; H, harmful association with outcome.

Controls: N, no controls; SC, some controls; MC, multiple controls.

Appendix B: Review of Research Examining the Relationship Between Religion and Well-Being Outcomes

Outcome/investigators	Type	Method	N	Population	Location	Religious variable	Controls	Findings
WELL-BEING								
Alexander F (1991)	CS	S	156	CDA, E	Southern CA	ORA, NORA	N	B
Althauser (1990)	CS	C	274	CM (Methodist)	Southern US	IR, ER	SC	B
Anson (1990a)	PC	C	639	CDA, E	Israel	Observance of religious rituals	MC	M
Anson (1990b)	CS	R	105 vs. 125	Kibbutz members	Israel	Religious vs. secular	MC	B
Apel (1986)	CS	C	260	CM, R	Midwest US	ORA	N	B
Ayele (1999)	CS	C	100/55	Physicians/MP	Richmond, VA	NORA, IR	MC	B
Beckman (1982)	CS	S	719	CDA, E, 100%F	Southern CA	SR	MC	B
Bienenfeld (1997)	CS	C	89	R, E, 100%F	Ohio	RCm	MC	B
Blazer (1976)	PC	C	272	CDA, E N.	Carolina	SR, ORA, miscellaneous	N	B
Blaine (1995)	CS	C	144	CS	Buffalo,	NY SR, ORA, miscellaneous	N	B
Bulman (1977)	CS	C	29	MP (paralyzed)	Chicago	Religious scale	MC	NA
Burgener (1994)	CC	C	84 vs. Cs	Caregivers	New York	ORA, NORA	N	B
Cameron (1973)	CS	C	144	Handicapped	Michigan	SR (value of religion)	N	NA
Chamberlain (1988)	CS	C	188	CDA, 100%F	New Zealand	IR-like scales	SC	NA
Coke (1992)	CS	C	166	CDA, 100%B, E	New York	ORA, SR	MC	B
Coleman (1999)	CS	C	117	MP, B, AIDS	Los Angeles	SWB	N	B
Cutler (1976)	CS	R	438 and 395	CDA, E	National US	CM	MC	B
Decker (1985)	CS	C	100	MP, 90% M, A	Northwest US	SR	N	B
Doyle (1984)	CS	R	2,306	CDA, E	National US	SR	SC	B
Edwards (1973)	CS	R	507	CDA, E	Virginia	ORA	MC	B
Ellison CG (1989)	CS	R	1,500	CDA	National US	D, ORA, NORA, SR	MC	B
Ellison CG (1990)	CS	R	997	CDA	National US	D, ORA, NORA, SR	MC	B
Ellison CG (1991)	CS	R	997	CDA	National US	D, ORA, NORA, SR	MC	B
Emmons (1998)	CS	C	315	CS, CDA	Davis, CA	Spiritual striving	SC	B

(Continued)

Appendix B (*Continued*)

Outcome/investigators	Type	Method	N	Population	Location	Religious variable	Controls	Findings
Farakhan (1984)	PC	C	30	E, CDA, 100%F	Missouri	D, ORA	N	B
Feigelman (1992)	CS	R	20,000+	CDA	National US	D (disaffiliates)	MC	NA
Francis LF (1997)	CS	C	50	CDA, E	Wales	ORA, NORA	N	NA
Frankel (1994)	CS	C	299	CS	Ontario, CA	D, RB	N	B
Gee (1990)	CS	R	6,621	CDA	Canada	ORA, D	SC	B
Glik (1986, 1990a)	CC	C	93/83/137	New Age/Charisma/MP	Maryland	NewAge vs. Char vs. MP	MC	B
Graney (1975)	PC	S	60	E, CDA, 100%F	Midwest US	ORA	N	B
Guy (1982)	CS	S	1,170	E, CDA	Memphis, TN	ORA	N	B
Hadaway (1978)	CS	R	2,164	CDA	National US	D, ORA, SR	MC	B
Harvey (1987)	CS	R	11,071	CDA>40 y	Canada	SR	SC	B
Hater (1984)	CS	S	1,174	PP (opiod addicts)	National US	ORA, SR	MC	B
Heisel (1982)	CS	C	122	E, CDA, 100%B	New Jersey	ORA, NORA, E	SC	B
Hills (1998)	CS	C	230	CDA	Oxfordshire, ENG	RE	N	M
Hunsberger (1985)	CS	C	85	CDA, E	Ontario, Can	ORA, SR, RB	N	B
Inglehart (1990)	CS	R	169,776	CDA	14 western	ORA, SR	—	B
Jamal (1993)	CS	S	325	CDA (Muslims)	US & Canada	SR	SC	B
Poloma (1990)	CS	R	560	CDA	Akron, OH	RE, ORA, NORA, O	MC	M
Poloma (1991)	CS	R	560	CDA	Akron, OH	RE, CM, NORA	MC	M
Reyes-Ortiz (1996)	CS	S	55	MP	Richmond, VA	RC, NORA	N	B
Rayburn (1991)	CS	C	254	R, F	United States	Women relig (Ca,P,J)	SC	B
Reed K (1991)	CS	R	1473	CDA	National US	Strength of affil	SC	B
Reed P (1986)	CC	C	57 vs. Cs.	MP (terminal)	Southeast US	Scale	N	B
Reed P (1987)	CC	C	100 vs. Cs	MP (terminal)	Southeast US	Scale	N	B
Riley (1998)	CS	C	216	MP	Ann Arbor, MI	SWB, FACT-SP	N	B
Ringdal (1995,1996)	PC	S	253	MP (cancer)	Norway	RB	SC	B
Rogalski (1987)	CS	C	120	CDA, E	Los Angeles	SR	MC	B
Rosen (1982)	CS	C	148	CDA ,E	Georgia	RC	N	B
Schwartz (1997)	CS	S	46	Yale medical student	New Haven, CT	ORA	N	B

Study			N	Sample	Location	Measure		
Shaver (1980)	CS	U	2,500	F (Redbook)	National	US SR	N	M
Shuler (1994)	CS	C	50	Homeless, F	Los Angeles	ORA, NORA, RC	N	B
Singh (1982)	CS	R	1,459	CDA, E	National US	ORA	MC	B
Spreitzer (1974)	CS	R	1,547	CDA	National US	ORA, SR	MC	B
Marannell (1974)	CS	C	109	CS	Mid/South US	Religious dimensions	N	H
Markides (1983)	CS	R	338	CDA, 70%Mex	Texas	ORA, NORA, SR	MC	B
McClure (1982)	CS	C	233	CDA, CM	Southwest US	Religious activities	N	B
McGloshen (1988)	CS	—	226	F, E	Midwest US	ORA	MC	B
McNamara (1979)	CS	R	2,164	CDA	National US	SR, ORA, D, CM	SC	B
Mercer (1995)	CS	C	107	Accident victims	—	SR, ORA, RC	N	B
Moberg (1953)	CS	C	219	E, NH	Minnesota	CM	MC	NA
Moberg (1956)	CS	C	219	E, NH	Minnesota	CM, ORA, NORA	MC	B
Moberg (1965)	CS	C	5,000	E, CDA	MN, SD, ND,MO	CM, ORA	MC	B
Moberg (1984)	CS	C	1,081	CDA	US & Sweden	SWB scale	N	B
Moos (1979)	CS	C	122	Alcoholics	Palo Alto, CA	Moral-religious subscales	N	B
Morris D (1991)	CS	R	400	E, CDA	Indiana	ORA	MC	B
Musick (1996)	PC	R	2,623	E, CDA	North Carolina	ORA, NORA	MC	B
O'Connor (1990)	CS	C	176	E, NH	Quebec, Can	IR scale (French)	N	B
O'Reilly (1957)	CS	R	210	CDA, E, Catholic	Chicago	ORA	N	B
Ortega (1983)	CS	R	4,522	CDA	Northern AL	ORA	MC	B
Pfeifer (1995)	CC	C	44 vs. 45	Cs PP	Switzerland	IR, ER, miscellaneous	N	B
Pollner (1989)	CS	R	3,072	CDA	National US	ORA, NORA, RE	MC	B
Poloma (1989)	CS	R	560	CDA	Akron, OH	NORA, RE	MC	M
St. George (1984)	CS	R	3362	CDA	National US	ORA, SR, RB	MC	B
Steinitz (1980)	CS	R	1493	CDA, E	National US	ORA, SR, RB	SC	B
Tellis-Nayak (1982)	CS	R	259	CDA, E	National US	ORA, SR	MC	B
Thomas (1992)	CS	R	5629	CDA	National US	ORA, SR	MC	B
Tix (1997)	PC	S	239	Renal Transplants	Minnesota	RC, D	MC	B
Toseland (1979)	CS	R	871	CDA, E	National US	ORA	MC	NA

(Continued)

Appendix B (*Continued*)

Outcome/investigators	Type	Method	N	Population	Location	Religious variable	Controls	Findings
Usui (1985)	CS	R	704	CDA, E	Kentucky	ORA	MC	B
Walls (1991)	CS	C	98	CDA, CM, B	Pennsylvania	RB, ORA, NORA	MC	NA
Weiss (1990)	CS	C	226	Hare Krishna (HK)	United States	HK religiosity	N	B
Willits (1988)	PC	—	1650	CDA	Pennsylvania	ORA, RB	MC	B
Zautra (1977)	CS	R	454	CDA	Salt Lake City	Religious participation	SC	NA
HOPE/PURPOSE/MEANING								
Acklin (1983)	CC	C	26 vs. 18 Cs	MP (recurrent CG)	Atlanta, GA	IR/ER, ORA	N	B
Blaine (1995)	CS	C	144	CS	Buffalo, NY	SR, ORA, Misc	N	B
Bohannon (1991)	CS	C	272	Bereaved parents	Midwest US	D, ORA	SC	B
Bolt (1975)	CS	C	52	CS	Michigan	IR, ER	N	B
Burbank (1992)	CS	C	57	E, CDA	Rhode Island	SR	N	NA
Burns (1991)	CT	C	37 vs. 15	Cs Alcoholics	Virginia	Spiritual awareness (Step 11 spiritual)	—	B
Carroll (1993)	CS	C	100	AA members	Southern CA	EWB, RWB, SR	SC	B
Carson (1988)	CS	C	197	Nursing Students	Baltimore, MD	EWB, RWB, SR	SC	B
Carson (1990)	CS	C	65	MP (HIV+ men)	Baltimore, MD	SWB EWB,RWB	MC	B
Carver (1993)	PC	C	59	MP breast CA	Miami, FL	RC	MC	NA
Chamberlain (1988)	CS	C	188	CDA, 100%F	New Zealand	IR-like scale	N	B
Crandall (1975)	CS	C	86	CS	Idaho	IR, ER	N	B
Dember (1989)	CS	C	106	CS	—	RC	MC	NA
Ellis J (1991)	CS	C	100	CS	Tennessee	EWB, RWB	N	B
Fox (1995)	CS	C	22	MP (breast CA)	North Ireland	RWB	N	NA
Herth (1989)	CS	C	120	MP (cancer)	Illinois	SR	N	B
Idler (1997a)	CS	R	2,812	CDA, E	New Haven, CT	ORA, SR	MC	B
Jackson (1988)	CS	C	98	CM, B	Washington, DC	IR, RB, ORA	SC	B
Jacobson (1977)	PC	C	57	Alcoholics, PP	DePaul, WI	IR/ER	N	B
Kass (1991)	PC	C	83	MP	Boston, MA	INSPIRIT	SC	B
Moberg (1984)	CS	C	1,081	CDA	US & Sweden	SWB scale	N	NA

Study								
Richards D (1990)	CS	C	292	CDA	National US	Universal force	N	B
Richards D (1991)	CS	C	345	CDA	National US	ORA, RB, ORA	SC	B
Ringdal (1995, 1996)	PC	S	253	MP (cancer)	Norway	RB	SC	B
Sanders (1979/80)	CS	S	102 vs. 107Cs	Bereaved	Florida	ORA	MC	B
Sethi (1993, 1994)	CS	C	623	CM	United States	D, ORA, SR, RB	MC	B
Tellis-Nayak (1982)	CS	R	259	CDA, E	New York	D, RB, ORA, RE	MC	B
Vandercreek (1991)	CS	C	160/150	MP/CDA, F	Columbus, OH	ORA	SC	B
Veach (1992)	CS	C	148	CS & health pros	Nevada	Spiritual Exp	N	B
Zorn (1997)	CS	C	114	CDA, E, F	Wisconsin	RWB	SC	B
SELF-ESTEEM								
Bahr (1983)	CS	R	500	HS	Middletown, IN	D, ORA, RB	MC	NA
Benson P (1973)	CS	C	128	HS, 100% M	Michigan	RB, ORA, NORA	MC	M
Commerford (1996)	CS	C	83	NH, E	New York City	ORA, NORA, IR	MC	NA
Ellison CG (1993)	CS	R	1,933	CDA, B	National US	ORA, NORA	MC	B
Ellison CG (1990)	CS	R	1,344	CDA, B	National US	RC (prayer)	N	H
Fehr (1977)	CS	C	120	CS	Cincinnati, OH	Relig values, O	SC	NA
Jenkins (1988)	CS	C	62	MP (cancer)	Indiana	RC	SC	B
Jensen L (1995)	CS	—	3,835	CS	UT, TX WI, ID	D, "religiosity"	MC	B
Krause (1989)	CS	R	2,107	CDA, B	National US	ORA, NORA	MC	B
Krause (1992)	CS	R	448	CDA, E, B	National US	ORA, NORA, SR	MC	B
Krause (1995)	CS	R	1,005	CDA, E	National US	ORA, NORA, RC	MC	B
Maton (1989)	CS	C	81/68	Bereaved parents HS	Maryland	Spiritual support	MC	B
Meisenhelder (1986)	CS	R	163	CDA, F, married	Boston	D, SR	MC	B
Nelson P (1989)	CS	C	68	E, CDA	Texas	IR/ER scale	N	B
O'Connor (1990)	CS	C	176	E, NH	Quebec, Can	IR scale (French)	N	B
Plante (1997)	CS	C	102	CS	California	SR, NORA, ORA, RC	N	NA
Russo (1997)	PC	R	4,150	CDA, F	National US	D, ORA	SC	NA
Ryan (1993)	CS	C	105,151,34	CS, CM	New York	IR, ER, O, Q, RC	N	B

(Continued)

Appendix B (*Continued*)

Outcome/investigators	Type	Method	N	Population	Location	Religious variable	Controls	Findings
Sherkat (1992)	CS	C	156	CDA (bereaved)	Southeast	US D, ORA, NORA	MC	B
Smith C (1979)	CS	C	1,995	AD (Catholic)	5 countries	IR, ER, Q, Misc	SC	B
Watson P (1985)	CS	C	127/194	CS	Tennessee	0 IR, ER, Q, Misc	SC	B
Weltha (1969)	CS	C	565	CS	Iowa	Relig attitude scale	N	M
Wickstrom (1983)	CS	C	130	Cs (Christian)	4 US states	IR, ER	MC	NA
EDUCATIONAL ATTAINMENT								
Bankston (1996)	RS	C	402	AD Vietnamese-American	New Orleans	ORA	MC	B
Brown (1991)								B
Darnell (1997)	PC	R	1,135	Students	national	Fundamentalism	MC	H
Freeman (1986)	CS	R	2,358/4,961	Young BM/WM	Boston, Chi, Phil	ORA	MC	B
Hummel (1983)	CS	C	20	Private HS seniors, F	Pittsburgh	SR	MC	B
Johnson (1995)	CS	C	200	BM eighth graders	Mississippi	ORA	MC	B
Johnson B (2000)	CS	R/R	2,358/4,961	Young BM/WM B	Boston, Chi, Phil	ORA	MC	B
Keysar (1995)	CS	R	19,274	Adult women	National	Religious identification	MC	B
Koubek (1984)	RS	S	44	Assembly of God Youth	Northern Illinois	ORA, SR, RC	N	B
Lehrer (1999)	CS	R	1,313/1,831	Born between 1945–1960	Male	D	SC	M
Regnerus (2000)	CS	R	4,434	HS students	National	D, ORA,	MC	B
Regnerus (2001)	CS	R	9,771	HS students	National	D, ORA,	MC	B
Sanders (1995)	RS	C	800	BM eighth graders	Southeastern US	Church support	MC	B
Scharf (1998)	CS	R	201	HS students	National	Religiosity	MC	B
Sherkat (1999)	PC	R	1,135	Young adults	National	Fundamentalism	MC	M

Study	Type	Sampling	N	Population	Location	Religious variables	Findings	Controls
Thomas (1990)	CS	R	4,000	HS students	Utah	ORA, SR, RC	B	MC
Velez (1985)	PC	R	3,169	HS seniors	National	Denomination	B	MC
Wood (1988)	D	C	52	Relig private HS students	Rural-suburban	Moral-religious values	B	SC
Zern (1989)	D	C	251	College students	Northeastern US	ORA, SR, RC	B	SC

Type: CS, cross-sectional; PC, prospective cohort; RS, retrospective; CT, clinical trial; Exp, experimental; CC, case control; D, descriptive; CR, case report; Q, qualitative.

Method (sampling): R, random (probability or population-based sample); S, systematic sampling; C, convenience/purposive sample.

N: number of subjects in sample; Cs, controls.

Population: C, children; Ad, adolescents; HS, high school students; CS, college students; CDA, community dwelling adults; E, elderly; MP, medical patients; PP, psychiatric patients; NHP, nursing home patients; CM, church members; R, religious or clergy; F, female; M, male; B, black; W, white.

Location: city, state, or country.

Religious variables: ORA, organizational religious activities (religious attendance and related activities); NORA, (scripture study); SR, subjective religiosity; RCm, religious commitment; IR, intrinsic religiosity; ER, extrinsic religiosity; Q, quest; SWB, spiritual well-being; R, religious coping; M, mysticism; O, orthodoxy; RB, religious belief; RE, religious experience; CM, church membership; D, denomination; SDA, Seventh-Day Adventist.

Findings: NA, no association; M, mixed evidence; B, beneficial association with outcome; H, harmful association with outcome.

Controls: N, no controls; SC, some controls; MC, multiple controls.

10 Focused on Their Families: Religion, Parenting, and Child Well-Being

W. Bradford Wilcox

University of Virginia

The historical, social, and theological ties that bind religion and the family to one another run deep (Christiano 2000; Greven 1988). But these ties are by no means without controversy. In recent years, scholars have increasingly drawn attention to religious commitments to patriarchy and parental authority to argue that religion exerts a baleful influence on parents and, by extension, their children. Accordingly, this essay sets out to answer a basic question: Does religion foster the seedbeds of parental virtue or parental vice?

A growing, but largely speculative, literature by religious scholars, psychologists, and sociologists asserts that religion, particularly conservative Protestantism, fosters an authoritarian and abusive approach to parenting. In 1991, Princeton Theological Seminary professor Donald Capps delivered a presidential address to the Society for the Scientific Study of Religion titled "Religion and Child Abuse: Perfect Together." Capps argued that the religious endorsement of corporal punishment—found, for example, in evangelical Protestant advice books like James Dobson's *Dare to Discipline* (1970)—encourages parents to adopt an abusive parenting style. In a similar vein, John Gottman (1998), the noted family psychologist, has written, "As the religious right gains strength in the United States, there is also a movement of some fathers toward authoritarian parenting in childrearing patterns of discipline" (p. 183). And sociologists Julia McQuillan and Myra Max Ferree (1998) have argued that "the religious right" is an influential force "pushing men toward authoritarian and stereotypical forms of masculinity and attempting to renew patriarchal family relations" (p. 213).

Taken together, this literature makes two central claims. First, religion, especially conservative Protestantism, promotes an abusive or authoritarian parenting style. As Baumrind's (1971) seminal work on parenting suggests, an *authoritarian* parenting style is marked by a harsh and erratic approach to discipline, minimal expressions of affection, and low levels of parental responsiveness. Second, this literature also suggests that religion, especially conservative Protestantism, promotes a *patriarchal* style of parenting among men characterized by, among other things, low levels of paternal warmth and involvement. These two styles of parenting have been linked to negative child and adolescent outcomes (Amato, 1998; Amato & Rivera, 1999; Baumrind, 1971; Maccoby & Martin, 1983; Thomson, Hanson, & McLanahan, 1994).

This perspective, however, is based on virtually no empirical research (but see Wilcox, 1998). Moreover, the sociological theory of James Coleman suggests that religious institutions should have a largely beneficial effect on parents—especially in comparison with the other institutional actors that parents regularly encounter in the social world. There are also good theoretical reasons to hypothesize that parents with orthodox religious convictions, including conservative Protestant parents, will be particularly motivated to devote themselves to their children. Indeed, after briefly outlining a theoretical perspective on the link between religion and parenting, I proceed to show that evangelical parents and fathers, and religious parents more generally, come closer to typifying the *authoritative* style of parenting that Baumrind and others have linked to a range of positive outcomes among children and adolescents (Amato & Booth, 1997; Baumrind, 1971; Maccoby & Martin, 1983; Thomson et al., 1994).

Religion, Orthodoxy, and Parenting: A Theoretical Perspective

The work of James Coleman, who is best known for his contributions to a theory of social capital, suggests a number of reasons why religious institutions may play a salutary role in promoting an authoritative approach to parenting. In analyzing the institutions that influence children, Coleman (1990) distinguishes between two types of institutional actors: *primordial* institutions (e.g., religious bodies and families) and *purposive* institutions (e.g., corporations and state welfare agencies). He argues that primordial institutions generally have a more beneficial effect on children than do purposive institutions because the former tend to treat children as ends in themselves, whereas the latter tend to treat children in instrumental terms. I extend his argument to reflect on the ways in which religion as a primordial institution may have a more beneficial impact on parents than the purposive institutions that parents also encounter in the social world.

Primordial institutions have three characteristics that may be beneficial for parenting. First, they are organized around a collective belief system that stresses a particular vision of the good life and a range of virtues that help their members realize this good. In the case of religious actors, members are encouraged to serve God and neighbor and to acquire virtues such as truthfulness, fortitude, and charity that enable them to live out the collective goals of their community. More specifically, the generic and parent-related moral beliefs advanced by religious institutions help motivate parents to make the considerable sacrifices of time, willpower, and energy that are required to form good character in their children (Ammerman, 1997; Wilcox, 2002).

Second, primordial institutions have a long-term time horizon that leaves them with a profound stake in the moral character of their members. Because their members tend to be involved for a lifetime, primordial institutions have an inherent interest in cultivating virtues in their members—especially young members—that make them good institutional citizens. This is especially true of religious institutions because they are trying to pass on a body of religious belief and practice from one generation to the next. In Coleman's words, "This creates an intrinsic interest of the religious body in the kind of person the child is and will become" (1990, p. 600). In particular, religious institutions have a strong interest in promoting an ethic of intensive, sacrificial parenting that will lead the rising generation to faith.

Third, primordial institutions foster intergenerational closure. This means that primordial actors such as churches promote social ties between children, parents, and other adults in the community. These close ties allow adults to offer support and sanction for community-defined norms about parenting. These ties are also an important source of social support for parents when they are facing serious difficulties of a familial (e.g., disabled child) or extrafamilial (e.g., unemployment) nature (Ellison, 1994). Thus, religion should promote better parenting insofar as it connects parents to social networks that reinforce religious and community parenting norms and help parents deal with the stresses of family life.

By contrast, purposive institutions tend to have mixed effects on parents and children. First, unlike primordial institutions, purposive institutions are not organized around a collective belief system. As commercial or public institutions organized around narrow goals such as profit or the provision of a social service, purposive actors do not focus on an encompassing vision of the good life; indeed, in a liberal pluralistic society, public institutions are unable to endorse a specific vision of the good life. This means that purposive institutions cannot supply parents with a belief system that might motivate them to make considerable sacrifices on behalf of their children. So, for instance, a welfare agency may offer a parenting skills class to recipients but will refrain from offering a comprehensive moral vision of the parenting enterprise for fear of upsetting the religious and moral convictions of one part of the population or another.

Second, purposive institutions do not take a long-term view of the persons they deal with, either because they deal with them only over a short period of time or because they are at some social distance from them. Thus, they have no incentive to foster virtue in the persons they influence because they do not have to maintain direct contact with them on an ongoing basis. Thus, purposive institutions have no need to foster parental virtue. Take the entertainment industry, which exerts a massive influence on American family life. The industry aims to make a profit by offering programming that attracts the attention of consumers who have no long-term or personal connection to the company that produces the programming. Thus, entertainment companies have no institutional stake in the effects their programming may have on parents. Consider this exchange between a mother and Jerry Springer on his nationally syndicated talk show:

> JERRY SPRINGER: Mom, why are you going out with him?
> MOM: Because I love him.
> SPRINGER: How could you love him? He slept with your twelve-year-old daughter!...
> You don't see anything wrong in this story? What about your daughter? She's hurt.
> MOM: I love Amber... And I want both Amber and Glen to be in my life. And... if Amber can't accept it, then she can just stay living with her father and she can stay out of my life.
> SPRINGER: You're saying that to your own daughter? What's wrong with you? That's your daughter. That's your flesh and blood.
> MOM: It's just the way it is. I'm not going to be miserable because her and her father want things their way. (Hewlett & West, 1998, p. 126)

Clearly, *The Jerry Springer Show* offers a venal portrait of parenting, regardless of Springer's gestures in the direction of the high road. But the reason Universal Studios produces programming like this is that it is popular and profitable and the company has no direct, long-term contact with the consumers who watch it.

Purposive institutions also do not foster intergenerational closure. Given their short-term focus on narrowly defined ends, they have no need to bring adults and children into relationship with one another in the ongoing pursuit of a collective good. Thus, purposive actors like corporations and public bureaucracies are unable to furnish the social networks that can be so helpful to parents. *The Jerry Springer Show*, for example, may bring children and adults together in the limited sense that they are all watching the same show. But this virtual community does not offer any social ties marked by solidarity, reciprocity, or obligation.

For all these reasons, Coleman's theory suggests that any type of religion should have largely beneficial effects on parents. But particular forms of religion may be more likely to promote good parenting. Specifically, orthodox religion is more likely to promote good parenting than other forms of religion. Orthodox religion is committed to an objective, constant, and definable body of religious and moral truths. In the words of James Davison Hunter (1991), orthodoxy defines "a consistent, unchangeable measure of value, purpose, goodness, and identity, both personal and collective. It tells us what is good, what is true, how we should live, and who we are" (p. 44). Moreover, the strong, distinctive beliefs promoted by orthodox religions usually engender a sacrificial ethic on behalf of their faith among their adherents that translates into higher levels of religious participation, financial support for religious activities, and adherence to the moral teachings of the faith (Smith 1998; Stark & Finke 2000).

This chapter focuses on three different types of orthodox religious groups in the United States: conservative Protestants, traditional Catholics, and Orthodox Jews. Conservative Protestants believe that the Bible is the literal word of God and is therefore the authoritative guide to religious and moral truth. Traditional Catholics believe that biblical revelation and sacred tradition, as interpreted by the magisterium (teaching authority) of the Roman Catholic Church, provide all necessary truth about faith and the moral life. Orthodox Jews believe that the Torah is the revealed word of God and that the Talmud (the record of rabbinic discussions on Jewish law, ethics, customs, and legends) provides an authoritative guide to the beliefs and practices required by the Torah of all faithful Jews.

Why might orthodox religionists be better parents? First, the intensity of their religious belief motivates them to devote more time and energy to forming the religious character of their children than other parents. Second, the moral teaching embodied in their traditions places great stress on the obligations of parenthood. Third, they tend to have tight social networks that provide high levels of social support and normative integration. Finally, the dramatic cultural revolution that swept the United States after the 1960s, a revolution that challenged religious and moral beliefs dear to orthodox religious believers, prompted many conservative Protestants, traditional Catholics, and Orthodox Jews to devote themselves even more to parenting for fear that outside influences—from peers to teachers to the media—would undercut their religious and moral convictions. In a word, orthodox religionists have come to see the family as the first line of defense against a larger culture they see as debased and debasing.

Before I can examine the relationship between religion and parenting, I must define good parenting at greater length. As noted earlier, psychological theory suggests that an authoritative style of parenting, characterized by high levels of warmth and sufficient discipline, is best for children. Specifically, an affectionate approach to parenting is important for engendering self-respect and social competence among children and for minimizing the likelihood of anxiety and antisocial behavior among children. But this affectionate approach must also be supplemented with a firm approach to discipline whereby parents set limits and rules for their children and back up those expectations with consistent rewards and sanctions. Children who benefit from this warm but firm style of parenting do better on a range of different social and psychological outcomes—from juvenile delinquency to depression (Baumrind, 1971; Chase-Lansdale & Pittman, 2002; Maccoby & Martin 1983).

There are also three important social-structural dimensions that foster good parenting: family structure, intergenerational closure, and the quantity of time that parents spend with their children. Children benefit from ties with significant adults—especially their parents—that extend over time and are characterized by high levels of interaction. Such ties give parents countless opportunities to influence their children and to attend to the ongoing religious, moral, social, and intellectual development of their children. They also provide parents with a long-term horizon that makes them more likely to attend to the long-term interests of their children and a retrospective view of their children that allows them to link events in the children's past to their present behavior and outlook (Coleman, 1990).

This is one of the reasons why family structure is so important. Generally, in cases of divorce and out-of-wedlock birth, one parent, typically the father, stops having regular contact with his or her children a few years after the divorce or out-of-wedlock birth (Cooksey & Fondell, 1996; Furstenberg, 1988; Popenoe, 1996). Accordingly, this parent loses the long-term, day-in, day-out perspective and contact with his or her child that is so helpful in fostering good parenting. Furthermore, single parents tend to have less affectionate interaction with their children and provide less firm and consistent discipline compared with parents in an intact, married family, largely because of the stresses associated with single parenthood. These two factors help explain why children who grow up outside an intact, married family are less likely to benefit from the authoritative parenting of two parents and, consequently, face a higher risk of a range of negative psychological and social outcomes (Amato & Rivera, 1999; Carlson, 1999; Chase-Lansdale & Pittman, 2002; McLanahan & Carlson, 2002; McLanahan & Sandefur, 1994).

The structure of the ties that parents have with other adults and children in their children's social world is also very important. Children benefit from intergenerational closure in their social networks (Coleman, 1990). In this case, closure means that parents know who their children are friends with, and they know the adults with whom their children spend time outside the home. Such closure allows parents (1) to stay abreast of developments in their children's lives and (2) to reinforce norms by monitoring their children's peer groups and by relying on other adults in their social network to support their values. Children who have parents who can rely on their social networks to reinforce their beliefs are more virtuous (Chase-Lansdale & Pittman, 2002; Hagan, MacMillan, & Wheaton, 1996).

The depth of ties between parent and child is integral to establishing a child's sense of self-respect and a child's identification with the virtues and values espoused by his or her parents. Although the quality of the time parents spend with their children is important, it is also important for parents to spend a high quantity of time with their children. This time allows parents to interact with their children in a wide range of settings and circumstances, to monitor the behavior and development of their children in a consistent manner, and to develop a "secure attachment" with their children over the life course. For these reasons, greater parental involvement is associated with a range of positive outcomes for children (Amato, 1998; Amato & Booth, 1998; Chase-Lansdale & Pittman, 2002; Hagan et al., 1996).

Religious Discourse about Parenting

The parenting advice found in most religious traditions promotes, in the main, the virtues and values that are conducive to an authoritative parenting style and to a good social environment for parenting. Furthermore, a close reading of evangelical Protestant advice books does not suggest that fathers are encouraged to take a distant, "stereotypical" approach to parenting. The following citations from traditional Catholic, conservative Protestant, and Orthodox Jewish sources are indicative of the general tenor of religious parenting advice, especially among orthodox religious groups in the United States.

In *Lifeline*, James Stenson, a traditional Catholic, argues that parents must make considerable sacrifices if they seek to raise children who are virtuous and faithful. They must demonstrate to their children that they are capable of living out virtues such as faith, fortitude, and temperance, and they must teach those virtues to their children:

> [T]here seems to be an economic law in children's upbringing: You either pay now or you pay later. Parents who sacrifice to live these virtues themselves, and lead their children to do the same, can later see their children grow into exceptional men and women, the delight of their parents' later lives. But those parents... who neglect their children's character formation throughout childhood, can spend their later lives in bitter disappointment. This happens all too often. Just look around you. (Stenson, 1996, pp. 28–29)

Moreover, in Stenson's view, the stakes that parents face are particularly profound because parenting plays a crucial role in setting children on a path to heaven or hell. Accordingly, he argues that God will hold parents accountable for the job they did in raising their children: "God calls every parent to responsibility. He will hold you answerable for the eternal destiny of your children" (p. 17). Thus, not only does Stenson encourage a sacrificial ethic among parents, he also invests that ethic with transcendent significance of the utmost importance.

James Dobson, president of Focus on the Family, is the most prominent parenting expert in the conservative Protestant world. He draws on his doctoral training in child development and his evangelical faith to advocate parenting that combines a strict approach to discipline with an affectionate approach to nondisciplinary situations. For instance, in *The Strong-Willed Child*, Dobson writes:

> Healthy parenthood can be boiled down to those two essential ingredients, love and control, operating in a system of checks and balances. Any concentration on love to the exclusion of control usually breeds disrespect and contempt. Conversely, an authoritarian and oppressive home atmosphere is deeply resented by the child who feels unloved or even hated. To repeat, the objective for the toddler years is to strike a balance between mercy and justice, affection and authority, love and control. (1978, p. 61)

As this passage suggests, Dobson supports an approach to parenting that seems to conform largely to the authoritative style of parenting advocated by leading developmental psychologists like Diana Baumrind. However, drawing upon biblical teaching about discipline and parental authority (e.g., Proverbs 13:24; Ephesians 6:1), Dobson has also been a vocal proponent of the parental use of corporal punishment, especially in cases where young children are being disobedient. His support of corporal punishment, and parental authority more generally, has led many scholars to suspect that his advice, and the advice offered by other conservative Protestant experts, promotes an authoritarian approach to parenting.

It is important to note, however, that Dobson and other experts in this subculture argue that spanking should be applied judiciously and that parents should refrain from angry outbursts that, in their view, harm children and undermine children's respect for their parents' authority. In Dobson's words: "Parents often use anger to get action instead of using action [spanking] to get action [compliance]... Trying to control children by screaming is as utterly futile as trying to steer a car by honking the horn" (1992, p. 36). Moreover, Dobson (1978) also argues that parents' most important disciplinary responsibility is to set clear and consistent rules for their children: "The most important step in any disciplinary procedure is to establish reasonable expectations and boundaries in advance.... Once a child understands what is expected, he should then be held accountable for behaving accordingly" (pp. 29–30). Only when children engage in "willful defiance" are they to be spanked (p. 37). Thus, conservative Protestant experts do not offer parents an indiscriminate license to engage in abusive parenting behavior; rather, they encourage parents to adopt a strict approach to parenting that encompasses clear rules, strong expectations of obedience, and a willingness to rely on spanking but not yelling.

Orthodox Jewish leaders also offer extensive parenting advice to Jewish parents. Two passages from a parenting column written by Rabbi Y. Y. Rubinstein of Ezras Torah Yeshiva are suggestive of this genre. In the first selection, he quotes from a nineteenth-century Jewish text that stresses the importance of parental oversight:

> And as for you, Jewish parents, do not forget that it was at the time when you were young that the decline began. Sin has made giant steps since you were young; keep guard over your children! Some already move in the direction of this sin in the tenth, ninth, eighth year. Test the schools, the playmates, the servants, the friends of the house! Know that vice enters into the circle of youth by every way. Become the friends of your children! Give them early warning! Stand by their side in their battle! (Rubinstein, 2002)

Here, Rubinstein is making the point that parents need to monitor the children and adults that their children spend time with so as to protect them from engaging in practices that Judaism deems immoral. Later, Rubinstein warns parents that they must treat their spouse with love and affection, and that they must do all they can to avoid divorce. He argues that the quality and the stability of Jewish marriages are enormously consequential for the happiness of Jewish children:

> When I see young people who are in bad shape religiously or emotionally I always wonder "What is the home like?" Often "Unhappy" kids are the products of "Unhappy" parents... The greatest gift that we can give our children is a happy home. The Torah provides the advice to make that ambition a reality. (Rubinstein, 2002)

In sum, the family-related discourse produced by orthodox religious groups exhorts parents to high levels of parental affection, involvement, and oversight, and also urges them to take a strict approach to discipline. These religious traditions also stress the importance of marital stability, which has important effects on parenting. Most important, this religious discourse imbues the parenting enterprise with transcendent significance. But what impact, if any, does this religiously grounded discourse have on parenting behaviors? I turn to this question in the next section.

Data Analysis

The empirical analysis is based on data taken from two different surveys—the National Survey of Families and Households (NSFH), sponsored by the University of Wisconsin-Madison, and the Survey of Adults and Youth (SAY), sponsored by Princeton, Columbia, and New York universities. The NSFH surveyed more than 13,000 adults in the period 1987–1988 and offers extensive information on a range of religious, economic, demographic, and family matters (Sweet, Bumpass, & Call, 1988). The NSFH analysis relies on a subsample of 5,300 respondents who were parents of school-age children (ages 5 to 18). SAY, which oversampled residents in urban and suburban America, surveyed more than 6,000 parents and adolescents (ages 10 to 18) in the period 1998–1999. SAY incorporates information on a range of sociocultural phenomena; SAY also is the first parenting survey to ask respondents detailed information about their religious identity (Center for Research on Child Wellbeing, 2002). Taken together, these surveys provide a good portrait of the influence that religion has on parenting.

I turn first to the data and results from the NSFH. The empirical analysis is based on logistic regression models that provide estimates of the impact of religion on a range of parenting outcomes, after controlling for relevant socioeconomic factors. For the NSFH, I conducted separate analyses of fathers and mothers in an effort to evaluate the charges of "patriarchal" and "stereotypical" behavior directed against conservative Protestant men.

For independent variables, I focused on two religious measures. To construct a measure of theological conservatism, I used a two-item scale based on respondents' agreement with the following statements: (1) "The Bible is God's word and everything happened or will happen exactly as it says" and (2) "The Bible is the answer to all important human problems." The 41% of parents who agreed with both of these statements were coded as theological conservatives—most of whom are conservative Protestants. Because the NSFH did not ask questions about specifically Catholic or Jewish beliefs, I am not able to determine how religious orthodoxy in these two traditions influences parenting using this survey. Parents were also asked how often they attended church. The 35% of parents who indicated that they attend church once a week or more than once a week were coded as weekly attendees.

The four dependent variables are based on the following questions. Parents were asked how often they spanked their child, how often they yelled at their child, and how often they praised and hugged their child. Responses ranged from 1 (*never*) to 4 (*very often*). Parents were also asked how often they participated in a range of one-on-one activities (from reading with their child to taking their child on outings). Responses ranged from 1 (*never or rarely*) to 6 (*almost every day*). I then divided the parents into two groups: those who scored in the top third (or, in the case of praising and hugging, the top half) of the relevant measure and those who did not. (Because spanking and yelling are viewed as negative behaviors, they are reverse-coded.) Thus, Figures 1 through 4 indicate whether theologically conservative fathers and mothers are more or less likely to end up in the top third of the parenting population in the measure under study.

Figure 1 indicates that theologically conservative fathers and mothers are both less likely than other parents to end up in the top third of parents who report never spanking their school-age children. Theologically conservative mothers are 23% less likely to end up in this group than other mothers, and theologically conservative fathers are 25% less likely to end up in this group than other fathers. A similar pattern emerges among the weekly attending parents, where weekly attending mothers are 27% less likely to end up in this group than other mothers, and weekly attending fathers are 25% less likely than other mothers to end up in this group. Thus, Figure 1 indicates that parents who are theologically conservative or weekly attendees are significantly more likely than other parents to resort to spanking when it comes to disciplining their children (see also Ellison et al., 1996). This would seem to offer some evidence in support of the thesis that conservative Protestant parents, and religious parents more generally, are authoritarian parents.

Figure 2 shows that theological conservatism and weekly church attendance is associated with lower rates of yelling on the part of both mothers and fathers of school-age children. Theologically conservative mothers and fathers are, respectively, 46% and 33% more likely to end up in the top third of parents who report never or seldom yelling at their children. Likewise, mothers and fathers who attend church at least once a week are, respectively, 41% and 60% more likely to be in the group of parents who rarely yell. These findings run contrary to the authoritarian thesis, because they show that conservative

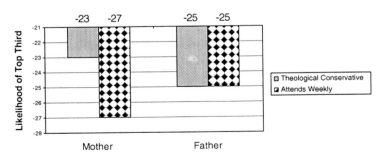

Figure 1. Low levels of parental spanking

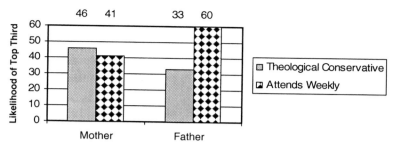

Figure 2. Low levels of parental yelling

Protestant parents, and religious parents more generally, are less likely to resort to the angry verbal outbursts that are associated with abusive, authoritarian parenting.

Figure 3 indicates that theologically conservative and weekly attending parents are significantly more likely to report praising and hugging their school-age children. Specifically, mothers and fathers who are theologically conservative are, respectively, 27% and 29% more likely than other parents to be among the top half of parents who report praising and hugging their children very often. Mothers and fathers who attend church at least once a week are, respectively, 28% and 45% more likely than low-attending parents to end up in this group. These findings also run contrary to the authoritarian thesis, insofar as they show that theologically conservative and high-attending parents are more affectionate with their children than are other parents.

Figure 4 shows that weekly attending parents are significantly more likely to end up among the top third of parents who report the most one-on-one interaction with their school-age children. Specifically, mothers and fathers who attend church at least once a week are, respectively, 37% and 41% more likely than other parents to be highly involved with their children. Theologically conservative fathers, but not mothers, are also 39% more likely than other

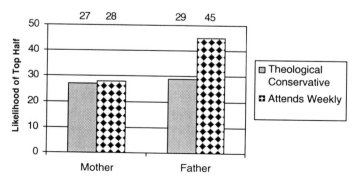

Figure 3. High levels of parental praising and hugging

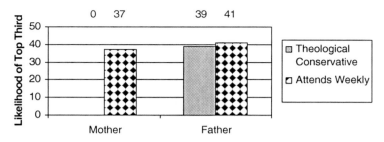

Figure 4. High levels of parental one-on-one interaction

fathers to be highly involved with their children. Thus, Figure 4 provides additional evidence that conservative Protestantism and church attendance are not associated with an authoritarian approach to parenting.

Taken together, Figures 1 through 4 suggest that conservative Protestant parents, as well as religious parents in general, come closer to approximating an authoritative approach to parenting rather than an authoritarian approach. Although they are more likely to use corporal punishment, they are less likely to yell at their school-age children and more likely to praise and hug their children. Theologically conservative fathers are also more likely to be involved in one-on-one activities with their school-age children. Thus, the NSFH suggests that religiously active and theologically conservative parents combine a strict but controlled approach to discipline with a warm, engaged style of parenting in nondisciplinary situations.

Figures 1 through 4 also provide little evidence that conservative Protestant men take a "patriarchal" and "stereotypical" approach to parenting that distances them from their children. Indeed, theologically conservative and high-attending fathers are more involved and expressive with their school-age children than other fathers. Although they spank their children more often than other fathers, they also yell at them less often. Thus, in many ways, high-attending and theologically conservative fathers come closer to approximating the iconic "new man" than do other fathers.

The Survey of Adults and Youth allows us to broaden this empirical portrait of religion and parenting by incorporating detailed religious identity measures for Jews and Catholics, as well as for Protestants. In the logistic regression results that follow, parents who indicate a religious identity are compared with those who indicate no religious identity. I also compare parents who attend religious services weekly with those who do not. The analyses control for a range of factors—from education to race—that might otherwise confound the relationship between religion and parenting. Most of the results examine the likelihood that a parent of a particular religious background will end up in the top third of parents in the relevant outcome.

With respect to independent variables, I relied on parent reports of religious identity and religious attendance. Specifically, parents were asked

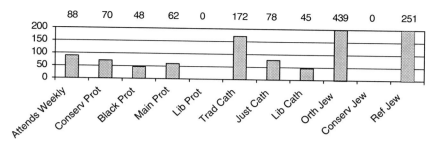

Figure 5. Likelihood of living in intact, married families

to report their religious identity, if any, from "evangelical Protestant" to "Orthodox Jew." I used their self-identifications to classify parents into the following religious groups: conservative Protestant (which includes self-described "evangelical" or "fundamentalist" Protestants), black Protestants, mainline Protestants, liberal Protestants, traditional Catholics, "just" Catholics, liberal Catholics, Orthodox Jews, Conservative Jews, Reform Jews, and no religious identity.[1] Parents who reported attending religious services once a week or more were coded as weekly attendees.

I focus on four dependent variables in SAY. First, I rely on demographic information to determine whether the adolescents in the survey were living in intact, married families at the time of the survey. Second, to tap inter-generational closure, I rely on three questions posed to adolescents asking them if their parents knew their friends and the parents of their friends and had some kind of regular contact with them. The third variable measures the extent to which parents set rules for seven different areas—from television to chores. The fourth variable measures parental involvement in five different domains—from homework help to sports.

Figure 5 indicates that religion is generally associated with family stability. Specifically, parents of adolescents who attend religious services weekly are 88% more likely to live in intact, married families than those who do not attend weekly. Moreover, virtually all parents who indicate a religious identity are more likely to live in intact families compared with parents who indicate no religious identity. Figure 5 indicates that traditional Catholics, Reform Jews, and Orthodox Jews are especially likely to live in intact families. These parents are, respectively, 172%, 251%, and 439% more likely than nonreligious parents to live in intact families. Thus, Figure 5 suggests that religious parents are more likely to offer their children the benefit of growing up in intact, married homes. Figure 5 also indicates that the most orthodox parents from each tradition—that

[1] Parents who identified themselves as "secular Jews" were no different from parents who identified themselves as "no religious identity" in the analyses that follow. Thus, I included secular Jews in the none category, which is also the comparison category. These analyses do not include parents who indicated an Islamic, Mormon, or other religious identity.

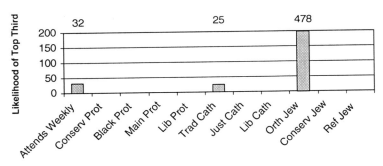

Figure 6. High levels of interaction with children's friends and parents

is, conservative Protestants, traditional Catholics, and Orthodox Jews—score higher than other parents in their religious tradition.

Figure 6 shows that parents of adolescents who attend church or synagogue weekly are 32% more likely than other parents to score in the top third of intergenerational closure. This means that they are more likely to know and have contact with their children's friends and the parents of their children's friends. Likewise, traditional Catholics and Orthodox Jews are, respectively, 25% and 478% more likely to score high on intergenerational closure. Thus, high-attending parents, as well as traditional Catholic and Orthodox Jewish parents, seem better able to monitor and control the social environment of their children. Thus, Figure 6 indicates that attendance and orthodoxy are, once again, associated with a superior parenting environment.

Figure 7 indicates that parents who attend weekly are 29% more likely to register in the top third of parental rule setters. This means that such parents set rules for their adolescents in more domains than other parents. Furthermore, conservative and liberal Protestant parents are, respectively, 24% and 32% more likely than parents with no religious identity to score in the top third of rule setters. By contrast, parents from the Reform Jewish tradition are 51% less likely to end up in this group. This means that high-attending parents,

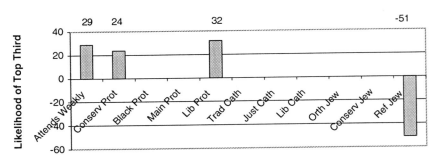

Figure 7. Parents who report lots of rules

conservative Protestant parents, and liberal Protestant parents are more likely than most parents to set rules for their adolescents, whereas Reform Jews are less likely to set rules for their teenagers. Thus, Figure 7 suggests that Protestant parents are more inclined to rely on rules, which is in keeping with the classic Protestant focus on parental authority.

Figure 8 shows that parents who attend weekly are 83% more likely than other parents to score in the top third in the SAY measure of parental involvement. This means that they spend more time in activities like homework help, volunteering with their teenage children, and playing sports with them. Figure 8 also shows that conservative Protestant, black Protestant, traditional Catholic, "just" Catholic, and Orthodox Jewish parents are more involved with their children than nonreligious parents. Once again, orthodox parents are the most involved parents in their respective traditions. Specifically, conservative Protestant, traditional Catholic, and Orthodox Jewish parents are, respectively, 50%, 66%, and 404% more likely to score in the top third of parental involvement.

In general, Figures 5 through 8 reveal that religious orthodoxy and attendance are associated with significantly higher investments in parenting and with better parenting environments. Parents who attend church or synagogue weekly scored consistently higher on every parenting outcome. The most orthodox religious groups—conservative Protestants, traditional Catholics, and Orthodox Jews—were also more likely to score positively on the various dimensions of parental social capital. This means that high-attending and orthodox religious parents are more likely than other parents to provide their children with stable and closed social ties, high levels of social control, and an intense parenting style. It is interesting to note, however, that conservative Protestant parents do seem to approach discipline differently than traditional Catholics and Orthodox Jews. Conservative Protestants rely on rules more, perhaps in keeping with their history of legalistic individualism. By contrast, traditional Catholics and Orthodox Jews rely more on closed social networks; that is, they exercise control over their children by making sure they are associating with the right crowd.

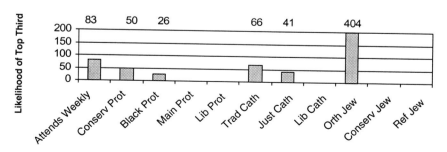

Figure 8. High levels of parental involvement

Conclusions

This chapter suggests that parents who are deeply religious—that is, who hold orthodox religious beliefs and practice their faith regularly—stand a better chance of creating the kind of home environment and practicing the parental virtues that promote character in their children. On average, they make considerable sacrifices to spend time with their children, to discipline their children in a spirit of self-control, to keep their marriages together, to deal with their children in an affectionate way, and to oversee their children's social life. Given the fact that virtually every parenting outcome associated with religious practice and orthodoxy has been shown to have a beneficial effect on children, these sacrifices should translate into higher levels of religious, moral, social, and psychological well-being among children who grow up in religious homes.

The one exception to this trend is that conservative Protestant and high-attending parents are more likely to use corporal punishment, which is generally associated with antisocial behavior and psychological distress (Straus, Sugarman, & Giles-Sims, 1997). On the other hand, other studies suggest that corporal punishment has a negative effect on children only when it is combined with low levels of parental affection and involvement (Baumrind, 1997; Larzelere, 1996). Thus, even on this parenting dimension, the high levels of involvement and affection demonstrated by religious parents may outweigh any negative effects associated with corporal punishment. Thus, I find little evidence to support the thesis articulated by leading family scholars, including John Gottman, that conservative Protestantism—or any other major American religious tradition, for that matter—promotes an authoritarian parenting style characterized by high levels of corporal punishment, low levels of parental warmth, and low levels of parental responsiveness. Indeed, in most respects, highly religious parents, including conservative Protestant parents, come close to approximating the authoritative parenting style generally associated with positive child outcomes.

Indeed, this essay lends additional evidence in support of Coleman's theoretical claim that primordial institutions such as religion play a beneficial role in the lives of children (see also Wilcox, 2002). Undoubtedly, the structural features of primordial religious institutions—for example, their social closure and long-term time horizon—play an important role in cultivating the seedbeds of parental virtue. But their strong collective belief systems also play a central role in motivating parents to sacrifice on behalf of their children. Given their profound interest in transmitting faith from one generation to the next, religious parents recognize that they have to sacrifice so that their children will embrace their faith as adults. Furthermore, dramatic shifts in our culture have spurred conservative Protestants, traditional Catholics, and Orthodox Jews to rededicate themselves to a family-centered way of life, a way of life that they believe is threatened by secularism, commercialism, and immorality. In a word, religious parents—especially orthodox ones—are attempting to shore up faith and family by focusing on their own families.

References

Amato, P. R. (1998). More than money? Men's contributions to their children's lives. In A. Booth & A. C. Crouter (Eds.), *Men in families: When do they get involved? What difference does it make?* (pp. 241–278). Mahwah, NJ: Erlbaum.

Amato, P. R., & Booth, A. (1997). *A generation at risk: Growing up in an era of family upheaval.* Cambridge, MA: Harvard University Press.

Amato, P. R., & Rivera, F. (1999). Paternal involvement and children's behavior problems. *Journal of Marriage and the Family, 61,* 375–384.

Ammerman, N. T. (1997). Golden rule Christianity: Lived religion in the American mainstream. In D. D. Hall (Ed.), *Lived religion in America: Toward a history of practice* (pp. 196–216). Princeton, NJ: Princeton University Press.

Baumrind, D. (1971). Current patterns of parental authority. *Developmental Psychology Monographs, 4,* 1–102.

Baumrind, D. (1997). Necessary distinctions. *Psychological Inquiry, 8,* 176–182.

Capps, D. (1991). Religion and child abuse: Perfect together. Presidential address of the Society for the Scientific Study of Religion. *Journal for the Scientific Study of Religion, 31,* 1–14.

Carlson, M. J. (1999). *Family structure, father involvement and adolescent behavioral outcomes.* Unpublished doctoral dissertation, University of Michigan, Ann Arbor.

Center for Research on Child Wellbeing. 2002. *Survey of Adults and Youth.* Available at http://crcw.princeton.edu/crcw/spy2.htm. Retrieved April 24, 2002.

Chase-Lansdale, P. L., & Pittman, L. D. (2002). Welfare reform and parenting: Reasonable expectations. In M. K. Shields (Issue Ed.), *The future of children: The impact of welfare reform on children.* Los Altos, CA: Center for the Future of Children, The David and Lucile Packard Foundation.

Christiano, K. J. (2000). Religion and the family in modern American culture. In S. K. Houseknecht & J. G. Pankhurst (Eds.), *Family, religion, and social change in diverse societies* (pp. 43–78). Oxford: Oxford University Press.

Coleman, J. (1990). *Foundations of social theory.* Cambridge, MA: Harvard University Press.

Cooksey, E. C., & Fondell, M. M. (1996). Spending time with his kids: Effects of family structure on fathers' and children's lives. *Journal of Marriage and the Family, 58,* 693–707.

Dobson, J. C. (1978). *The strong-willed child.* Wheaton, IL: Tyndale House.

Dobson, J. C. (1992). *The new dare to discipline.* Wheaton, IL: Tyndale House.

Ellison, C. G. (1994). Religion, the life stress paradigm, and the study of depression. In J. S. Levin (Ed.), *Religion in aging and health: Theoretical foundations and methodological frontiers* (pp. 78–121). Newbury Park, CA: Sage.

Ellison, C. G., Bartkowski, J. P., & Segal, M. L. (1996). Conservative Protestantism and the parental use of corporal punishment. *Social Forces, 74,* 1003–1029.

Furstenberg, F. F., Jr. (1988). Good dads–bad dads: Two faces of fatherhood. In A. Cherlin (Ed.), *The changing American family and public policy* (pp. 193–218). Washington, DC: Urban Institute Press.

Gottman, J. M. (1998). Toward a process model of men in marriages and families. In A. Booth & A. Crouter (Eds.), *Men in families* (pp. 149–192). Mahwah, NJ: Erlbaum.

Greven, P. (1988). *The Protestant temperament: Patterns of child-rearing, religious experience, and the self in early America.* Chicago: University of Chicago Press.

Hagan, J., MacMillan, R., & Wheaton, B. (1996). New kid in town: Social capital and the life course effects of family migration on children. *American Sociological Review, 61,* 368–385.

Hewlett, S. A., & West, C. (1998). *The war against parents.* New York: Houghton Mifflin.

Hunter, J. D. (1991). *Culture wars: The struggle to define America.* New York: Basic Books.

Larzelere, R. E. (1996). A review of the outcomes of parental use of nonabusive or customary physical punishment. *Pediatrics, 98,* 824–828.

Maccoby, E. E., & Martin, J. A. (1983). Socialization in the context of the family: Parent-child interaction. In E. M. Hetherington (Ed.), *Handbook of child psychology: Vol. 4. Socialization, personality, and social development* (4th ed., pp. 1–101). New York: Wiley.

McLanahan, S. S., & Carlson, M. J. (2002). Welfare reform, fertility and father involvement. In M. K. Shields (Issue Ed.), *The future of children: The impact of welfare reform on children* (pp. 147–165). Los Altos, CA: Center for the Future of Children, The David and Lucile Packard Foundation.

McLanahan, S. S., & Sandefur, G. (1994). *Growing up with a single parent*. Cambridge, MA: Harvard University Press.

McQuillan, J., & Ferree, M. M. (1998). The importance of variation among men and the benefits of feminism for families. In A. Booth & A. Crouter (Eds.), *Men in families* (pp. 213–226). Mahwah, NJ: Erlbaum.

Popenoe, D. (1996). *Life without father: Compelling new evidence that fatherhood and marriage are indispensable for the good of children and society*. New York: Free Press.

Rubinstein, Y. (2002, April). Happy families. Available at http://www.torah.org/features/par-kids/families.html. Retrieved June 22, 2006.

Smith, C. (1998). *American evangelicalism: Embattled and thriving*. Chicago: University of Chicago Press.

Stark, R., & Finke, R. (2000). *Acts of faith: Explaining the human side of religion*. Berkeley and Los Angeles: University of California Press.

Stenson, J. (1996). *Lifeline: The religious upbringing of your children*. Princeton, NJ: Scepter Press.

Straus, M. A., Sugarman, D., & Giles-Sims, J. (1997). Spanking by parents and subsequent antisocial behavior of children. *Archives of Pediatric Adolescent Medicine, 151*, 761–767.

Sweet, J. A., Bumpass, L. L., & Call, V. (1988). *The design and content of the National Survey of Families and Households* (NSFH Working Paper No. 1). Madison: University of Wisconsin, Center for Demography and Ecology.

Thomson, E., Hanson, T. L., & McLanahan, S. S. (1994). Family structure and child well-being: Economic resources vs. parent socialization. *Social Forces, 73*, 221–224.

Wilcox, W. B. (1998). Conservative Protestant childrearing: Authoritarian or authoritative? *American Sociological Review, 63*, 796–809.

Wilcox, W. B. (2002). Religion, convention, and paternal involvement. *Journal of Marriage and Family, 64*, 780–792.

11 Minding the Children with Mindfulness: A Buddhist Approach to Promoting Well-Being in Children

Julie E. Thomas

Youngstown State University

Lisa A. Wuyek

St. Joseph's Healthcare

The Basic Tenets of Buddhist Philosophy

"Buddhism is a system of thought, a religion, a spiritual science and a way of life which is reasonable, practical and all-embracing. For 2,500 years it has satisfied the spiritual needs of nearly one-third of mankind. It appeals to those in search of truth because it has no dogmas, satisfies the reason and the heart alike, insists on self-reliance coupled with tolerance for other points of view. It embraces science, religion, philosophy, psychology, mysticism, ethics and art, and points to man alone as a creator of his present life and sole designer of his destiny." This statement by the eminent British judge Christmas Humphreys (as cited in Chodron, 1990, p. 195) captures the all-encompassing nature of Buddhism.

To begin with, let us briefly review the founder of this ancient tradition. The historical Buddha, Prince Siddhartha, was born in the sixth century BCE to the royal couple of Kapilavastu of the Sakya clan. In spite of being provided with all the comforts befitting his status, he gave up his princely robes to seek out the solutions to life's fundamental questions. These questions pertained to the nature of life and death and to finding a way out of suffering so that he could teach it to others. Siddhartha studied under the great meditation masters of his time, accomplished all they had taught, and still felt his fundamental questions had not been answered. He then for 6 years sought realizations through asceticism and once again abandoned this path when he realized that all it did was weaken his body. Finally, while sitting under a Bodhi tree in the village of Bodhgaya in northern India, he vowed not to get up until he had attained enlightenment. It is said that after overcoming many internal doubts and external obstacles at dawn of the full moon in the fourth lunar month, Siddhartha succeeded in freeing his mind of all defilement and obscurations and—in realizing his true potential—he became the fully enlightened Buddha (Chodron, 1990). The word *Buddha* is not a personal name. It is a state that we can attain. It means "awakened," "blossomed," "enlightened" (Thurman, 1998).

There are a variety of Buddhist traditions, some of the most prominent being Theravada and the branches of Mahayana Buddhism, which includes Pure Land, Zen, and Vajrayana (Chodron, 1990). Although each tradition has its unique flavor, none of them believes that there is a Creator or God who is separate and apart from the rest of creation. What these traditions do hold in common is that each of us has the seed of the Buddha or the capacity to awaken and attain enlightenment within him or her. Our essential or true nature is referred to as *Buddha nature*. It is considered to be clear and compassionate, like the blue sky. Just as clouds occasionally obscure the sky, similarly our ignorance and misconceptions obscure the clarity and compassion of our Buddha nature (McDonald, 1984). The Four Noble Truths, furthermore, are the cream of the Buddha's teaching. These, Buddhists believe, are the facts of existence and something to be practiced and realized, rather than understood intellectually (Nhat Hanh, 1998). Because a more detailed discussion of the Four Nobel Truths is beyond the scope of this chapter, we will focus on the concept of *Bodhichitta* as an approach to promoting child well-being.

Bodhichitta: The Heart of Transformation

This concept, though hard to translate, is a very important one in Buddhism. *Bodhi* means "awake," "enlightened," or "completely open." *Chitta* means "mind," "heart," or "attitude." (Buddhists do not differentiate between the heart and the mind.) As Chödrön (2001) explains, the completely open heart and mind of bodhichitta is often referred to as "the soft spot, a place as vulnerable and tender as an open wound, raw as a broken heart" (p. 4). It is equated in part with the ability to love and to feel compassion.

Very often in our intimate relationships, as Chödrön (2001) astutely suggests, we tend to put up protective walls made of opinions, prejudices, and other barriers built on a deep fear of being hurt. These walls are further fortified by emotions of all kinds: anger, craving, indifference, jealousy, envy, arrogance, and pride. The soft spot is the opening, the crack in the walls that we erect.

Those who train wholeheartedly in awakening bodhichitta (i.e., the ability to keep our hearts and minds open to tenderness, to experience heartbreak, pain, and uncertainties without shutting down) are called *bodhisattva warriors*. These individuals can then enter challenging situations and interpersonal relationships in order to alleviate suffering. Bodhichitta also refers, in the words of Chödrön (2001), to the willingness to cut through personal reactivity and self-deception, to the dedication to uncovering the basic undistorted energy of bodhicitta and awakening courage and love. Just as alchemy changes any base metal into gold, bodhichitta along with mindfulness can, if we let it, transform any activity, word, or thought into a vehicle for awakening our compassion.

The ability for transformation thus lies within the mind, and the key to the mind is *meditation*. This, in turn, raises the question: What is meditation?

The Role of Meditation

There is a great deal of misunderstanding about meditation. It is not simply sitting in a particular posture or breathing a particular way. It is not spacing out or running away or gazing at your navel. Although the best results may come about when we meditate in a quiet place, we can also meditate while working, walking, or making dinner. Meditation, thus, is the activity of mental consciousness (including feelings, memories, and dreams). It involves one part of the mind observing, analyzing, and dealing with the rest of the mind. It can take many forms: concentrating single-pointedly on an object, understanding a personal problem, generating love for all humanity, praying to an object of devotion, or communicating with our own inner wisdom. Through meditation we can recognize our mistakes and adjust our mind to think and react more realistically and honestly. We learn to have fewer unrealistic expectations of people and things around us and therefore meet with less disappointment; relationships improve and life becomes more stable and satisfying. We develop a sense of spaciousness and clarity about what is going on around us. Transforming the mind or our habits, however, is a slow and gradual process. Whereas there are many short-term gains, the ultimate aim of meditation is to awaken a very subtle level of consciousness and to use it to discover reality, directly and intuitively (McDonald, 1984). This state of mind is the enlightened state. Furthermore, love, compassion, joy, and equanimity are the very nature of an enlightened person. As Thich Nhat Hanh (1998) indicates, they are the four aspects of true love within us and within others. These are referred to as the *four limitless qualities* and the *four immeasurable minds* and are the *aspiration practices* in which a bodhisattva trains.

It is important to note at the outset that these aspiration practices differ from affirmations. Examples of the latter are "I am good and only good things will come to me." They are a way of telling yourself, as Chödrön (2001) succinctly points out, that you are feeling fine in order to hide the fact that you secretly have fears. In aspiration practices, the intent is not to hide our true feelings. It is simply expressing a willingness to open our hearts and move closer to our fears, a willingness that then becomes helpful in increasingly difficult relationships. It helps us to remain steadfast with our experience, whatever it may be.

Let us look at each of these qualities in more detail and see how it relates to parenting.

Bodhisattva Training: Its Relevance to Parenting and Children's Well-Being

Parenting, Myla and Jon Kabat-Zinn (1997) observe, is one of the most challenging, demanding, and stressful—yet one of the most important—endeavors that human beings are faced with. It profoundly influences the minds and hearts and overall well-being of children. Yet, parents often come to this task with very little preparation, training, or understanding of the inner experiences of parenting. Parenting requires one to stay very much in the present moment to sense what may be needed. In other words, it requires one to become mindful. Moreover, when inner resources get depleted, one has to find effective and healthy ways to replenish them without doing so at the expense of one's children. Furthermore, very often despite their best intentions, parents tend to run more or less on automatic pilot to the extent that they are chronically preoccupied and fatigued, as well as invariably too pressed for time to be in touch with the richness of the present moment. These factors may result all too commonly in missed opportunities, resentment, blame, and a sense of isolation and alienation on all sides. Furthermore, the Kabat-Zinns point out that our culture does not place great value on parenting as valid and honored work. This further underscores the reason to have a larger framework to examine and understand the work of parenting. Mindfulness provides framework by which parents can relate to both their inward and outward experiences.

Mindful parenting thus involves keeping in mind what is truly important as we go about the activities of daily living with our children. It means remembering to bring moment-to-moment nonjudgmental attention and openness into one's interactions with children. It is seeing one's children clearly and listening to and trusting one's heart. To cultivate mindfulness requires conscious, sustained effort, attention, and a willingness to be authentic, awake, and attuned (M. & J. Kabat-Zinn, 1997). This process has profound benefits for both children and parents.

An awareness and understanding of the four limitless qualities, which are based on mindfulness, can further deepen our understanding about relationships, including the parent–child relationship.

Love versus Attachment: What's the Difference?

Buddhists refer to *love* as the wish for others and ourselves to be happy and to have the causes of happiness. Love is recognizing others' kindness and faults and, in spite of that, being focused on others' welfare without having an ulterior motive to fulfill our self-interest. Thus, the practice of *maitri* or *loving-kindness* is training to be honest, loving, and compassionate. This practice is first directed to our own self. We begin to cultivate a clear-seeing kindness rather than self-denigration. Cultivating unconditional loving is an important step, without which it is very difficult to genuinely feel unconditional love for others. We first touch the soft spot or the bodhicitta within ourselves, recognize without judgment how we erect barriers between ourselves and others, and discern how we obstruct our innate capacity to love without an agenda (Chödrön, 2001). This type of training is particularly crucial in our role as parents and caretakers.

Love is often confused with what Buddhists refer to as *attachment*. Attachment can exaggerate others' (e.g., our spouses' or children's) good qualities and makes us crave to be with them. As a result, we tend to ride an emotional roller coaster—feeling good when we are with them and miserable without them. Attachment is clearly linked with expectations of what others should be or do: "I love you if ..." Very often, however, these expectations tend to be based on superficial qualities and our own projections and are not realistic (Chodron, 1990).

Moreover, we tend to have fixed concepts of what relationships should be, including romantic relationships and parent–child relationships. We often forget that these concepts are only an opinion. Thus, when others do not live up to our expectations, we are disappointed or angry. Or we may cajole our spouses and children into becoming what we expect them to be or nag or boss them to make them feel guilty. We can also become possessive of our spouse or children. When we are attached, we often do not give others a choice because we feel we know what will make them happy. This tendency leads to further deterioration in our relationships and creates misery within the family. For example, when a child misbehaves, an argument or a quarrel often ensues, as the child has not lived up to the parent's fixed expectation. On the other hand, if a parent were more open and flexible and recognized that her or his child was constantly changing, the parent could be more effective in helping the developing child (Chodron, 1990).

Attachment is thus based on our emotional cravings, which makes us continuously cling to and seek something from others. These cravings, in turn, leave us feeling emotionally tied to the other and obligated to perform a certain role rather than experiencing a sense of freedom to be the persons we are. These cravings are believed to be the result of our ignorance, which tends to obscure the bodhimind. It is also the result of not recognizing the truth of *impermanence and egolessness*.

Compassion versus Burnout: One Does Not Lead to the Other

Whereas love is wishing others to have happiness, compassion is the wish for others to be free from suffering. Genuine compassion, again, is not the same as attachment, as it is not merely an emotional response based on projections and expectations. It is a firm commitment founded on reason and deep concern for the needs of others (Chödrön, 2001). Again, compassion is a critical component of parenting.

For example, the mother's mental state can affect the physical and mental well-being of her unborn child. The central importance of love and compassion continues throughout childhood. A child feels happy and protected when he or she has a caretaker who is open and affectionate. In school, true concern for students' overall well-being by their teachers is as important as their academic education. A doctor's compassion and warmth very often can be curative more so than his or her degree or technical skill (Tenzin Gyatso, 2001). Thus, the connections based on love and compassion play a critical role in a child's and family's well-being, illustrating furthermore how closely our sense of well-being is dependent on each other.

Compassion, however, is considered to be more challenging than loving-kindness, because, as Chödrön (2001) makes clear, it takes courage to open to our own suffering and failures; that is, to recognize our biases and attitudes that tend to create and perpetuate our suffering and that of our spouse and children. It involves a willingness to accept all aspects of ourselves and others, the positive and negative qualities, empathy and cruelty. Genuine compassion, moreover, is a relationship whereby we do not create a separation or distance from those in distress. True compassion strips these away, for only when we know our own darkness are we present in the darkness of others (Chödrön, 2001). This does not mean, however, that one suffers in the same way as the person who is suffering.

Children who grow up with parents who are empathic and feel parental acceptance of a wide range of their behaviors and feelings feel free in turn to express a whole range of feelings themselves. Moreover, they tend to demonstrate caring and concern for those who are hurt or distressed (M. & J. Kabat-Zinn, 1997).

Compassion, moreover, is not the same as "idiot compassion," which Chödrön (2001) describes as the tendency to avoid conflict so that we look good by saying yes when we should say a definite no. It is important to recognize when to say enough and to set clear boundaries in our intimate relationships. It does not mean giving permission to others (including our family members) to walk all over us or to put us down.

The bodhisattvas or compassionate practitioners of the Buddhist path are, according to Tenzin Gyatso (2001), "wisely selfish people" because they recognize that the more one's activities and thoughts are focused and directed to the fulfillment of others' well-being, the greater the personal benefits. This involves recognition of *interdependence*, which according to the Buddhists is a fundamental law of nature.

Joy: The Ability to Rejoice for Others and Ourselves Without Jealousy

Rejoicing in ordinary things is the third limitless quality and is not sentimental or trite. Joy (*mudita*), Chödrön (2001) suggests, helps us drop our complaints and allows us to connect with the inner strength of basic goodness by recognizing the fortunate conditions that are present in our lives. Joy is learning to appreciate what we have in any given moment and to rejoice in our own well-being and our children's laughter and delight and their well-being. Joy is filled with peace and contentment, and, unlike jealousy or envy, we take pleasure in the happiness and good fortune of others. This is again important to us in our role as caretakers, because, in addition to teaching us to celebrate life, joy keeps us from being overwhelmed by suffering. Furthermore, it also helps us to model this quality for our children.

Equanimity or Nonattachment—Not the Same as Detachment

Equanimity (*upeksha*) is a profound quality of mindfulness that cultivates the ability to let go. With equanimity, we can acknowledge that things are as they are, even though we may wish otherwise. Acceptance is an inner orientation that acknowledges that things are as they are, whether they are the way we want them to be or not, no matter how terrible they may be or seem to be at certain moments. It allows us to accept the things that we have no control over, and it allows us to have the courage to remain open in the face of adversity (Bennett-Goleman, 2001). As M. and J. Kabat-Zinn (1997) point out, too many times parents do not accept their children for who they are. These authors also emphasize that when children feel their parents' acceptance for their lovable selves as well as for their difficult, repulsive, and exasperating selves, it frees them to become more balanced and whole. For it is in honoring their whole selves that inner growth and healing can take place. At the same time, the Kabat-Zinns caution that being open and accepting does not mean being naive or passive.

Equanimity can also be referred to as the wisdom of equality, that is, cultivating the vast mind that does not narrow reality into for or against, likes and dislikes, "us" against "them." It involves learning to let a larger perspective emerge by practicing mindfulness. We do our best to soften, stretch our hearts, which allows the barriers to come down and stops us from becoming rigid and inflexible. Equanimity requires learning to extend our kinship to family members and others who suffer the same kind of aggression or craving. We do this because we begin to realize we are all in the same boat and interconnected (Chödrön, 2001).

Equanimity, furthermore, is not emotional indifference. In fact, emotional upheavals are very often the context in which one learns compassion and equanimity. In other words, as parents we learn to engage with the emotional challenges our children present to us. Thus, equanimity is the courage to be fully engaged with whatever comes to our door and growing in the ability to dwell in places that may be emotionally difficult and uncomfortable for us. This quality does not deaden us but paradoxically brings us completely alive. In this way, we evolve from being limited to limitless (Chödrön, 2001).

Impermanence, Non-self, and Interdependence: Their Pertinence
to Parenting

The Buddha taught that everything is impermanent—plants and flowers,
furniture, people, political regimes, feelings, thoughts. Impermanence is the
law of nature, but it does not necessarily lead to suffering. For example, without
impermanence, children would not grow up to be adults. What makes us suffer
is incorrect thinking—*wishing things to be permanent*. Recognizing the reality of
impermanence, on the other hand, teaches us the importance of respecting and
valuing the present moment and fully appreciating what we do have at any
given time (Nhat Hanh, 1998). This is particularly true in our role as parents.
The time we have with our children is limited as they leave when they get
older, or owing to separation or death. Our awareness of the fleetingness of
life teaches us, as the Kabat-Zinns (1997) write, to live in the present moment
as fully as possible with our children. It reminds us to express our love and
affection and to rejoice in our children while feeling at the same time the
certainty of life arising and life passing.

Non-self, or egolessness, is also a very important concept and often misun-
derstood. Non-self is not a doctrine or a philosophy or the advocating of
nothingness or nihilism. Part of the misunderstanding of this concept lies in
the various definitions of the terms *ego* and *self*. If we consider the ego, as
Welwood (2000) does, in its functional domain (i.e., its capacity to organize
and manage both internal and external functioning in the world), we could
consider it as a kind of business manager or agent that masters the way of the
world. We can view it as a theoretical construct or a *fabricated self* that serves
a useful explanatory function. The problem arises when we believe that this
manager *is* who we are. Buddhism considers the fixation on the "I" as the center
around which human life revolves to be extremely problematic. When this
conceptualized "I," based on identifications and conditioned beliefs, becomes
the command center of the psyche—the knower, the controller, and the doer—
this cuts us off from more authentic knowing and actions that arise from our
true nature. Our true nature reveals a vast expanse of being and awareness
that is egoless—not owned or controlled by this bounded, controlling sense of
self (Welwood, 2000).

Furthermore, we often get attached to the feeling of an independent, static,
unchanging, solid, and substantial "I," self, or ego. According to Thurman
(1998), this is the biggest intuitive lie known to human consciousness. This "I,"
as he points out, is not just that we are selfish; we perceive it as the one sure
thing, the *only* thing we can count on. This in turn leads to grasping, anger,
and hatred and a separation from the other, because the bottom line is what
"I" want or desire. Yet when we examine this seemingly objective and easily
identifiable "I," we have a hard time finding it. If the self or "I" does not exist
in the way I think, then I will have to acknowledge that my habitual way of
sensing myself is in error. I begin to recognize that the self or "I" does not
exist apart from others. It is, moreover, constantly changing and fluid.

On the other hand, Buddhists do not deny that there is continuity to our lives. We are like a river that is constantly flowing and changing and is not separate or static, whether within one lifetime or from one lifetime to the next. Hence, Thich Nhat Hanh (1998) somewhat facetiously states that instead of saying "Happy Birthday," what we should really say is "Happy Continuation Day." In that sense there is no birth and death: Life is an endless continuum without beginning and ending.

Non-self or egolessness thus helps us to recognize that happiness is not an individual matter. It helps us to loosen our grip and relax, particularly in our intimate relationships, because we begin to realize the importance of staying open, flexible, and attentive, not only to our own needs but also to those of others. Thus, in a family dispute, egolessness may involve the parent and the adolescent or the spouses recognizing the importance of each understanding the other better rather than insisting that their way is the right and only way. Running away does not necessarily help either, as you realize that you carry the problem with you, and these problems tend to manifest wherever you are.

Interdependence, another key and related concept, is the recognition that nothing comes into being without something else. All events and incidents are so intimately linked with the fate of others that people and human activities cannot be conceived apart from the existence of other people. This is a fundamental law of nature and is very evident in our familial relationships (Nhat Hanh, 1998). Moreover, according to Daniel Stern (as cited in M. & J. Kabat-Zinn, 1997), the small, repeated exchanges that take place between parent and child form the basis for the most fundamental lessons of emotional life. This points to the importance of parents engaging wholeheartedly in this dance of interconnectedness that in turn is vital to their children's well-being.

In some instances, however, strong emotions obscure our ability to see things clearly and to relate effectively. This in turn raises the question as to how we handle difficult emotions such as sadness and anger.

Healing Difficult Emotions

Tulku Thondup (1996) discusses four meditation techniques we can use to strengthen our healing: (1) seeing or visualizing each emotion or problem as an image; (2) thinking of each with its name; (3) feeling the qualities of the healing image; and (4) believing in its effectiveness. These techniques are based on the understanding that thoughts gain power as they take shape in our mind. Seeing makes things vivid and immediate to us. When we name something, we empower it and relate it to ourselves through the power of thought. When we feel something, we become wholly absorbed in it. When we believe in the power and effectiveness of something, it becomes a reality.

For example, when dealing with the emotion of sadness, it is helpful to realistically and calmly acknowledge or be mindful of the feelings that are present—for example, that sadness exists. In other words, rather than engaging in denial or repression, one invites the difficult emotion to surface so that we can release it. This approach may also help locate a place in the body where the feeling is concentrated. We then visualize it, for example, as a dark cloud, which enables our mind to touch this unhealthy point with healing energies. The process of visualizing, feeling, naming, and believing—but not dwelling— in the reality of our sadness helps us get hold of what is wrong so that we can then cure it directly. We also at the same time can visualize healing energy as, for example, light, wind, rain, or a deity. We then feel the power of that presence filling us with energy. Finally, you need to trust that the sadness you experience in this case is in the image of the clouds and that the source of power is indeed present and can heal. Although one has to be realistic about what meditation can really do to change the world around us, it does help us to change our attitudes and feelings, which can give us a measure of peace and calm. This, in turn, may improve the situation or the way others in the family act toward us (Thondup, 1996).

Anger is one of the more deadly enemies that exist within us and can cause a great deal of anguish. It can, as Nawang Gehlek (2001) points out, take different forms, such as impatience, irritation, a tantrum, or hatred. Anger at oneself or self-hatred is seen to develop over time. Initially, it may appear as dissatisfaction, perhaps because of an unfulfilled desire. As the unfulfilled desire grows stronger, our sense of failure and incompetence increases, which turns into anger and then into hatred and self-destructive acts. Part of the reason for getting stuck in hatred is that we believe we have permanently ruined everything for ourselves or we see ourselves as hopelessly bad. As we know from our earlier discussion, though, nothing is permanent, and each of us has the seed of the Buddha nature within us.

Furthermore, our tendency to blame others, particularly in our familial relationships, makes it hard for us to see our role in the situation and to recognize how we may be contributing to it. The antidote to anger, Buddhists believe, is patience—not in the sense of waiting things out so much as refraining from hurting and harming and, in fact, pushing yourself to care for yourself and others. Patience in that sense is not weak, as it is totally engaged, focused, and concentrated. Patience along with enthusiasm can create interest in life and work, which in turn results in joy (Nawang Gehlek, 2001).

To move from anger to patience, however, takes time, particularly as strong negative emotions can be overpowering. For this reason, it is helpful, first, to find out if your anger is valid or not. If you cannot make that determination, the suggestion is to take a diversion such as a walk, sitting in a calm, beautiful space, such as in nature, and allowing your heavy thoughts to lift away. Once the anger has been weakened, there is ample opportunity to do something else (Nawang Gehlek, 2001). Thus, mindfulness or awareness of our feelings of anger is key as it helps us take care of this strong emotion in a manner that is not harmful to us or to other members of our family.

Teaching Children to Live Mindfully

Thich Nhat Hanh (1994) recommends arranging a "breathing room" in the house where we can be alone to practice just breathing and smiling in difficult moments. The little room can be regarded as an embassy of the Buddha. It must be respected and should not be violated by anger or shouting. When a child is about to be shouted at, she or he can take refuge in that room. Neither parent can shout at her or him anymore. The parent or other family members can also use this room when they begin to experience irritation or annoyance or feel a tempest is brewing. This further models for the child the practice of peace and reconciliation. Children, moreover, to calm down when they feel anger, fear, or frustration, can use the following short poem composed by Nhat Hanh:

> Breathing in, I calm body and mind.
> Breathing out, I smile.
> Dwelling in the present moment,
> I know this is the only moment. (as cited in Oshima-Nakade, 1994, p. 107)

Another simple poem by Nhat Hanh (1994) can be shared with children to teach them about breathing mindfully:

> In, out
> Deep, slow
> Calm, ease
> Smile, release
> Present moment, wonderful moment. (as cited in Oshima-Nakade, 1994, p. 177)

In other words, Nhat Hanh believes it is possible for children to participate in mindful living and that they should be invited to be copractitioners.

Storytelling, as Mobi Warren (1994) mentions, is another ancient and universal technique for sharing the teachings of the Buddha. Stories often speak across ages, enabling children and adults to share a common learning experience and explore the many facets of Buddhism together. The Jataka are traditional stories of the past animal lives of the Buddha that provide a wonderful resource for persons interested in using storytelling in their own families.

A Literature Review of Empirical Research into Some Buddhist Concepts

There have been more empirical studies focusing on Buddhism—and elements of Buddhism—than one might initially expect. What follows is a representative sampling of those empirical studies; it is by no means a comprehensive literature review but rather a basic guide to the major areas on which such research has focused thus far.

The notion that one's beliefs and overall psychological state affect one's physical health is by no means new. Borysenko's 1987 book addressed that very topic; she found study after study linking one's beliefs to one's physical health, documenting, for instance, the fact that high levels of chronic stress, as well as chronic feelings of helplessness, contribute to ill health. She reported that such a mental state can throw off one's endocrine balance and "depletes the brain of the vital neurotransmitter norepinephrine, the chemical in our brains that is necessary for feelings of happiness and contentment" (p. 21). Interestingly, chronic feelings of helplessness can be worse than the effects of chronic stress. In the 1970s, researcher and psychologist Jay Weiss set up two groups of rats, each exposed to the same stressor: an electrical shock. The first group could stop the shocks by rotating a wheel; the second group had no control at all. Those rats without control developed ulcers twice as large as those rats that could manipulate the shock (as cited in Borysenko, 1987, p. 21).

Another finding discussed in Borysenko's work relates to the field of psychoneuroimmunology, which explores the interconnections of the body. A group of hormonal "messengers"—neuropeptides—is secreted by the brain, immune system, and nerve cells in several other organs. The areas of the brain controlling emotion reportedly are "particularly rich in receptors for these chemicals." In addition, "the brain also has receptor sites for molecules produced by the immune system alone—the lymphokines and interleukins. What we see, then, is a rich and intricate two-way communication system linking the mind, the immune system, and potentially all other systems, a pathway through which our emotions—our hopes and fears—can affect the body's ability to defend itself" (p. 13).

On a different front, behavior modification also occupies a fairly good-sized part of research on Buddhism. For instance, Shapiro and Zifferblatt (1976) compared and contrasted Zen meditation and behavioral self-management techniques, using both naturalistic observation and experimental analysis, in the hopes of discovering clinical implications. When these authors broke down the process of Zen meditation, they defined it as "a sequence of behaviors involving certain cues and consequences, and thereby under explicit contingency arrangements" (p. 519), which was strikingly similar to the way in which behavioral self-management strategies were defined. Shapiro and Zifferblatt demonstrated the inherent similarity between meditation and behavioral modification. Further, they concluded that a combination of the two techniques could lead to both rehabilitative and preventive benefits.

Mikulas (1978) confirmed the link between Buddhism and behavior therapy and the potential benefits of combining the two:

> Behaviorism minimizes the use of theoretical constructs ... likewise, Buddha avoided metaphysical speculation and generally advised people on the real problems in daily living. Behaviorism focuses on the objective study of observable behaviors; Buddhism encourages each person to observe objectively ... one's own consciousness. Behavior modification ... has given great emphasis to self-control; in Buddhism the person must help himself/herself, especially since there is no savior. Behavior modification procedures, including relaxation training and biofeedback (Brown, 1975), help the client get in touch with and control bodily functions related to physical and psychological health; Buddhist mindfulness practices similarly help the practitioner discriminate subtle cues from the body. (p. 60)

The meditative component of Buddhism has perhaps provoked more research than any other. Lehrer, Sasaki, and Saito focused their 1999 study on Zazen meditation and cardiac variability. Learned control of cardiac variability may be connected with improved autonomic health; there is evidence that those skilled in the practice of slowed breathing and meditation, such as Zen monks, may be able to control their heart rate variability and, in turn, benefit their health. High cardiac variability suggests "more active homeostatic reflexes" (Lehrer et al., 1999, p. 813) and may be an indicator of adaptive capacity. Low variability, however, is often found in those suffering from ill health or psychological conditions, such as panic disorder, generalized anxiety disorder, or depression. The study suggested that learned control over cardiac variability could benefit those with emotional disorders and those with risk factors for cardiac disease. The study also noted that Eastern religious practices and slowed respiration have been proved effective in treating asthma, drug addiction, and hypertension.

In addition, such practices have also proved useful in the treatment of anxiety disorders. One early study that is particularly representative of this research trend is that of Goldman, Dormitor, and Murray (1979). These researchers trained a Zen meditation treatment group in the meditative process for 1 week in the laboratory, and all groups were instructed to keep logs of their experience. Measures of anxiety—including the State-Trait Anxiety Inventory and the Epstein-Fenz Manifest Anxiety Scale—indicated a decrease in anxiety for both the meditation group and the control group. Interestingly, locus of control and gender were not related to outcome results, but volunteer status was, suggesting that motivation influenced outcome.

Shapiro, Schwartz, and Bonner (1998) conducted a similar study in which they examined the effects of mindfulness-based stress reduction. For 8 weeks, participants were involved in a meditation-based stress-reduction intervention. The study's findings suggested that the meditation-based intervention could reduce anxiety and psychological distress, as well as increase empathy and spiritual awareness.

The link between Zen meditation and John Smith's ABC Relaxation Theory was explored in Gillani and Smith's (2001) study. ABC (Attentional Behavioral Cognitive) Relaxation Theory holds that all relaxation techniques are influenced by relaxation states ("R-states"; i.e., Disengagement, Energized, Mental Quiet, Prayerful), relaxation beliefs, and relaxation dispositions, motivations, and attitudes. For instance, "progressive muscle relaxation consistently evokes Disengagement and Physical Relaxation whereas breathing exercises and yoga stretching evoke R-states Energized and Aware" (p. 840). Meditation, the researchers concluded, was connected to R-states Mental Quiet, Mental Relaxation, and Timeless/Boundless/Infinite. The study also noted that "mindfulness Zen," which is a "blend of yoga, breathing, imagery, progressive muscle relaxation, and Zen ... may well be effective for problems such as anxiety with complex etiologies" (p. 845).

Perhaps one of the best-known therapies with a Buddhist connection is Marsha Linehan's Dialectical Behavior Therapy (DBT) for individuals with borderline personality disorder. Linehan herself acknowledges the influence of Eastern spirituality and meditation: "The DBT tenets of observing, mindfulness, and avoidance of judgment are all derived from the study and practice of Zen meditation" (Linehan, 1993, pp. 20–21). In addition, DBT uses metaphors and storytelling—both important components of Buddhism—to teach dialectical thinking and to open up possibilities of new behaviors and new meanings for patients.

DBT also makes great use of mindfulness skills, derived from the meditation skills found in Eastern spirituality. Three "what" and three "how" mindfulness skills are taught early on in therapy. The "what" skills are observing, describing, and participating; the "how" skills, which assist in the performance of the "what" skills, are taking a nonjudgmental stance, focusing on one thing in the moment, and being effective. In therapy, clients are also introduced to the three "primary states" of mind: reasonable mind, emotion mind, and wise mind. To attain wise mind—the integration of the reasonable and emotion minds—Linehan has patients "follow their breath (attend to their breath coming in and out), and after some time try to let their attentional focus settle into their physical center, at the bottom of their inhalation. That very centered point is 'wise mind.' Almost all patients are able to sense this point" (p. 215).

Other studies focus less on therapy and more on psychosocial factors of meditation. For instance, Thananart, Tori, and Emavardhana (2000) conducted a study in Thailand on the psychosocial changes in male adolescents who were participating in a 6-week Buddhist ordination program. The participants were all novices; the authors' goal was to examine what the behavioral and emotional consequences were to those participating in the Buddhist program. A control group was also assessed after 6 weeks in an intense English-language course. It was found that those adolescents in the Buddhist program were more likely to have changes in their behavioral and emotional states that were highly positive and enduring. These results are based on self-report questionnaires and parental questionnaires, which asked each adolescent and his parents to rate the adolescent on psychosocial characteristics (e.g., responsibility, helping behavior, degree of concentration) and on both behavior (e.g., being respectful) and emotional control (e.g., mood, distractibility). The questionnaires were completed at three intervals: prior to the program, after program completion, and at a 6-month follow-up. Thananart et al. found large, statistically significant changes in behavior and emotional control for the adolescents in the Buddhist program; reports from adolescents and parents in that program were equivalent to each other. Although there were behavioral and emotional changes in the control group, they were described as "small, nonsignificant . . . [and] were of much lower magnitude" (p. 289).

Because the adolescents in Thananart et al. were asked to rate themselves, the study raises interesting questions about the effect of Buddhist meditation on self-concept. Haimerl and Valentine (2001) explored that issue. They predicted that practicing meditation would develop several levels of the self-concept, specifically, the interpersonal, intrapersonal, and transpersonal dimensions.

Previous studies suggested that practicing meditation led to an increase in internal locus of control and self-actualization (Hjelle, 1974). Haimerl and Valentine separated their groups of meditators into three categories: prospective (those who had not meditated before the study but planned to); beginner (those who had fewer than 2 years of experience); and advanced (those with more than 2 years). Participants took the Temperament and Character Inventory (TCI) to assess self-concept dimensions. It was found that advanced meditators scored "significantly higher" than prospective meditators on all three self-concept dimensions. "The results ... demonstrated that scores on the intrapersonal, interpersonal, and transpersonal levels of the TCI were a positive function of meditation experience, suggesting that progress in Buddhist meditation leads to significant growth in these components of personality" (p. 44).

One other area of research into Buddhism is the exploration of Buddhism's effect on "counseling behaviors." Leung's 1973 study focused on two such behaviors: "the ability to have empathic understanding of the client and the ability to respond selectively to client statements during a counseling interview" (p. 227). The study looked at meditative deep breathing and external concentration as means of developing these desired counseling behaviors. Twenty undergraduates used as controls received no such training; the 37 participants who were trained in meditative breathing and external concentration significantly increased their abilities in both empathic understanding and selective responding.

These empirical studies thus show evidence that applying some of the Buddhist concepts to one's life can have a positive outcome on a person's well-being, a fact that Buddhist practitioners around the world have known for 2,500 years.

References

Bennett-Goleman, T. (2001). *Emotional alchemy: How the mind can heal the heart.* New York: Harmony Books.

Borysenko, J. (1987). *Minding the body, mending the mind.* New York: Bantam.

Brown, B. B. (Ed.). (1975). *The biofeedback syllabus: A handbook for the psychophysiologic study of biofeedback.* Springfield, IL: Thomas.

Chödrön, P. (2001). *The places that scare you: A guide to fearlessness in difficult times.* Boston: Shambhala.

Chodron, T. (1990). *Open heart, clear mind.* Ithaca, NY: Snow Lion.

Gillani, N. B., & Smith, J. C. (2001). Zen meditation and ABC Relaxation Theory: An exploration of relaxation states, beliefs, dispositions, and motivations. *Journal of Clinical Psychology, 57,* 839–846.

Goldman, B. L., Dormitor, P. J., & Murray, E. J. (1979). Effects of Zen meditation on anxiety reduction and perceptual functioning. *Journal of Consulting and Clinical Psychology, 47*(3), 551–556.

Haimerl, C. J., & Valentine, E. R. (2001). The effect of contemplative practice on intrapersonal, interpersonal, and transpersonal dimensions of the self-concept. *Journal of Transpersonal Psychology, 33,* 37–52.

Hjelle, L. A. (1974). Transcendental meditation and psychological health. *Perceptual and Motor Skills, 39,* 623–628.

Kabat-Zinn, M. & J. (1997). *Everyday blessings: The inner work of mindful parenting.* New York: Hyperion.

Lehrer, P., Sasaki, Y., & Saito, Y. (1999). Zazen and cardiac variability. *Psychosomatic Medicine, 61,* 812–821.

Leung, P. (1973). Comparative effects of training in external and internal concentration on two counseling behaviors. *Journal of Counseling Psychology, 20*(3), 227–234.

Linehan, M. M. (1993). *Cognitive-behavioral treatment of borderline personality disorder.* New York: Guilford.

McDonald, K. (1984). *How to meditate: A practical guide.* Somerville, MA: Wisdom Publications.

Mikulas, W. L. (1978). Four noble truths of Buddhism related to behavior therapy. *Psychological Record, 28,* 59–67.

Nawang Gehlek, R. (2001). *Good life and good death: Tibetan wisdom on reincarnation.* New York: Riverhead Books.

Nhat Hanh, T. (1994). Meditation practices for children. In S. Eastoak (Ed.), *Dharma family treasures: Sharing Buddhism with children* (pp. 97–101). Berkeley, CA: North Atlantic Books.

Nhat Hanh, T. (1998). *The heart of the Buddha's teaching: Transforming suffering into peace, joy and liberation.* New York: Broadway Books.

Oshima-Nakade, M. B. (1994). The Poem. In S. Eastoak (Ed.), *Dharma family treasures: Sharing Buddhism with children* (pp. 107–108). Berkeley, CA: North Atlantic Books.

Shapiro, D. H., & Zifferblatt, S. M. (1976). Zen meditation and behavior self-control: Similarities, differences, and clinical implications. *American Psychologist, 31*(7), 519–532.

Shapiro, S. L., Schwartz, G. E., & Bonner, G. (1998). Effects of mindfulness-based stress reduction on medical and premedical students. *Journal of Behavioral Medicine, 21*(6), 581–599.

Tenzin Gyatso, the Fourteenth Dalai Lama. (2001). *The compassionate life.* Somerville, MA: Wisdom Publications.

Thananart, M., Tori, C. D., & Emavardhana, T. (2000). A longitudinal study of psychosocial changes among Thai adolescents participating in a Buddhist ordination program for novices. *Adolescence, 35,* 285–293.

Thondup, T. R. (1996). *The healing power of mind: Simple meditation exercises for health, well-being and enlightenment.* Boston: Shambhala.

Thurman, A. F. (1998). *Inner revolution: Life, liberty and the pursuit of real happiness.* New York: Riverhead Books.

Warren, M. (1994). Storytelling Dharmas. In S. Eastoak (Ed.), *Dharma family treasures: Sharing Buddhism with children* (pp. 103–106). Berkeley, CA: North Atlantic Books.

Welwood, J. (2000). *Toward a psychology of awakening: Buddhism, psychotherapy, and the path of spiritual and personal transformation.* Boston: Shambhala.

V
The Changing Connections
of Adolescence

12 The Psychobiology of Adolescence

Linda Patia Spear

Binghamton University

In studies of brain development, the focus is often on the rapid growth of the brain before birth and for the first few years thereafter during which the rapidly growing infant begins to interact with and learn about the world. But brain development is a lifelong process. New nerve cells are formed into adulthood (van Praag et al., 2002), and throughout life the brain retains the ability to alter its microstructure based on life experiences (Greenbush, Cohen, & Juraska, 1999; Kleim et al., 1998). For the most part, the magnitude of brain remodeling and plasticity is relatively modest after infancy, with one notable exception: adolescence. Adolescence is a time of rapid physical change that includes periods of abrupt growth and the emergence of secondary sexual characteristics, along with sometimes striking changes in mood and behavior. Although these changes in body appearance and behavior are more obvious, they are no more dramatic than the physiologic changes occurring internally in the adolescent, transitions that include substantial increases in hormone release as well as a dramatic metamorphosis of brain. The magnitude of these brain alterations is difficult to fathom. For instance, it has been estimated that as many as 30,000 connections (synapses) between nerve cells may be lost *per second* during portions of the pubertal/adolescent period across the entire cortical region of primate brain (Rakic, Bourgeois, & Goldman-Rakic, 1994). Before reviewing some of the major characteristics of this brain metamorphosis during adolescence, the stage will first be set by defining adolescence and considering the potential evolutionary underpinnings of this developmental transition.

Adolescence, Behavior, Hormones, and Evolution

What Is Adolescence?

The adolescent period subsumes the gradual transformation from young/ dependency to maturity/independency. This time period is not synonymous with puberty, with the pubertal processes of sexual maturation (including increases in sex hormones and development of secondary sexual characteristics) occurring during a relatively restricted interval within the broader adolescent period. There is no single indicator signaling the beginning or end of adolescence; consequently, precise boundaries of this period are difficult to draw. In humans, the age range from 12 to 18 years is typically considered to be prototypical adolescence, with less agreement in the "gray zones" outside this age range. Some researchers consider the entire second decade as adolescence (Petersen, Silbereisen, & Sörensen, 1996), with ages up to 25 years being considered as late adolescence by others (Baumrind, 1987). There are substantial differences across individuals in the time course of adolescence, with this timing varying with nutritional status (delayed with lower body fat; Frisch, 1984), gender (later in males than females; Savin-Williams & Weisfeld, 1989), as well as sociocultural values and economic conditions (Enright, Levy, Harris, & Lapsley, 1987).

Adolescence Within an Evolutionary Context

The attainment of sexual maturation within a context of more mature, genetically related individuals presents a challenge for species: to avoid inbreeding. Inbreeding is problematic for survival, given that offspring derived from the mating of closely related individuals have lower viability associated with the enhanced prospects for expression of recessive genes that are lethal or that reduce fitness or fecundity (see Bixler, 1992, for discussion). Emigrating from the home area to territory far from genetically related individuals is one strategy to avoid such "inbreeding depression" that has been used successfully by many species (Bixler, 1992; Moore, 1992). Indeed, in the vast majority of species of birds and mammals (including humans in preagricultural societies), male adolescents, female adolescents, or both emigrate away from the home territory prior to reproducing (Keane, 1990; Schlegel & Barry, 1991).

Behaviors that serve to facilitate emigration by sexually emergent adolescents may have been retained by many species to avoid inbreeding and enhance species survival and viability. Some such behaviors may include shifts in social affiliation, increases in risk taking/sensation seeking, and perhaps alterations in vigilance.

Social Behavior

Adolescents from various species exhibit increased social interactions with peers, sometimes along with increases in parental conflicts (e.g., Csikszentmihalyi, Larson, & Prescott, 1977; Primus & Kellogg, 1989; Steinberg, 1989). Shifts in social affiliation may facilitate movement away from the home area, with exploration and emigration sometimes occurring in the company of same-sexed chums. Such increases in social affiliations likely serve other functions as well, for instance, helping adolescents to develop new skills and social support (see Galef, 1977; Harris, 1995).

Risk Taking

In addition to alterations in social affiliations, adolescents from a broad array of species, including humans, also exhibit increases in behaviors broadly classified as risk taking or sensation/novelty seeking (Adriani, Chiarotti, & Laviola, 1998; Trimpop, Kerr, & Kirkcaldy, 1999). An adolescent-associated increase in risk taking has been suggested to serve a number of potentially adaptive functions, such as increasing the probability of reproductive success among males of a variety of species, including humans (Wilson & Daly, 1985). Increases in risk taking and the seeking of novel stimuli would also provide the impetus to explore new and broader areas away from the home, hence facilitating emigration.

Increases in adolescent risk taking, although perhaps an evolutionarily adaptive mechanism for species to avoid inbreeding, may nevertheless occur at considerable cost to individual adolescents. Risk taking and emigration into new regions with uncertain resources and unknown threats are fraught with danger. Even in modern societies where emigration is no longer common, engaging in risk-taking and sensation-seeking behaviors is, well, risky. Indeed, mortality rates are higher during adolescence than at most other ages across a variety of species, including humans (e.g., Crockett & Pope, 1993; Irwin & Millstein, 1992). It could be argued that in human adolescents from modern industrialized societies, these behaviors may reflect more a burden from our ancestral past than behaviors of current adaptive relevance. Yet, moderate amounts of risk taking have been suggested to represent "developmentally appropriate experimentation" for human adolescents, with adolescents who engage in moderate amounts of risk taking being more socially competent than both low and frequent risk takers (Shedler & Block, 1990). Thus, although risk taking may have been (and arguably may still be) beneficial to some extent, high levels of risk taking may be detrimental and even life-threatening, both for the adolescent as well as for others who are affected by the adolescent's behavior.

Eating and Sleeping

Adolescents of a variety of species not only exhibit alterations in social behavior and increased risk-taking and sensation-seeking behaviors but also alterations in other behaviors as well. Associated with the adolescent spurt in growth is an increase in consummatory behavior and metabolic rate, an effect that is evident across a variety of species, including humans (not withstanding cultural pressure for dieting and excessive thinness among female adolescents) (Ganji & Betts, 1995; Nance, 1983; Post & Kemper, 1993). Adolescents not only eat more, but they also sleep less (Levy, Gray-Donald, Leech, Zvagulis, & Pless, 1986). This decline in time spent sleeping is accompanied by a phase delay— a preference for waking and going to bed later than younger individuals (Carskadon, Vieira, & Acebo, 1993). Although undoubtedly influenced in part by sociocultural factors, there appears to be a biological component to this phase shift in that this predilection to stay up late is also evident in adolescents of other species (e.g., rats: Alföldi, Tobler, & Borbély, 1990).

Positive Affect

Adolescents also appear to differ from individuals at other ages in the way in which they respond to motivational stimuli. Relative to younger or older individuals, human adolescents exhibit an increase in negative affect and depressed mood (e.g., Larson & Asmussen, 1991). Adolescents also report experiencing and expecting to experience positive situations as less pleasurable than other aged individuals. Between late childhood and adolescence, the number of reports of feeling happy decline by 50%; even when engaged in the same activities, adolescents judge them to be less pleasurable than do adults (Larson & Richards, 1994). This decrease in the amount of positive affect that they obtain from stimuli may lead adolescents to seek new positive reinforcers via engaging in risk-taking behaviors, including drug taking.

Drug Use

Indeed, some degree of exploratory drug use is normative during adolescence (Shedler & Block, 1990). According to the National Institute on Drug Abuse 2000 Monitoring the Future study, high school seniors report that approximately 50% have tried marijuana/hashish, 62% have smoked cigarettes, and 80% have tried alcohol. Although drug experimentation differs from drug misuse and should not be so construed (Crome, 1999), some adolescent drug use is excessive, with 10% of 8th graders, 21% of 10th graders, and 31% of 12th graders reporting that they were drunk on one or more occasions during the past month.

"Raging Hormones"—Or Are They?

Puberty, or the process of attaining sexual maturation, occurs sometime during the adolescent period. And it has long been assumed that hormonal changes associated with the pubertal process are a major contributor to behavioral change during adolescence. Indeed, puberty is associated with considerable alterations in hormone release, with rising levels of pituitary release of luteinizing hormone (LH) and follicle-stimulating hormone (FSH) precipitating increases in hormones released from the gonads, predominately testosterone from the testes in males and estrogen from the ovaries in females (for review, see Brooks-Gunn & Reiter, 1990). Other hormone changes are also evident, including increases in release of growth hormone (e.g., Brook & Hindmarsh, 1992), as well as a rise beginning prepubertally in a number of adrenal androgens (Parker, 1991). Postpubertal increases in normative levels of the stress-related hormone cortisol have also been reported (see Cicchetti & Walker, 2001) and have been suggested to reflect in part greater vulnerability to or exposure to stressors during adolescence (see Walker & Walder, 2003).

Common folklore has often assumed that the "raging hormones" of adolescence are responsible for many of the age-specific behavioral peculiarities of adolescence. The data to date do not support a strong association. The evidence shows at best only small, direct effects of androgens and estrogens on human adolescent behavior (e.g., Graber & Brooks-Gunn, 1996), including some association of adrenal androgens with particular adjustment problems in adolescence (Susman & Ponirakis, 1997). Even in laboratory animals, with their arguably stronger relationship between hormone levels and behavior than seen in humans (for discussion, see Coe, Hayashi, & Levine, 1988), behavioral change during adolescence may not be necessarily dependent on developmental increases in pubertal hormones (Coe et al., 1988; Smith, Forgie, & Pellis, 1998). It may be too simplistic to search for direct relationships between particular gonadal hormones and specific behaviors. Hormones may interact with psychological variables, social context, and a diversity of changes occurring in the adolescent brain to affect adolescent behavior.

Adolescence: Universality versus Individual Differences

Undergoing the challenging transition from immaturity to maturity is associated with behavioral change along multiple dimensions. Although the emphasis in the preceding discussion has been on general similarities in certain types of adolescent behavior across species, it is obvious that certain adolescent characteristics are unique to humans, to specific cultures, or even to specific individuals. For instance, within human populations, sociocultural factors may influence expression of adolescent characteristic features; in cultures where behavioral change during adolescence is disruptive to other aged individuals, a more tumultuous adolescence may result than in cultures where these age-specific attributes are more congruent with cultural norms and values (Schlegel & Barry, 1991). Even in the same cultural setting, adolescents who undergo the growth spurt and pubertal transformation unusually early or late in adolescence may be exposed to different pressures than adolescents undergoing these transitions more normatively; such timing has been shown to correlate with behavior in a gender-specific manner (for review and discussion, see Graber, Petersen, & Brooks-Gunn, 1996).

Recognizing individual, cultural, and species differences in expression of certain adolescent behaviors need not belie appreciation of particular underlying behavioral features that bear similarity across adolescents of a variety of species. And to the extent that common evolutionary pressures have led adolescents of a variety of species to exhibit certain shared behavioral attributes (e.g., increases in risk taking and affiliation with peers), these behavioral features may reflect similar underlying biological substrates. Indeed, as discussed in the following section, the brains of adolescents from a variety of species undergo dramatic change during adolescence. And as we shall see, brain regions undergoing particularly marked change during adolescence are also the very ones that are critical for influencing common behavioral features of adolescents.

The Changing Adolescent Brain

The adolescent brain is a brain in metamorphosis. As the relatively inefficient brain of the juvenile/child is sculpted during adolescence into the adult brain, many brain connections are lost as some others are added. The magnitude of these changes is considerable. For instance, by the end of adolescence, there is a decline by almost 50% in the average number of connections to neurons in some regions of primate neocortex (Bourgeois, Goldman-Rakic, & Rakic, 1994; Rakic et al., 1994); similar declines in connections (synapses) between neurons have been reported in the human neocortex (Huttenlocher, 1979). This dramatic loss in connectivity bears some similarity to the pruning of nonfunctional synapses seen during the prenatal and early postnatal period after an early overproduction of synapses and has been suggested to reflect plasticity as the brain is restructured to meet the demands of adolescence (Rakic et al., 1994). Yet, the pruning during adolescence may not reflect the culling of nonfunctional synapses but rather the culling of synapses maintained for years and presumably playing some functional role in juvenile brain before their adolescent demise (Spear, 2003). More synaptic connections are not necessarily better; some forms of mental retardation are associated with elevated numbers of synapses (Goldman-Rakic, Isseroff, Schwartz, & Bugbee, 1983).

Adolescent Decline in Brain Energy

Pruning of cortical synapses may be one mechanism by which the relatively inefficient brain of the child becomes sculpted during adolescence into a leaner, more efficient, and less energy-consuming adult brain. Prior to adolescence, stimuli activate relatively broad regions of cortex. Adolescence is associated with a decline in the amount of cortical brain tissue activated during cognitive tasks (e.g., Casey, Giedd, & Thomas, 2000) and an increase in the extent to which left and right cortical regions can process information independently (Merola & Liederman, 1985). The brain utilizes more energy in early childhood than in adolescence and adulthood, with measures reflecting the energy needed for brain activity (glucose or oxygen utilization; blood flow) peaking early in childhood and declining to reach adult levels during adolescence in humans (for review, see Chugani, 1996) as well as other species (e.g., rats: Tyler & van Harreveld, 1942; cats: Chugani, 1994). Changes in the relative size of particular brain regions are evident as well, with adolescent-associated declines in relative volume of "gray matter" (neuronal cell body regions) in some cortical regions contrasting with gender-specific increases in volumes of a number of subcortical brain regions such as the amygdala and hippocampus (Giedd, Castellanos, Rajapakse, Vaituzis, & Rapoport, 1997).

Adolescent Transformations in Prefrontal Cortex and Cognition

The nature of adolescent-associated brain transformations depends on the region of brain under investigation. Among the brain regions undergoing considerable transformation during adolescence across a variety of species are frontal brain regions such as the prefrontal cortex (PFC), a brain region critical for a variety of complex cognitive functions, including the so-called executive function tasks. Increases in frontal activation during a variety of cognitive tasks have recently been reported during adolescence (Luna et al., 2001; Rubia et al., 2000), findings interpreted to suggest that improvements in cognitive function, judgment, and insight during adolescence may be related to maturation of circuitry integrating frontal regions with other brain areas (Luna et al., 2001). Anatomic data provide evidence of structural changes in PFC during adolescence in a variety of species. Relative volume of the gray matter (cellular component) of the PFC declines during adolescence in species ranging from humans (Jernigan, Trauner, Hesselink, & Tallal, 1991) to rats (van Eden, Kros, & Uylings, 1990). Neurons typically communicate with each other at synaptic connections by means of chemical messengers called neurotransmitters; this chemical input to neurons in the PFC undergoes substantial change during adolescence. Among the synapses being pruned during adolescence are those that receive input from an abundant excitatory neurotransmitter, glutamate (Zecevic, Bourgeois, & Rakic, 1989); in contrast with this developmental decline in excitatory input, input to PFC from an important inhibitory neurotransmitter, dopamine (DA), increases during adolescence both in primates (Rosenberg & Lewis, 1994) and rodents (Kalsbeek, Voorn, Buijs, Pool, & Uylings, 1988).

Adolescence, Dopamine, Reward, and Affect

During adolescence, alterations in DA input are evident not only in PFC but in other brain regions as well. The cells releasing DA in frontal brain regions such as the PFC are located some distance away in the core of the brain (in regions called the ventral tegmental area and substantia nigra) and send long projections (called axons) forward to make synaptic connections in a variety of forebrain regions. During adolescence, there are developmental alterations in the functioning of DA systems that project to PFC (called the mesocortical

DA system) as well as those that project to other brain areas, including the striatum (mesostriatal DA system) and limbic regions including the nucleus accumbens and amygdala (mesolimbic DA system). These age-related changes in mesolimbic and mesocortical DA projection systems may be of particular relevance to adolescents given the importance of these systems in modulating social behaviors, risk taking, and the rewarding effects of drugs, novelty, and other reinforcing stimuli (Koob, Robledo, Markou, & Caine, 1993; Le Moal & Simon, 1991).

One way these DA systems are considerably remodeled during adolescence is in terms of a notable decline in DA receptors—that is, receptive regions on the neurons receiving DA input that sense the presence of DA and modify the neurons' activity accordingly. This DA receptor decline is particularly notable in the striatum, where these receptors may decline by one third to one half or more between childhood and adulthood in humans (Montague, Lawler, Mailman, & Gilmore, 1999; Seeman et al., 1987) and rodents (Tarazi & Baldessarini, 2000; Teicher, Andersen, & Hostetter, 1995). Although the data are more mixed for DA receptors in mesolimbic and mesocortical regions, there is some evidence in rodents that a similar, albeit milder, ontogenetic decline may be seen in accumbens (Tarazi & Baldessarini, 2000; Tarazi, Tomasini, & Baldessarini, 1998, 1999), whereas DA receptors in the PFC remain elevated through adolescence, declining only in adulthood (Andersen, Thompson, Rutstein, Hostetter, & Teicher, 2000).

During adolescence, there also appears to be a developmental shift in balance between mesocortical and mesolimbic DA projection systems, systems that generally act in opposition and compete with each other to influence behavior (Whishaw, Fiorino, Mittleman, & Castaneda, 1992). In terms of DA input to PFC, rates of synthesizing and utilizing DA are greater in the PFC of early adolescent than late adolescent rodents (Andersen, Dumont, & Teicher, 1997; Boyce, 1996), a pattern consistent with the suggestion that increases in DA input to PFC during adolescence (Leslie, Robertson, Cutler, & Bennett, 1991; Rosenberg & Lewis, 1994, 1995) may be followed by a compensatory decline in activity of this DA system late in adolescence. The converse ontogenetic pattern was observed in the mesolimbic DA system, with rates of DA synthesis and utilization being lower early in adolescence and increasing later in adolescence (Andersen et al., 1997; Boyce, 1996). This shift in balance might become even more pronounced by exposure to stressors early in adolescence, given that mesocortical DA systems are extremely sensitive to stressor activation relative to mesolimbic and striatal DA systems (e.g., Dunn, 1988).

This suggestion of a developmental shift in DA balance between mesocortical and mesolimbic DA systems, albeit largely derived from basic animal research (see Spear, 2000), could potentially have implications for human adolescents. Mesolimbic brain regions (and their mesocortical modulators) have been implicated in modulating the rewarding effects of drugs, social stimuli, novelty, and other reinforcing stimuli (e.g., Berridge & Robinson, 1998; Koob et al., 1993), with the accumbens paying a particularly critical role in this regard (Schultz, 1998). Functional insufficiencies in so-called mesolimbic

DA "reward pathways" have been linked to a reward deficiency syndrome in humans (Gardner, 1999), with individuals with this syndrome "actively seek[ing] out not only addicting drugs but also environmental novelty and sensation as a type of behavioral remediation of reward deficiency" (p. 82). To the extent that there is a shift in the balance away from mesolimbic DA activity during early adolescence, might young adolescents exhibit a very mild and transient version of a "reward deficiency syndrome"? In this regard, it is interesting that reports of feeling "very happy" drop by 50% between childhood (5th grade) and early adolescence (7th grade), with adolescents also reporting situations as less pleasurable than adults (Larson & Richards, 1994). A transient early adolescent decline in mesolimbic DA activity could potentially provide a partial anatomic substrate for this affective change.

Alterations in Other Neural Systems During Adolescence

Adolescent-associated transformations of brain are not limited to alterations in PFC and in DA projections to this and other forebrain regions. For instance, adolescent rodents exhibit substantially lower rates of utilization of the neurotransmitter serotonin in the accumbens than younger or older animals (Teicher & Andersen, 1999); these findings are of particular interest in that a number of characteristics associated with low serotonin activity—including anxiety, greater negative affect, increased alcohol drinking—are reminiscent of those frequently observed in adolescents.

In contrast with the developmental decline in DA receptors, other neurotransmitter receptors increase substantially during adolescence. For example, cannabinoid receptors undergo considerable maturation during the adolescent period (Belue, Howlett, Westlake, & Hutchings, 1995), with cannabinoid agonists (including the active ingredients in marijuana) inducing clear-cut behavioral effects in late adolescent and adult, but not preadolescent, rodents (Fride & Mechoulam, 1996a, 1996b).

The adolescent amygdala is an area of considerable recent interest. In addition to an old and complex literature implicating developmental changes in the amygdala in the timing of puberty (for review, see Moltz, 1975), there is evidence for substantial alterations in amygdala activity and in its processing of emotional and stressful stimuli during adolescence in both laboratory animals (Kellogg, Awatramani, & Piekut, 1998; Terasawa & Timiras, 1968) and humans (Killgore, Oki, & Yurgelun-Todd, 2001; Thomas et al., 2001). The recent functional magnetic resonance imaging (fMRI) data in humans, however, are as confusing as they are intriguing, with findings that adolescents show less (Killgore et al., 2001), more (Thomas et al., 2001), or equivalent (Pine et al., 2001) left amygdala activation than adults when looking at faces with emotional context. In the latter study, however, differences did emerge between adolescents and adults in the patterns of cortical activation during processing of the emotional stimuli (Pine et al., 2001), emphasizing the potential importance of multiple brain regions in adolescent-associated changes in emotional processing.

Another area that is currently receiving much attention is the cerebellum and the neural circuitry connecting this region with the forebrain. Although functions attributed to the cerebellum have traditionally focused on balance and motor control, lesions of the cerebellum have been shown to disrupt performance on executive function tasks and affect regulation (e.g., Schmahmann & Sherman, 1998). These deficits are more typical of damage to mesocortical and mesolimbic brain regions and may emerge due to lesion-induced disruptions of circuits that interconnect the cerebellum with a number of forebrain regions, including the PFC (Middleton & Strick, 2000, 2001). Although limited developmental data are available at present, expression of this syndrome may intensify around adolescence, with deficits characteristic of this syndrome being more apparent in older than younger individuals within a 3- to 16-year age span (Levisohn, Cronin-Golomb, & Schmahmann, 2000). Data such as these have precipitated substantial interest in potential developmental transformations in cerebellum during adolescence, and relevant findings are likely to accumulate rapidly.

Adolescent Brain Transformations: Implications for Stress Responsiveness, Psychological Functioning, and Lasting Drug Effects

As outlined above, although some of the transformations occurring in adolescent brain involve processes of growth, much is regressive, with a loss of up to one half of the neural connections in some brain regions along with a decline in overall amount of energy used by the brain. Among the brain regions undergoing particularly pronounced transformations are forebrain regions receiving projections from DA neurons, including the PFC, accumbens, and amygdala. And as briefly reviewed earlier in this chapter, these mesocortical and mesolimbic systems include brain circuitry critical for modulating risk-taking and novelty-seeking behaviors as well as attributing rewarding value to a variety of stimuli, including social peers, drugs, and other reinforcers. Given the pronounced developmental changes occurring in these brain regions during adolescence, it would be extraordinary if adolescents did not differ from other aged individuals in their behavior along these dimensions. Indeed, these dramatic adolescent-associated transformations in brain may have evolved in part to facilitate social and risk-taking behaviors serving to foster emigration (and hence minimize inbreeding—discussed earlier), as well as behaviors easing the transition into adulthood.

Stress Responsiveness

There may be a number of ancillary consequences of these neural alterations as well. Many of the brain regions undergoing notable restructuring during adolescence are sensitively activated by stressors (e.g., mesocortical and mesolimbic DA systems; see Dunn, 1988). And as discussed above, any adolescent-associated shift to greater mesocortical than mesolimbic DA transmission early in adolescence would be expected to be exacerbated further by stressors (see Spear, 2000), given the greater sensitivity of the DA projections to PFC (Dunn, 1988). Indeed, adolescence appears to be an unusually stressful life stage for adolescents of a variety of species, not only in terms of the number of stressful events but also with respect to certain physiologic reactions to stressors (for review, see Spear, 2000). Along with this apparent alteration in stress responsiveness, it is interesting that adolescence has also been associated with a relative equalization of certain health risks associated with lower socioeconomic status (West, 1997), including levels of the stress-related hormone cortisol (Lupien, Ménard, Lussier, McEwen, & Meaney, 1998). That is, notable health inequities associated with low socioeconomic status (SES) that are evident during childhood largely disappear from approximately 12 to 19 years of age, reemerging subsequently in adulthood (West, 1997). Interestingly, the adolescent abatement of the SES difference in baseline levels of cortisol seems to be associated with an elevation in cortisol levels of the higher SES group up to levels characteristic of the lower SES group, raising the possibility that the stresses of adolescence could contribute to this transient, adolescent equalization of health.

Psychological Functioning

Another potential ancillary consequence of the developmental transformations in adolescent brain may be age-related alterations in the expression of psychopathology and signs of brain damage. In some cases, symptomatology may partially abate or resolve completely during adolescence. For example, Tourette syndrome tends to improve considerably during adolescence (Kurlan, 1992), and only about 10% of individuals with childhood epilepsy continue to have epileptic episodes in adolescence (see Saugstad, 1994). A similar lessening of symptomatology is seen in rhesus monkeys after early lesions of the orbital frontal area of the brain; lesion-associated deficits evident early in life resolve considerably as animals reach maturity (Goldman, 1971).

More common than a resolution of symptoms during adolescence is the opposite—with consequences of some types of brain damage or other early insults (Flores, Wood, Liang, Quirion, & Srivastava, 1996; Goldman, 1971; Kellogg, 1991; Lipska & Weinberger, 1993b) as well as overt symptomatology of some psychological disorders emerging only during adolescence. For instance, eating disorders show a substantial increase during adolescence, particularly among females (Brooks-Gunn & Attie, 1996). Rates of depressive disorders likewise increase considerably during adolescence, from an incidence rate of clinical depression of about 1% in children to adult-typical incidence rates of 8% by 19 years of age (Kutcher & Sokolov, 1995). A gender difference in depression incidence also emerges during adolescence, with greater prevalence rates in females emerging in adolescence and continuing into adulthood (for review, see Ge, Lorenz, Conger, Elder, & Simons, 1994). Adolescents may vary from individuals of other ages in the neurochemical (Kutcher & Sokolov, 1995) and hormonal (Puig-Antich, 1987) correlates of this depression, although the precise physiologic substrates leading to the increasing incidence of depression among adolescents (particularly female adolescents) remain to be determined.

Perhaps the best-known example of an adolescent-onset disorder is schizophrenia. Despite growing evidence that schizophrenia is a disorder of fetal development (for review, see Bunney & Bunney, 1999) associated with an early disruption in nerve cell migration (Akbarian et al., 1993), typical features of this disorder are not fully expressed until at least adolescence. Researchers have surmised that the sculpting of brain during adolescence may expose underlying neural deficiencies and result in the emergence of symptoms (Lipska & Weinberger, 1993a, 1993b), or that developmental alterations in stress-sensitive forebrain regions may increase vulnerability to stressors, precipitating symptom expression (Bogerts, 1989).

Lasting Effects of Adolescent Drug Use?

Many of the brain regions undergoing developmental change during adolescence are very sensitive to activation by alcohol and other drugs, raising the possibility that use of these substances during adolescence could alter developmental processes ongoing in these brain regions. Several studies in laboratory animals have supported this possibility with adolescent exposure to ethanol. Chronic exposure to ethanol recently has been reported to induce substantially more ethanol-induced brain damage in regions including the PFC (Crews, Braun, Hoplight, Switzer, & Knapp, 2000), greater cognitive disruptions (Osborne & Butler, 1983), and greater sensitivity to later ethanol-induced memory disruptions (White, Ghia, Levin, & Swartzwelder, 2000) in adolescent than adult rats. Human adolescents with alcohol use disorders or alcohol dependence have been reported to exhibit neuropsychological impairments, including memory retrieval deficits (Brown, Topert, Granholm, & Delis, 2000), and to have smaller hippocampal volumes (De Bellis et al., 2000) than comparison subjects. It remains to be determined, however, whether the reported associations between these outcomes and alcohol use are causally related to alcohol exposure or reflect other risk factors and whether such use reflects a greater probability of alcohol problems and alcoholism in adulthood.

Conclusions

Recognizing commonalities in behavior, brain, and physiologic function among adolescents across a variety of species can lead to an appreciation that some fundamental behavioral proclivities of adolescents may be biologically influenced, with evolutionary roots. The dramatic metamorphosis occurring in adolescent brain is particularly pronounced in brain regions critical for modulating the reinforcing qualities of stimuli such as social peers, drugs, and risky situations. A developmental shift in balance of relative activity between these brain regions may lead to a temporary and mild "reward deficiency syndrome," leading adolescents to find typical reinforcers less pleasurable than at other ages and encouraging them to explore new potential reinforcers through risk taking and the use of alcohol and other drugs.

Given the massive metamorphosis of adolescent brain, it seems unrealistic not to expect adolescents to behave differently. Rather than working to modify the fundamental behavioral predispositions of adolescents, a more realistic strategy may be to help them channel their proclivities in ways that enable them to conquer this critical developmental transition while avoiding long-term costs to themselves or others.

References

Adriani, W., Chiarotti, F., & Laviola, G. (1998). Elevated novelty seeking and peculiar d-amphetamine sensitization in periadolescent mice compared with adult mice. *Behavioral Neuroscience, 112,* 1152–1166.

Akbarian, S., Bunney, W. E., Jr., Potkin, S. G., Wigal, S. B., Hagman, J. O., Sandman, C. A., et al. (1993). Altered distribution of nicotinamide-adenine dinucleotide phosphate-diaphorase cells in frontal lobe of schizophrenics implies disturbances of cortical development. *Archives of General Psychiatry, 50,* 169–177.

Alföldi, P., Tobler, I., & Borbély, A. A. (1990). Sleep regulation in rats during early development. *American Journal of Physiology, 258,* R634–R644.

Andersen, S. L., Dumont, N. L., & Teicher, M. H. (1997). Developmental differences in dopamine synthesis inhibition by (±)-7-OH-DPAT. *Naunyn-Schmiedeberg's Archives of Pharmacology, 356,* 173–181.

Andersen, S. L., Thompson, A. T., Rutstein, M., Hostetter, J. C., Jr., & Teicher, M. H. (2000). Dopamine receptor pruning in prefrontal cortex during the periadolescent period in rats. *Synapse, 37,* 167–169.

Baumrind, D. (1987). A developmental perspective on adolescent risk taking in contemporary America. In C. E. Irwin Jr. (Ed.), *Adolescent social behavior and health* (pp. 93–125). San Francisco: Jossey-Bass.

Belue, R. C., Howlett, A. C., Westlake, T. M., & Hutchings, D. E. (1995). The ontogeny of cannabinoid receptors in the brain of postnatal and aging rats. *Neurotoxicology and Teratology, 17,* 25–30.

Berridge, K. C., & Robinson, T. E. (1998). What is the role of dopamine in reward: Hedonic impact, reward learning, or incentive salience? *Brain Research Reviews, 28,* 309–369.

Bixler, R. H. (1992). Why littermates don't: The avoidance of inbreeding depression. *Annual Review of Sex Research, 3,* 291–328.

Bogerts, B. (1989). Limbic and paralimbic pathology in schizophrenia: Interaction with age- and stress-related factors. In S. C. Schulz & C. A. Tamminga (Eds.), *Schizophrenia: Scientific progress* (pp. 216–226). Oxford: Oxford University Press.

Bourgeois, J.-P., Goldman-Rakic, P. S., & Rakic, P. (1994). Synaptogenesis in the prefrontal cortex of rhesus monkeys. *Cerebral Cortex, 4,* 78–96.

Boyce, W. T. (1996). Biobehavioral reactivity and injuries in children and adolescents. In M. H. Bornstein & J. L. Genevro (Eds.), *Child development and behavioral pediatrics* (pp. 35–58). Mahwah, NJ: Erlbaum.

Brook, C. G., & Hindmarsh, P. C. (1992). The somatotropic axis in puberty. *Endocrinology and Metabolism Clinics of North America, 21,* 767–782.

Brooks-Gunn, J., & Attie, I. (1996). Developmental psychopathology in the context of adolescence. In M. F. Lenzenweger & J. J. Haugaard (Eds.), *Frontiers of developmental psychopathology* (pp. 148–189). New York: Oxford University Press.

Brooks-Gunn, J., & Reiter, E. O. (1990). The role of pubertal processes. In S. S. Feldman & G. R. Elliott (Eds.), *At the threshold: The developing adolescent* (pp. 16–53). Cambridge, MA: Harvard University Press.

Brown, S. A., Tapert, S. F., Granholm, E., & Delis, D. C. (2000). Neurocognitive functioning of adolescents: Effects of protracted alcohol use. *Alcoholism: Clinical and Experimental Research, 24*, 164–171.

Bunney, W. E., Jr., & Bunney, B. G. (1999). Neurodevelopmental hypothesis of schizophrenia. In D. S. Charney, E. J. Nestler, & B. S. Bunney (Eds.), *Neurobiology of mental illness* (pp. 225–235). New York: Oxford University Press.

Carskadon, M. A., Vieira, C., & Acebo, C. (1993). Association between puberty and delayed phase preference. *Sleep, 16*, 258–262.

Casey, B. J., Giedd, J. N., & Thomas, K. M. (2000). Structural and functional brain development and its relation to cognitive development. *Biological Psychology, 54*, 241–257.

Chugani, H. T. (1994). Development of regional brain glucose metabolism in relation to behavior and plasticity. In G. Dawson & K. W. Fischer (Eds.), *Human behavior and the developing brain* (pp. 153–175). New York: Guilford.

Chugani, H. T. (1996). Neuroimaging of developmental nonlinearity and developmental pathologies. In R. W. Thatcher, G. R. Lyon, J. Rumsey, & N. Krasnegor (Eds.), *Developmental neuroimaging: Mapping the development of brain and behavior* (pp. 187–195). San Diego, CA: Academic Press.

Cicchetti, D., & Walker, E. F. (2001). Stress and development: Biological and psychological consequences. *Development and Psychopathology, 13*, 413–418.

Coe, C. L., Hayashi, K. T., & Levine, S. (1988). Hormones and behavior at puberty: Activation or concatenation? In M. R. Gunnar & W. A. Collins (Eds.), *Minnesota Symposia on Child Development: Vol. 21. Development during the transition to adolescence* (pp. 17–41). Hillsdale, NJ: Erlbaum.

Crews, F. T., Braun, C. J., Hoplight, B., Switzer, R. C., III, & Knapp, D. J. (2000). Binge ethanol consumption causes differential brain damage in young adolescent rats compared with adult rats. *Alcoholism: Clinical and Experimental Research, 24*, 1712–1723.

Crockett, C. M., & Pope, T. R. (1993). Consequences of sex differences in dispersal for juvenile red howler monkeys. In M. E. Pereira & L. A. Fairbanks (Eds.), *Juvenile primates: Life history, development, and behavior* (pp. 104–118). New York: Oxford University Press.

Crome, I. B. (1999). Treatment interventions—Looking towards the millennium. *Drug and Alcohol Dependence, 55*, 247–263.

Csikszentmihalyi. M., Larson, R., & Prescott, S. (1977). The ecology of adolescent activity and experience. *Journal of Youth and Adolescence, 6*, 281–294.

De Bellis, M. D., Clark, D. B., Beers, S. R., Soloff, P. H., Boring, A. M., Hall, J., et al. (2000). Hippocampal volume in adolescent-onset alcohol use disorders. *American Journal of Psychiatry, 157*, 737–744,

Dunn, A. J. (1988). Stress-related activation of cerebral dopaminergic systems. *Annals of the New York Academy of Sciences, 537*, 188–205.

Enright, R. D., Levy, V. M., Jr., Harris, D., & Lapsley, D. K. (1987). Do economic conditions influence how theorists view adolescents? *Journal of Youth and Adolescence, 16*, 541–549.

Flores, G., Wood, G. K., Liang, J.-J., Quirion, R., & Srivastava, L. K. (1996). Enhanced amphetamine sensitivity and increased expression of dopamine D2 receptors in postpubertal rats after neonatal excitotoxic lesions of the medial prefrontal cortex. *Journal of Neuroscience, 16*, 7366–7375.

Fride, E., & Mechoulam, R. (1996a). Developmental aspects of anandamide: Ontogeny of response and prenatal exposure. *Psychoneuroendocrinology, 21*, 157–172.

Fride, E., & Mechoulam, R. (1996b). Ontogenetic development of the response to anandamide and Δ-(9)-tetrahydrocannabinol in mice. *Developmental Brain Research, 95*, 131–134.

Frisch, R. E. (1984). Body fat, puberty and fertility. *Biological Reviews, 59*, 161–188.

Galef, B. G., Jr. (1977). Mechanisms for the social transmission of food preferences from adult to weanling rats. In L. M. Barker, M. Best, & M. Domjan (Eds.), *Learning mechanisms in food selection* (pp. 123–148). Waco, TX: Baylor University Press.

Ganji, V., & Betts, N. (1995). Fat, cholesterol, fiber and sodium intakes of US population: Evaluation of diets reported in 1987–88 Nationwide Food Consumption Survey. *European Journal of Clinical Nutrition, 49*, 915–920.

Gardner, E. L. (1999). The neurobiology and genetics of addiction: Implications of the reward deficiency syndrome for therapeutic strategies in chemical dependency. In J. Elster (Ed.), *Addiction: Entries and exits* (pp. 57–119). New York: Russell Sage Foundation.

Ge, X., Lorenz, F. O., Conger, R. D., Elder, G. H., Jr., & Simons, R. L. (1994). Trajectories of stressful life events and depressive symptoms during adolescence. *Developmental Psychology, 30*, 467–483.

Giedd, J. N., Castellanos, F. X., Rajapakse, J. C., Vaituzis, A. C., & Rapoport, J. L. (1997). Sexual dimorphism of the developing human brain. *Progress in Neuro-Psychopharmacology & Biological Psychiatry, 21*, 1185–1201.

Goldman, P. S. (1971). Functional development of the prefrontal cortex in early life and the problem of neuronal plasticity. *Experimental Neurology, 32*, 366–387.

Goldman-Rakic, P. S., Isseroff, A., Schwartz, M. L., & Bugbee, N. M. (1983). The neurobiology of cognitive development. In P. H. Mussen (Ed.), *Handbook of child psychology: Vol. 2. Infancy and developmental psychobiology* (pp. 281–344). New York: Wiley.

Graber, J. A., & Brooks-Gunn, J. (1996). Transitions and turning points: Navigating the passage from childhood through adolescence. *Developmental Psychology, 32*, 768–776.

Graber, J. A., Petersen, A. C., & Brooks-Gunn, J. (1996). Pubertal processes: Methods, measures, and models. In J. A. Graber, J. Brooks-Gunn, & A. C. Petersen (Eds.), *Transitions through adolescence: Interpersonal domains and context* (pp. 23–53). Mahwah, NJ: Erlbaum.

Greenbush, W. T., Cohen, N. J., & Juraska, J. M. (1999). New neurons in old brains: Learning to survive? *Nature Neuroscience, 2*, 203–205.

Harris, J. R. (1995). Where is the child's environment? A group socialization theory of development. *Psychological Review, 102*, 458–489.

Huttenlocher, P. R. (1979). Synaptic density of human frontal cortex: Developmental changes and effects of aging. *Brain Research, 163*, 195–205.

Irwin, C. E., Jr., & Millstein, S. G. (1992). Correlates and predictors of risk-taking behavior during adolescence. In L. P. Lipsitt & L. L. Mitnick (Eds.), *Self-regulatory behavior and risk taking: Causes and consequences* (pp. 3–21). Norwood, NJ: Ablex.

Jernigan, T. L., Trauner, D. A., Hesselink, J. R., & Tallal, P. A. (1991). Maturation of human cerebrum observed in vivo during adolescence. *Brain, 114*, 2037–2049.

Kalsbeek, A., Voorn, P., Buijs, R. M., Pool, C. W., & Uylings, H. B. M. (1988). Development of the dopaminergic innervation in the prefrontal cortex of the rat. *Journal of Comparative Neurology, 269*, 58–72.

Keane, B. (1990). Dispersal and inbreeding avoidance in the white-footed mouse, *Peromyscus leucopus*. *Animal Behaviour, 40*, 143–152.

Kellogg, C. K. (1991). Postnatal effects of prenatal exposure to psychoactive drugs. *Pre- and Peri-Natal Psychology, 5*, 233–251.

Kellogg, C. K., Awatramani, G. B., & Piekut, D. T. (1998). Adolescent development alters stressor-induced Fos immunoreactivity in rat brain. *Neuroscience, 83*, 681–689.

Killgore, W. D. S., Oki, M., & Yurgelun-Todd, D. A. (2001). Sex-specific developmental changes in amygdala responses to affective faces. *Neuroreport, 12*, 427–433.

Kleim, J. A., Swain, R. A., Armstrong, K. A., Napper, R. M. A., Jones, T. A., & Greenbush, W. T. (1998). Selective synaptic plasticity within the cerebellar cortex following complex motor skill learning. *Neurobiology of Learning and Memory, 69*, 274–289.

Koob, G. F., Robledo, P., Markou, A., & Caine, S. B. (1993). The mesocorticolimbic circuit in drug dependence and reward—A role for the extended amygdala? In P. W. Kalivas & C. D. Barnes (Eds.), *Limbic motor circuits and neuropsychiatry* (pp. 289–309). Boca Raton, FL: CRC Press.

Kurlan, R. (1992). The pathogenesis of Tourette's syndrome: A possible role for hormonal and excitatory neurotransmitter influences in brain development. *Archives of Neurology, 49*, 874–876.

Kutcher, S., & Sokolov, S. (1995). Adolescent depression: Neuroendocrine aspects. In I. M. Goodyer (Ed.), *The depressed child and adolescent: Developmental and clinical perspectives* (pp. 195–224). Cambridge: Cambridge University Press.

Larson, R., & Asmussen, L. (1991). Anger, worry, and hurt in early adolescence: An enlarging world of negative emotions. In M. E. Colten & S. Gore (Eds.), *Adolescent stress: Causes and consequences* (pp. 21–41). New York: Aldine de Gruyter.

Larson, R., & Richards, M. H. (1994). *Divergent realities: The emotional lives of mothers, fathers, and adolescents.* New York: Basic Books.

Le Moal, M., & Simon, H. (1991). Mesocorticolimbic dopaminergic network: Functional and regulatory roles. *Physiological Reviews, 71,* 155–234.

Leslie, C. A., Robertson, M. W., Cutler, A. J., & Bennett, J. P., Jr. (1991). Postnatal development of D1 dopamine receptors in the medial prefrontal cortex, striatum and nucleus accumbens of normal and neonatal 6-hydroxydopamine treated rats: A quantitative autoradiographic analysis. *Developmental Brain Research, 62,* 109–114.

Levisohn, L., Cronin-Golomb, A., & Schmahmann, J. D. (2000). Neuropsychological consequences of cerebellar tumour resection in children: Cerebellar cognitive affective syndrome in a paediatric population. *Brain, 123,* 1041–1050.

Levy, D., Gray-Donald, K., Leech, J., Zvagulis, I., & Pless, I. B. (1986). Sleep patterns and problems in adolescence. *Journal of Adolescent Health Care, 7,* 386–389.

Lipska, B. K., & Weinberger, D. R. (1993a). Cortical regulation of the mesolimbic dopamine system: Implications for schizophrenia. In P. W. Kalivas & C. D. Barnes (Eds.), *Limbic motor circuits and neuropsychiatry* (pp. 329–349). Boca Raton, FL: CRC Press.

Lipska, B. K., & Weinberger, D. R. (1993b). Delayed effects of neonatal hippocampal damage on haloperidol-induced catalepsy and apomorphine-induced stereotypic behaviors in the rat. *Developmental Brain Research, 75,* 213–222.

Luna, B., Thulborn, K. R., Munoz, D. P., Merriam, E. P., Garver, K. E., Minshew, N. J., et al. (2001). Maturation of widely distributed brain function subserves cognitive development. *Neuroimage, 13,* 786–793.

Lupien, S. J., Ménard, C., Lussier, I., McEwen, B., & Meaney, M. J. (1998, November). *Basal morning cortisol levels and cognitive function in children from low and high socioeconomic status.* Paper presented at the annual meeting of the Society for Neuroscience, Los Angeles, CA.

Merola, J. L., & Liederman, J. (1985). Developmental changes in hemispheric independence. *Child Development, 56,* 1184–1194.

Middleton, F. A., & Strick, P. L. (2000). Basal ganglia and cerebellar loops: Motor and cognitive circuits. *Brain Research Reviews, 31,* 236–250.

Middleton, F. A., & Strick, P. L. (2001). Cerebellar projections to the prefrontal cortex of the primate. *Journal of Neuroscience, 21,* 700–712.

Moltz, H. (1975). The search for the determinants of puberty in the rat. In B. E. Eleftheriou & R. L. Sprott (Eds.), *Hormonal correlates of behavior: A lifespan view* (pp. 35–154). New York: Plenum.

Montague, D. M., Lawler, C. P., Mailman, R. B., & Gilmore, J. H. (1999). Developmental regulation of the dopamine D1 receptor in human caudate and putamen. *Neuropsychopharmacology, 21,* 641–649.

Moore, J. (1992). Dispersal, nepotism, and primate social behavior. *International Journal of Primatology, 13,* 361–378.

Nance, D. M. (1983). The developmental and neural determinants of the effects of estrogen on feeding behavior in the rat: A theoretical perspective. *Neuroscience and Biobehavioral Reviews, 7,* 189–211.

Osborne, G. L., & Butler, A. C. (1983). Enduring effects of periadolescent alcohol exposure on passive avoidance performance in rats. *Physiological Psychology, 11,* 205–208.

Parker, L. N. (1991). Adrenarche. *Endocrinology and Metabolism Clinics of North America, 20,* 71–83.

Petersen, A. C., Silbereisen, R. K., & Sörensen, S. (1996). Adolescent development: A global perspective. In K. Hurrelmann & S. F. Hamilton (Eds.), *Social problems and social contexts in adolescence* (pp. 3–37). New York: Aldine de Gruyter.

Pine, D. S., Grun, J., Zarahn, E., Fyer, A., Koda, V., Li, W., et al. (2001). Cortical brain regions engaged by masked emotional faces in adolescents and adults: An fMRI study. *Emotion, 1,* 137–147.

Post, G. B., & Kemper, H. C. G. (1993). Nutrient intake and biological maturation during adolescence. The Amsterdam Growth and Health Longitudinal Study. *European Journal of Clinical Nutrition, 47,* 400–408.

Primus, R. J., & Kellogg, C. K. (1989). Pubertal-related changes influence the development of environment-related social interaction in the male rat. *Developmental Psychobiology, 22,* 633–643.

Puig-Antich, J. (1987). Sleep and neuroendocrine correlates of affective illness in childhood and adolescence. *Journal of Adolescent Health Care, 8,* 505–529.

Rakic, P., Bourgeois, J.-P., & Goldman-Rakic, P. S. (1994). Synaptic development of the cerebral cortex: Implications for learning, memory, and mental illness. In J. van Pelt, M. A. Corner, H. B. M. Uylings, & F. H. Lopes da Silva (Eds.), *Progress in brain research: Vol. 102. The self-organizing brain: From growth cones to functional networks* (pp. 227–243). Amsterdam: Elsevier.

Rosenberg, D. R., & Lewis, D. A. (1994). Changes in the dopaminergic innervation of monkey prefrontal cortex during late postnatal development: A tyrosine hydroxylase immunohistochemical study. *Biological Psychiatry, 36,* 272–277.

Rosenberg, D. R., & Lewis, D. A. (1995). Postnatal maturation of the dopaminergic innervation of monkey prefrontal and motor cortices: A tyrosine hydroxylase immunohistochemical analysis. *Journal of Comparative Neurology, 358,* 383–400.

Rubia, K., Overmeyer, S., Taylor, E., Brammer, M., Williams, S. C. R., Simmons, A., et al. (2000). Functional frontalisation with age: Mapping neurodevelopmental trajectories with fMRI. *Neuroscience and Biobehavioral Reviews, 24,* 13–19.

Saugstad, L. F. (1994). The maturational theory of brain development and cerebral excitability in the multifactorially inherited manic-depressive psychosis and schizophrenia. *International Journal of Psychophysiology, 18,* 189–203.

Savin-Williams, R. C., & Weisfeld, G. E. (1989). An ethological perspective on adolescence. In G. R. Adams, R. Montemayor, & T. P. Gullotta (Eds.), *Biology of adolescent behavior and development* (pp. 249–274). Newbury Park, CA: Sage.

Schlegel, A., & Barry, H., III (1991). *Adolescence: An anthropological inquiry.* New York: Free Press.

Schmahmann, J. D., & Sherman, J. C. (1998). The cerebellar cognitive affective syndrome. *Brain, 121,* 561–579.

Schultz, W. (1998). Predictive reward signal of dopamine neurons. *Journal of Neurophysiology, 80,* 1–27.

Seeman, P., Bzowej, N. H., Guan, H.-C., Bergeron, C., Becker, L. E., Reynolds, G. P., et al. (1987). Human brain dopamine receptors in children and aging adults. *Synapse, 1,* 399–404.

Shedler, J., & Block, J. (1990). Adolescent drug use and psychological health: A longitudinal inquiry. *American Psychologist, 45,* 612–630.

Smith, L. K., Forgie, M. L., & Pellis, S. M. (1998). The postpubertal change in the playful defense of male rats depends upon neonatal exposure to gonadal hormones. *Physiology and Behavior, 63,* 151–155.

Spear, L. P. (2000). The adolescent brain and age-related behavioral manifestations. *Neuroscience and Biobehavioral Reviews, 24,* 417–463.

Spear, L. P. (2003). Neurodevelopment during adolescence. In D. Cicchetti & E. F. Walker (Eds.), *Neurodevelopmental mechanisms in psychopathology* (pp. 62–83). Cambridge: Cambridge University Press.

Steinberg, L. (1989). Pubertal maturation and parent-adolescent distance: An evolutionary perspective. In G. R. Adams, R. Montemayor, & T. P. Gullotta (Eds.), *Advances in adolescent behavior and development* (pp. 71–97). Newbury Park, CA: Sage.

Susman, E. J., & Ponirakis, A. (1997). Hormones–context interactions and anti-social behavior in youth. In A. Raine, P. A. Brennan, D. P. Farrington, & S. A. Mednick (Eds.), *Biosocial bases of violence* (pp. 251–269). New York: Plenum Press.

Tarazi, F. I., & Baldessarini, R. J. (2000). Comparative postnatal development of dopamine D(1), D(2) and D(4) receptors in rat forebrain. *International Journal of Developmental Neuroscience, 18,* 29–37.

Tarazi, F. I., Tomasini, E. C., & Baldessarini, R. J. (1998). Postnatal development of dopamine and serotonin transporters in rat caudate-putamen and nucleus accumbens septi. *Neuroscience Letters, 254*, 21–24.

Tarazi, F. I., Tomasini, E. C., & Baldessarini, R. J. (1999). Postnatal development of dopamine D1-like receptors in rat cortical and striatolimbic brain regions: An autoradiographic study. *Developmental Neuroscience, 21*, 43–49.

Teicher, M. H., & Andersen, S. L. (1999, October). *Limbic serotonin turnover plunges during puberty.* Poster session presented at the annual meeting of the Society for Neuroscience, Miami Beach, FL.

Teicher, M. H., Andersen, S. L., & Hostetter, J. C., Jr. (1995). Evidence for dopamine receptor pruning between adolescence and adulthood in striatum but not nucleus accumbens. *Developmental Brain Research, 89*, 167–172.

Terasawa, E., & Timiras, P. S. (1968). Electrophysiological study of the limbic system in the rat at onset of puberty. *American Journal of Physiology, 215*, 1462–1467.

Thomas, K. M., Drevets, W. C., Whalen, P. J., Eccard, C. H., Dahl, R. E., Ryan, N. D., et al. (2001). Amygdala response to facial expressions in children and adults. *Biological Psychiatry, 49*, 309–316.

Trimpop, R. M., Kerr, J. H., & Kirkcaldy, B. (1999). Comparing personality constructs of risk-taking behavior. *Personality and Individual Differences, 26*, 237–254.

Tyler, D. B., & van Harreveld, A. (1942). The respiration of the developing brain. *American Journal of Physiology, 136*, 600–603.

van Eden, C. G., Kros, J. M., & Uylings, H. B. M. (1990). The development of the rat prefrontal cortex: Its size and development of connections with thalamus, spinal cord and other cortical areas. In H. B. M. Uylings, C. G. van Eden, J. P. C. De Bruin, M. A. Corner, & M. G. P. Feenstra (Eds.), *Progress in brain research: Vol. 85. The prefrontal cortex: Its structure, function and pathology* (pp. 169–183). Amsterdam: Elsevier.

van Praag, H., Schinder, A. F., Christie, B. R., Toni, N., Palmer, T. D., & Gage, F. H. (2002). Functional neurogenesis in the adult hippocampus. *Nature, 415*, 1030–1034.

Walker, E. F., & Walder, D. (2003). Neurohormonal aspects of the development of psychotic disorders. In D. Cicchetti & E. F. Walker (Eds.), *Neurodevelopmental mechanisms in psychopathology* (pp. 526–544). Cambridge: Cambridge University Press.

West, P. (1997). Health inequalities in the early years: Is there equalisation in youth? *Social Science and Medicine, 44*, 833–858.

Whishaw, I. Q., Fiorino, D., Mittleman, G., & Castaneda, E. (1992). Do forebrain structures compete for behavioral expression? Evidence from amphetamine-induced behavior, microdialysis, and caudate-accumbens lesions in medial frontal cortex damaged rats. *Brain Research, 576*, 1–11.

White, A. M., Ghia, A. J., Levin, E. D., & Swartzwelder, H. S. (2000). Binge pattern ethanol exposure in adolescent and adult rats: Differential impact on subsequent responsiveness to ethanol. *Alcoholism: Clinical and Experimental Research, 24*, 1251–1256.

Wilson, M., & Daly, M. (1985). Competitiveness, risk taking, and violence: The young male syndrome. *Ethology and Sociobiology, 6*, 59–73.

Zecevic, N., Bourgeois, J.-P., & Rakic, P. (1989). Changes in synaptic density in motor cortex of rhesus monkey during fetal and postnatal life. *Developmental Brain Research, 50*, 11–32.

13 Elders and Sons

David Gutmann

Northwestern University Medical School

The Powers of the Patriarchs

Across history and cultures, senior men—fathers, grandfathers, and tribal elders—have borne a great responsibility: the disciplining, the socializing, in effect, the humanizing of the young, particularly young males. For if young males are to be of any value to society or to themselves, at least two major transitions have to take place: They have to separate in the psychological sense from their mothers, so that they can join their peers and fathers in the work of men—the work that is typically done away from home and on the periphery of their communities. Even more difficult, young men, designed by evolution to take life, have to tame their potentially murderous aggression and predation, turning it from antisocial to prosocial ends. Senior men have until recently played vital roles in sponsoring these critical reversals. But it is no secret that—particularly under the influences of urbanity, modernity, and egalitarian political cultures—this corrective power of the elders has dwindled to the point where they can no longer maintain their own prestige, much less graduate young males to responsible manhood. Elder power is still observed in those few enclaves, usually religious and military, that uphold traditional virtues, teachings, and practices. But for the most part, the power to inspire, tame, and discipline the young, and especially young men, has passed out of the elders' hands, even out of the parents' hands, and has been largely conceded to the peer group, to the media that cater to its hectic fashions, and to charismatic "celebrities."

These changes, probably unparalleled in the history of our species, have many sources; but a major contributing factor has to do with the loss of totemic, moral, and social powers by senior males—including fathers. The nature of such powers, as well as their acquisition and employment by traditional elders, will be considered in the first half of this chapter. In the second half, we will review the consequences, particularly for the psychosocial maturation of young males, that follow the disempowering of the patriarchs.

The Animistic Conception of Power

Folk-traditional societies maintain different ideas about the sources and the proper uses of personal powers. Nevertheless, each such society conceives of itself as an island in a sea of vital but also dangerous energies. These forces reach the shores of the familiar, pragmatic world, but they stretch far beyond, into the disquieting realm of gods, devils, ghosts, and quasi-divine ancestors. So conceived, power gets into the mundane world, to sustain human beings, their societies, and the forms of nature, but it does not originate there; and the major task of the community is to ensure—through its rituals and consecrated individuals—a constant supply of the vital essence.

In the South Seas, the spiritual power that penetrates and enlivens the human realm was known as *Mana*. Although such vital forces, supernatural in their origin, are known by many names, and across a wide range of usually preliterate societies, I will use that term throughout. In the course of this brief essay, I will refer to a number of other beliefs and practices that have wide and often universal distribution across cultures. All of these, along with many others, are noted in Donald Brown's *List of Human Universals* , a compendium based on a comprehensive review of the available ethnographic evidence (Brown, 1991).

Like the idea of *soul*, Mana mingles the material and the insubstantial. Viewed animistically, Mana is stuff: It can be sold, transferred, or captured. In the traditional mind, Mana is not impersonal but exists in a dynamic relationship with mortals: It has intention and meaning in regard to those human agents and actions that defend against, acquire, or deploy such totemic powers.

The Power Bringers

In the folk-traditional society, ordinary individuals cannot by their own private efforts collect or generate the portions of Mana necessary to secure themselves and their dependents against the threats of hunger, illness, accident, or failure in warfare. Mana is always sacred, and it is always double-faced: It can uplift, energize, vivify, but it can also blast and destroy those targeted by its possessor, or those without proper ritual protection against it.

Such two-faced power is collected by those *unordinary* representatives of the community who can live on the borderline of the sacred, endure the toxic blast of its powers, fend off such evil aspects, while passing neutralized, benign Mana into the community for collective purposes. The power bringers are the true heroes of the traditional community: They are the unordinary figures who can overlap the ultimate sources of Mana, buffer and survive its toxic aspect, while allowing its good influences to flow into and sustain the pragmatic, daily world. Without these human bridges, the pragmatic world would be without substance, a place of shadows.

Generally, those who traffic on the dangerous cusp between the community and the supernatural need to comprise within themselves the paradoxical aspects of the power that they would manage. As metaphors of the double-edged powers, they must be both destructive and benevolent, in some cases both male and female, or both humble and arrogant. In short, the power bringers are, in some important sense, *strangers*: They inhabit this world and yet possess special qualities that distinguish them from the ordinary run of humanity. Across traditional cultures, the usual power brokers and collectors are the magician-chief, the warlock or sorcerer, the warrior who captures the power of enemy dead, and the hunter who slays the totem animal. For some cultures, the power bringer is what we would call the "madman" or the "epileptic," both of whom occupy space in this world but seem to speak the language of another.

Power Bringers: The Elders

Across traditional communities, old men are more likely than young men to meet the job description of the power bringer. Thus, older men are moving into the country of the stranger: Although still alive in this world, they will soon join the ancestors in their special power shed of the mythic past. They wear the uncanny aura of the corpse that they will become and so are naturally suited to deal with the ultimate strangers, the gods. Their milder temperament also fits the elders to deal with divinity. Young men are bold: Their task is to capture strength from enemy and from nature. Like Prometheus, who stole fire from the gods but ended up being eternally punished, young men might challenge and offend the supernaturals: They could bring down divine wrath rather than divine favor. But the milder senior man, who has taken on the androgyny of later life, is more apt to beseech their Mana from the gods, rather than fight them for it. Thus, my older informants among the Galilean Druse (the *Aqil*) would present a yearning, self-effacing, implicitly feminine face toward Allah. But the special access to God that their humble prayers won for them also earned them great social prestige, as patriarchal rulers. Their wrinkles were not the stigmata of age and weakness, but dueling scars from God. Clearly, their submissive face toward God is a precondition for their haughty face toward their juniors. Thus, even as they humble themselves before Allah, the Druse Aqil play the autocratic patriarch to their sons and wives, who knew them as the "Allah of the house." In this concrete instance, we see in microcosm the power-bringing role of the traditional elder: Because he touches Allah in the *Hilweh*, the prayer house, within his own house the Druse Aqil personifies Allah for others. Submitting to great power, he has gained some portion of it for himself and can pass it on to the deserving.

Incidentally, women are usually exempt from this particular calculus of power. As women bear within themselves the mystery, the power to create life, they are already, in men's eyes, divinely empowered and taboo. They have their own Mana stream and their own ways of bathing in it. They do not have to concern themselves with the power-grabbing, power-enticing games of men. It is mainly the older women, who have become barren but also "Manly-Hearted," who engage in the male-dominated rituals of power management. For the purposes of this chapter, I will stick with the masculine power themes.

Later, we will consider some of the rituals through which the power of patriarchal elders and fathers is passed on to their sons. But before we address the evolution of sons into fathers, and the role of strong elders in furthering that maturation, we should first consider the special trajectories of male development and the special challenges that males are called upon to face.

Separating from the Mother: The Father's Role

Erik Erikson once remarked (personal communication) that the central issue in human development is the unique vulnerability and protracted dependency of the human child. Any viable human group takes this special fragility into account. Thus, despite differences in their child-rearing goals, most societies maintain common understandings about the generic needs to be addressed by any child care regime. They recognize that, to thrive in body and in spirit, the vulnerable child must be assured of two kinds of parental nurturance: He or she must have assurance, first, of physical security and, second, of emotional security.

There is also a general recognition, across our species, that the same parent cannot provide both kinds of security, and that males and females have to be prepared, early in life, for their special child-rearing assignments. The child's physical security ultimately depends on activities carried out far from home: warfare, hunting (including the hunt for business and clients), and the cultivation of distant tillage. Men are generally assigned the task of providing physical security on the perimeter, not because they are more privileged, but because they are more expendable. Thus, in the hard calculus of species survival, there is typically an oversupply of males: One man can inseminate many females even into late adulthood, but women, on the average, can gestate only one child every 2 years or so during their relatively brief window of fertility. The surplus males, those over the number required to maintain replacement population levels, can be assigned to the dangerous, high-casualty "perimeter" tasks by which they underwrite the physical security of their families and communities. "When it comes to slaughter, you do not send your daughter" is one of our most predictable human rules; and there are very good reasons for it: Viable societies do not, during its brief season of fertility, expose the vulnerable uterus to machine-gun fire. Thus, women are generally assigned to secure areas, there to supply the formative experiences that give rise to emotional security in children.

This is a large generalization, but the cross-cultural record bears it out. Thus, George Murdoch's review (1935) of ethnographic data from 224 subsistence-level societies, indicates that any productive or military activity requiring a protracted absence from the home—hunting, trapping, herding, deep-sea fishing, offensive warfare—is performed almost exclusively by males. Activities carried out closer to home—dairy farming, erecting and dismantling shelters, harvesting, tending kitchen gardens and fowl—are sometimes exclusive to men, more often exclusive to women, but are in most instances carried out by both sexes. Hearthside activities, however, particularly those having to do with preserving and preparing food, as well as the care of young children, are almost exclusively the province of women.

Incontestably, men are creatures of the perimeter; and while they start out swaddled to their mothers in the home, they must eventually leave the nest for the extradomestic world. Later, as fathers they must reenter the home domain and eventually work out a schedule of movement, often on a daily basis, between some version of the periphery and the intimacies of the domestic zone.

Here, then, is a central paradox of masculine development: The "Golden Cord" tie to the mother is crucial at the beginning of life, but it must, at some critical point in development, be severed. The boy who persists beyond the proper season as a mother's son will be psychologically vulnerable to the otherwise routine separations inherent in living: In youth, he is at risk to become an addicted delinquent; as a father, he is likely to be an envious sibling rather than a "good-enough" parent to his own children; and as a spouse, his wife will be drained by his chronic neediness and put at risk by his violent rages toward women. In later life—if he makes it that far—he is at risk to be a depressed psychosomatic cripple and a drain on the health system.

But bear in mind that even in traditional settings, the patriarchs—fathers or elders—do not get to influence a son's development until the end of the neonatal period. At the outset of life, the mother–child merger (a continuation in psychological terms of the intrauterine umbilical link) is primary, and the father, as during the prenatal period, plays only an incidental role.

As Niles Newton has pointed out, the mother can devote herself almost exclusively to child care because she herself is being nurtured, "mothered," by her husband (Newton, 1973). The father's task is not to share the mother's chores but to maintain a protected, neutral zone, one in which his gratified and secure spouse, under the sway of the hormone oxytocin, can bring about the mother–child bond that fosters the infant's capacity for what Erik Erikson has called *basic trust* (Erikson, 1952). Assured of a stable maternal base, one that he can trust to be there even when he strays away, the infant can begin to explore his world and even provoke change in it. Thus, human development proceeds by paradox and in a dialectical fashion: The almost exclusive mother–child symbiosis that is so crucial in the first months of life prepares the baby for the period of early autonomy, when the child will practice psychological and physical separation from the mother. Alternating these out-migrations with episodes of rapprochement and return, the infant begins to develop the resources that will support his later, more protracted forays away from the mother.

In effect, the nursing mother sponsors the son's first steps toward separation from the mother, as well as his future alliance with the father.

Through her offices, the boy reaches a point where the "I–Thou" distinction appears, and the father—like himself, an entity distinct from the mother—acquires the tonus of reality, of unremitting and trustworthy "out there-ness." Thus, as the postnatal arrangement of the family—father tends mother, mother tends baby—begins to phase out, the traditional father, the father whose patriarchal qualities distinguish him from the mother, becomes a psychological constant, a fixed presence in the emotional life of the child. Such a loving but stern father spreads an umbrella of security under which the son can temporarily shelter, even as he continues to develop a distinct sense of self. Thus, the patriarchal father becomes, in the proper season, what the psychoanalysts call a "transitional object"—a kind of psychological halfway house. He provides a secure way station on the son's psychological voyage away from the mother and allows that risky but necessary evolution to go forward.

Becoming the Father's Son

Besides loosening the dependent connection to the mother, sons must—again with the aid of fathers and elders—cut their explicitly erotic tie to her and control the fierce competitive aggression that goes with it. After all, as Desmond Morris reminds us, fathers and sons are not too far away (on the evolutionary timescale) from a shared primate heritage of violent male-to-male, father-to-son rivalry for sexual possession of the reproductive females—including the son's mother and the father's mate (Morris, 1994). As a species, we are protected, by the incest taboo, against the wilder expressions of that competition, but the primate tendencies that we naked apes inhibit in our muscles are still conserved inside our heads, taking the form of potent and even murderous "Oedipal" dreams and fantasies.

The first generation of psychoanalysts—those reared in the more "tragic," European view of human affairs—carried out pioneering studies of this Oedipal theme in child development. In their account, little boys, charged high with untested illusions of omnipotence, are driven early on to challenge the strength and sexual prerogatives of the father. However, if they come up against true patriarchs, fathers who are neither antagonized nor intimidated by a small son's enmity (and who even relish him for his bold spirit, as a "chip off the old block"), these same little boys are quickly—and with real relief on their part—introduced to some basic propositions of the masculine reality principle: "You are not big, powerful, and supremely competent; instead, you are small, puny, and laughably unready. However, you show promise for better things. If you pay him proper respect, your powerful but concerned father will help you escape from your unfortunate condition." In other words, "If you can't lick 'em, join 'em." When (and if) they hear that message, young sons give up infantile, grandiose fantasies of co-opting the father's powers by violence in favor of a disciplined filial apprenticeship, built on identification with him and his powers. From then on, the boy's self-esteem will be based increasingly on experiences of real mastery, rather than hectic Superman fantasies. The quondam mother's son has switched allegiances and is ready for a psychological rebirth, as the father's son.

In short, having closed out his Oedipal rivalry, the son can unambiguously respect, emulate, and even love his father. He can willingly take instruction from him and from other authoritative elders: uncles, older brothers, teachers, and coaches. He has entered the so-called latency period—the time when the boy, no longer distracted by powerful appetites or fears, can devote himself to the rapid acquisition of new learning and new skills. The school, the team, the congregation of male peers becomes a world in its own right, a setting for new growth that supersedes the family.

The boy's post-Oedipal affection for the mother is, paradoxically, a consequence of the psychological separation that the father has helped to bring about. When boys no longer desperately *need* their mothers, they can more truly love them—and women in general—in a relatively uncomplicated, full-hearted way.

Rites de Passage: The Elders and the Pubertal Transition

Thus, latency entails an eased relation with both parents, but it is only a temporary calm before the storm of puberty shakes up the psychological status quo. The adolescent personality is subject to tectonic shocks as the pubertal body, marching to its own genetic drums, stumbles toward sexual maturity and adult physical powers. There is no mind–body dichotomy in human psychology, and the swelling, surgent, erotic body sends shock waves through the whole psychological system. Boys are rather suddenly tumbled, whether they like it or not, into adult bodies, even as their primitive emotional states are revived. For example, the Oedipal struggle with the father may be replayed, but now in a more dangerous form. The pubertal boy's challenge to the father is now more than the grandiose delusion of a physical and mental midget; now it is backed up by a body that can be quicker and more powerful than the slackening physique of his middle-aged father.

The disorderly transition to puberty is, of course, universal, but aggravated adolescent rebellion is not. Most viable cultures have developed fairly standard ways of ensuring that the biopsychological shake-up does not lead to individual pathology or to social crisis. Particularly in traditional societies, the whole age grade of male elders is mobilized to back up the father's threatened authority, to confirm the boy in the ways of men. The biological father helps the son achieve the first vital separation, from the mother; the collective fathers are mobilized to bring about the second great separation: from the family as a whole, and later from the physical precincts of the home community itself.

Typically, the collectivity of elders arranges an ordeal, a *rite de passage*, through which the pubertal son is consecrated to totemic sponsors and to the various patriarchal ideals. These rituals take as many forms as there are distinct cultures, but they always mark the point at which the elders pass on Mana to the young candidates for power. Like Mana itself, the rituals for acquiring it are double-natured. Before power can be exercised freely and even sadistically (as in war), it must be endured masochistically: The candidate must suffer, passively, the power that he would later use in an active way.

Thus, the young candidates for manhood must pay heavy dues of pain and terror to the elders and fathers before they are allowed to join their company as acknowledged men. The ordeals of passage can range from penile subincision with cowry shells as practiced by Papuan natives, to the Bar Mitzvah ceremonial of Orthodox Jews, and even to the doctoral oral exams of our graduate students. But in all cases, the young candidates are exposed to a trial, usually under the intense, critical gaze of the assembled elders, who monitor them for signs of weakness.

Leo Simmons reports many examples of the older man's awesome taboo powers, and the transmittal of these to adolescent males, the most striking coming from the Hottentot of Africa, among whom the old men initiate young men, who have passed their early life among women, into manhood (Simmons, 1945). The climax of the rite comes when the elder urinates on the candidate, who receives the urine with joy, rubbing it vigorously into his skin. His old sponsor then tells the candidate that he will increase and multiply and that his beard will soon grow. Clearly, in this case, even the urine of the old man has heroic power, the Mana of the patriarchal phallus through which it passed. In the most concrete sense, it "marinates" the young man with the powers of the senior man, thus bringing the lad in his turn to manhood.

Halfway around the world, the Sioux adolescent moved, by means of the vision quest, through privation to manly power. Carrying with him nothing of society's protection, the Sioux candidate went into the desert without food, clothing, or arms. He starved, he froze at night, he sang his death song. Finally, when he was delirious, his totem animal appeared to him in a vision and instructed him concerning his future powers and their proper use. Returning to the tribe, the candidate would submit his vision to the elders, who would evaluate it for authenticity. If in their judgment the vision represented a true communication from the immortals, then the candidate's ritual suffering had paid off: He knew his totem lodge, his place within the community, and the appropriate rituals that would link him with the power of his totemic sponsor. He was empowered to be a warrior, to join the rituals of his lodge, and to court women.

John Whiting and Irving Child found that the severity of the ordeal varied, across cultures, with the length of the breast-feeding period (Whiting & Child, 1953). The ritual marks a significant passage away from the mother; and as late weaning results in a strong maternal bond, a stringent ordeal is required to break it. By this token, if the boy is too visibly frightened or tearful, then he has not passed the test. He is still his mother's crybaby, a "mama's boy," and he has not been reborn—as a father's son and junior colleague—into the company of men. But if the lad endures with some grace and fortitude, then he has begun to make it as a man. He has been reborn as a son of the collective elders, as a protégé of taboo guardians, and as an age-grade brother of the initiates who have endured, with him, their people's basic training. Bonded to him through the ritual, these totem brothers represent the portion of the community that will go with him on his journeys beyond its borders.

Typically, a culture is founded on an origin myth: a story of how the people, at a time of trial and supreme danger, were sponsored, rescued, and made special by the intervention of usually supernatural but unquestionably *unordinary* beings. We think of Moses among the Israelites; Washington at Valley Forge; and nowadays, Martin Luther King Jr. and David Ben-Gurion. The typical puberty ritual replays this drama in a summarized form: Like his people in the origin myth, the candidate is in a liminal condition, a state of depletion, and if he survives the ordeal, it is because he too—like his people in the founding myth—has received strength from a totemic sponsor. As a young child, he became for a time the son of his father; now, as a youth, he becomes—through the ritual and the sponsorship of the elders—the protégé of some favoring deity whose "medicine" or Mana will provide the candidate with luck and protection on the road. He has been admitted into the Mana stream; receiving it as a boy, he can grow into a man. Later, as a father, he can pass on its effusions to his own sons.

Finally then, the rite of passage extends, for the candidate, the range of paternity: Now it reaches beyond the biological father, beyond the community elders, to include the ultimate fathers—the spiritualized ancestors and the gods. Knowing that he is securely tapped into the Mana stream, that he has assured resources, the son can look toward mating, marriage, and fatherhood for himself. Like his father before him, he can court a woman, he can attempt the frightening but exciting voyage into her body, and—secure in his manhood—he can return to the domestic world, the mother's world that he has recently "escaped." But this returnee is not a homesick and troublesome child; knowing that he can leave the domestic world and survive, he comes back as a mate and as a providing father. He can live again among the "mothers," and he can turn a woman into a mother, without becoming her child, without collapsing back into the "mama's boy" condition.

His passage into young manhood has inoculated the son against the dangers of the female in the world and in himself; and it also inoculates the community against masculine violence. In his passage toward manhood, the son's aggression has been transformed: Through the civilizing offices of his father, as backed up by the communal elders and totemic fathers, the son's potentially antisocial aggression has been given a positive, prosocial sign. In effect, the boy's aggression follows the general line of masculine evolution: As he moves his sights beyond the mother's domain, his aggressive potentials track with him and find new, nondomestic targets. From now on, his enemies will not be found in his own house, extended family, or significant community; these precincts he will preserve and protect as demilitarized zones, enclaves where his children and other dependents can feel secure. His enemies, if any, will come to him from outside his own house, from beyond the communal periphery—or he will forage beyond his own settlements to find them.

The Ebbing of Mana

In the city, and under conditions of modernity, there takes place a profound change in the social conception of power. It tends away from the animistic view and toward the modern, economic view. Under contemporary conditions, we lose the powerful idea of the bicameral distribution of power, of a distinction between a pragmatic world that is chronically bereft of vital powers and a numinous realm that is in all aspects taboo, composed entirely of Mana. As we have seen, under the sway of animism, the imbalance is compensated for, corrected by sanctified agents like the elders. These serve as bridgeheads between the two realms, transferring power from the Mana source to worthy recipients in the pragmatic, Mana-deprived world. But under contemporary conditions of urbanism and modernity, we override the distinction between the natural and supernatural domains, as well as the distinction between divine power and "ordinary" vigor. Under modern conditions, the energy that powers human affairs is believed to originate in persons, weapons, raw materials, and markets rather than gods; and its management calls for technical expertise, common sense, and hard-won experience rather than ritual preparation. The modern world needs mechanics and scientists to handle physical power; economists and politicians to handle social power; generals to handle war-making powers; but it has little need of sanctified power bringers. The Mana stream that spills from the gods, through elders and other anointed agents, into strong fathers and their respectful sons, dries up. Men can no longer count on the automatic transfer, across the generations, of the patrimony of power. Self-esteem is no longer guaranteed by anointed lineage, by ritual, or by filial obedience, but has to be rediscovered in each generation. Cut off from their charisma, the aged now show the repulsive side, rather than the awesome visage, of the stranger. The elders become "the aged," or cute but befuddled "Grandpa"; and fathers—when they stick around at all—become "Pops." Rather passive, unassuming, and often henpecked, they are transformed, at the very height of parenthood, into a version of the androgynous postparental father.

Absent Fathers and Mothers' Sons

Thus, in our times, legions of boys grow up under the ambiguous familial arrangements that are rapidly replacing normal fatherhood in America. What, as David Blankenhorn has asked, is the likely fate of sons who come of age without strong elders, without fathers, or with fathers who are little more than androgynous, ineffectual clones of the mother (Blankenhorn, 1995)? At least one consequence is clear: In the absence of compelling fathers, the mother's presence fills not only the outer domestic frame but also the son's interior psychic space. These fatherless boys are not likely, in their proper season, to win true psychological distance from their mothers.

True enough, the sons of patriarchal fathers can also be flawed, and precisely along the fault lines that gender feminists have catalogued: Besides being priggish, philistine, and unable to cry, they are distressingly prone to patronize and even diminish women. But despite all his pretensions, the patron is also a protector; and fathers' sons are for the most part reliable defenders of their mothers, wives, girlfriends, and daughters. When killing is the argument, they fight the men who come from the outside to hurt or kill their women and kids. Strong mothers build secure homes; fathers and fathers' sons maintain secure neighborhoods. But unfathered sons deploy their aggression indiscriminately: They can be murderously aggressive within the home as well as outside of it. They are prone to abuse, damage, and even kill their aging relatives, their wives, their kids, and their neighbors. Unfathered sons waste the homes and the neighborhoods that elders, mothers, fathers, and fathers' sons had once built.

As feminists have documented, men can be brutal toward women; but in this charge, no distinction is made between fathers' sons and mothers' sons. True enough, fathers' sons, the progeny of patriarchy, do show a talent and an appetite (particularly in wartime) for killing other men; but indiscriminate masculine violence against women is a guaranteed side effect not of patriarchy but of the unbuffered matricentric family. Without reliable fathers to oversee their timely separation from Big Mama, mothers' sons are left with little recourse but to hack violently at the Golden Cord.

Thus, boys who cannot achieve true psychological distance from the mother fall back instead on unreliable substitutes: physical distance and social distance. Physical distance they achieve by flight: from the mother's home to the streets, to the fighting gangs that rule them and, at the end of the day, to the all-male fraternity of the penitentiary. Social distance they gain through violence: Unable to finally split from the mother, they provoke her—through criminality, addictions, sexual exploitation, and physical threats—to the point where she bars them from her decent house. They use violence to drop out of the mother's cultural world, and off her scale of values; and once evicted to the streets, they turn to booze and drugs for the transient comfort that they can no longer take (nor expect to receive) from their mother's hand.

Through such desperate means, poorly fathered sons demonstrate—to their peers, to their mothers, and to themselves—that they are truly Men, and not needy little mamas' boys. Finally, by their physical violence and verbal raps on women they try, ineffectually, to kill off the unrelinquished "woman"—the psychic afterimage of the mother—within themselves.

Finally, in the absence of reliable fathers and elders, young men try to create their own puberty rituals. They self-administer their own ad hoc *rites de passage* and initiations. In the fathering society, the tests of manhood are administered by the male elders; and these trials are basic training for discipline, lawfulness, and manly productivity. But in the tests conducted by unsupervised gangs of adolescent males, the candidate usually proves his courage by violating some law of nature or of society; and the ritualized passage is not into responsible manhood but too often into the world of the criminal. Such rituals of passage are still preserved in the Mafia, where candidates for full membership as "made men" qualify by "making their bones"—that is, by killing a man. Thus, instead of curbing antisocial rebellion, the puberty rites of criminal and teenage gangs are designed to validate it.

Finally, then, despite their well-documented shortcomings, patriarchs—elders and fathers—are the best means our species has devised for managing the gravest threat to organized social life: male, particularly young male, violence. In our American case, the streets of the cities are being "Beirutized" by violence from sons without fathers and with only rudimentary superegos.

Mothers' Sons in Later Life

I do not mean to imply that all unfathered sons are fated to be wife abusers, muggers, or dopeheads. The majority manage to separate from the mother, at least in the social sense. For the most part, they seek and often find wives motherly enough to substitute for the actual mom. They marry women who will welcome a husband's special need for spousal mothering. In effect, these hungry men rediscover and re-create in their wives the "rapprochement" mother that they have never really relinquished (see Mahler & Pine, 1975). That is, they find in the nurturing wife an equivalent of the birth mother who delighted in their first exploratory steps but who also coaxed them back into her maternal embrace.

Such pleasant women can convert the mothers' sons—for a while at least—into good citizens and even into provident fathers. So long as the wife remains willing to mother her spouse, these at-risk men are reasonably content. But these mothers' sons are put at risk in the later years, when their postparental wives, who have raised their kids and paid their species dues, begin to defect from the mothering way (see Gutmann, 1994). These postparental wives still share the husband's bed and get the meals out, but their feelings toward their husbands have subtly changed: They are still willing to be the wife, but not the husband's mother. This straying older wife has imposed, on the husband, a separation from the mothering person that he himself has never before encountered, expected, or initiated.

This belated separation from "mom"/wife can precipitate, in vulnerable men, the much-debated "midlife crisis": To hold the wife's attention, to keep her in a nurturing posture, predisposed men can develop significant somatic symptoms. Through these, they signal to the wife, "If you don't want to take care of me, at least be caring toward my liver, or my heart." Their symptoms also bring them to the attention of clinic personnel, internists, and nurses. RNs can be, for such men, the final mother figures of the life cycle.

These men show us that, given favorable circumstances, early difficulties can be compensated, even for a long time; the down side is that they can eventually become pathogenic, sometimes so late in life that the original deficit can no longer be traced to its origins.

Thus, the early failures of maternal separation can bring on personal and social pathology across the life span. In their youth, the mothers' sons afflict others—and particularly women—with their rage; and in later life female caretakers can become victims of their aggravated dependency. This country's founding myth tells of a rebellion against monarchy, and so our American Society of Democratic Brothers has always been hostile to the patriarchal principle. Now we begin to realize the heavy costs, especially to women, of the unchecked matricentric principle that is arising to take its place.

The Restoration of Culture

A final word. Erik Erikson once remarked (personal communication) that deprivation per se is not psychologically destructive; it is only deprivation without meaning, without redeeming significance, that is psychologically destructive. Human cultures, whatever particular forms they might take, have a great and universal purpose: They provide the routine sacrifices of human parenthood with high significance and dignity. Without culture, as we can see all around us, children are at risk, and too often from their own resentful parents. But when the young man has been linked, through his father and through the rituals managed by the elders, to some part of the powerful myths on which his culture is founded, then he too can become an adequate father. Rather than seeming to intrude on his freedom, the state of fatherhood will grant him a special dignity, an *identity*, precisely because of the meaningful sacrifices that this condition demands.

Thus, when the elder appears as a permanent fixture of social life, culture in its more mythic, ritualized, and enduring aspects appears with him. As his stature is undercut, the cultural regulation of social life is correspondingly weakened. We have compelling evidence for this last assertion: As we in this society move away from participatory gerontocracy, as we undo the culture-tending role of male elders, we also move toward the condition of *deculturation*. When strong elders no longer tend culture and the extended family, then the unsupported, unbuffered, isolated nuclear family becomes the staging ground for various forms of spousal and child abuse. Thus, whereas the crisis of meaning and stability that comes with deculturation has special consequences for the aged and perhaps touches them first, it is finally revealed as a shared affliction that ends by damaging all of us, and particularly our children. An urgent task for our time is to enlist the elders in the great project of *reculturation*. If we remind them of the historic role that they have played in maintaining and conserving culture, we can perhaps mobilize at least some of them to work for its restoration.

References

Blankenhorn, D. (1995). *Fatherless America: Confronting our most urgent social issue.* New York: Basic Books.

Brown, D. E. (1991). *Human universals.* New York: McGraw-Hill.

Erikson, E. (1952). *Childhood and society.* New York: Norton.

Gutmann, D. (1994). *Reclaimed powers: Men and women in later life*. Evanston, IL: Northwestern University Press.

Mahler, M., & Pine, S. (1975). *The psychological birth of the human infant*. New York: Basic Books.

Morris, D. (1994). *The human animal*. London: BBC Books.

Murdoch, G. (1935). Comparative data on the distribution of labor by sex. *Social Forces, 15*, 551–553.

Newton, N. (1973). *Psychosocial aspects of the mother/father/child unit*. Paper presented at the meeting of the Swedish Nutrition Foundation, Uppsala.

Simmons, L. W. (1945). *The role of the aged in primitive society*. New Haven, CT: Yale University Press.

Whiting, J. W., & Child, I. (1953). *Child training and personality*. New Haven, CT: Yale University Press.

14 Spirituality and Resilience in Adolescent Girls

Lisa Miller

Columbia University

> Each of us has to figure out how we can pray to [G-d]. Everybody is different. For me, I do not say the usual prayers we learn in church. For me, I write. I write and write and write what is on my mind, and then [G-d] comes through. (Angelina, a 15-year-old minister's daughter)

Angelina's highly personal process of relating with the Divine reveals some normative hallmarks of adolescent spiritual development. Theologians and theoretical psychologists have identified adolescence as a period of "spiritual awakening" characterized by a search for meaning, an intensified capacity for spiritual experience, and a process of using this personal spiritual experience to question many of the religious beliefs and tenets learned in childhood (Fowler, 1981; Groeschel, 1983). Such a process of spiritual individuation clearly relies on the concomitant emergence of metacognition, identity work, and, more uniquely, a quest to know and achieve harmony with the Creator. The energy and focus given to spiritual understanding might also be viewed as more concentrated in adolescence. So, too, the great reward of better knowing the Creator emerges in adolescence.

> I had the most beautiful dream. I was in a library made of beautiful wood and it was showered with light. Lining the walls were books and books of knowledge about [G-d], and I knew that I was going to learn about Him. (Vivian, a 16-year-old Baha'i)

A growing body of quantitative research confirms as well as sheds further light on the developmental path of religiousness in adolescence. One line of quantitative research on developmental religiosity stems from Kendler, Gardner, and Prescott's (1997, 1999) twin studies of adult women. The researchers empirically derived three dimensions of religiousness: personal devotion (a direct personal relationship with the Divine), personal conservatism (close adherence to creed), and institutional conservatism (relative fundamentalism of religious denomination). These three dimensions of religiousness were replicated using confirmatory factor analysis in a nationally representative sample of adolescents (Miller, Davies, & Greenwald, 2000); the association between the former two dimensions was significantly higher in adolescents ($r = .77$) than in adults ($r = .33$), however, suggesting relatively less distinction between personal spirituality and creed in adolescence. In addition, compared with adults, a greater association was found among adolescents between religious denomination and personal devotion ($r = .37$ vs. $r = .18$) and personal conservatism ($r = .46$ vs. $r = .38$), respectively, indicating relatively less distinction in adolescents between personal religiousness and religious denomination.

The lesser distinction between the three dimensions of religiousness in adolescents potentially suggests that there is in childhood a process of mutual facilitation that necessarily precedes the articulation of distinct dimensions throughout adolescence. An example of mutual facilitation might be that involvement in a fundamentalist denomination encourages children to understand daily experience as part of G-d's plan, which in turn fosters a relationship with G-d, defined in the research literature as personal devotion. Kendler and colleagues (1997) found that approximately 29% of the differences between adults in strength of personal devotion are attributable to heritable factors. If personal devotion is in part determined by nonenvironmental factors, then participation in religious denomination may clarify, define, and augment an innate awareness of G-d. Subsequent differentiation between the three dimensions of religiousness closely parallels Fowler's (1981) theory of the Individuation Phase in the development of faith, a spiritual individuation process driven by reevaluation of religious beliefs based on personal religious experience.

Developmental Religiosity and Resilience

Further information on the developmental path of religiosity is gained through studies on religiosity and resilience against pathology or against the intergenerational transmission of pathology in high-risk samples of offspring.

Evidence for nonenvironmental contributions to spirituality in childhood includes the following: (1) as previously mentioned, twin studies show that 29% of the variance in personal devotion is attributable to heritability (Kendler et al., 1997); (2) child religiosity increases the level of personal religiosity in parents, suggesting that the child is not a tabula rasa upon which is inscribed parental religiosity; (3) normative rates of personal religiosity are found among children of parents with very low rates of personal religiosity, and religiosity carries customary protective qualities in these children (Miller, Weissman, Gur, & Adams, 2001); and (4) the process of religious socialization, underpinning mutual facilitation across dimensions of religiosity in childhood, appears highly resistant to distortion by parental pathology or aspiritual community norms.

How each of the three dimensions functions as a protective factor has received some investigation. Institutional conservatism (relative religious fundamentalism) has been associated with optimism (Sethi & Seligman, 1993), a sense of purpose (Pargament, 1997), a network of social support based on religious values (Koenig, 1998), clarification of personal responsibility (Pargament, 1997; Tix & Frazier, 1998), and the possibility for forgiveness and redemption after personal failure or interpersonal transgression (Park, Cohen, & Herb, 1990).

Personal conservatism (close adherence to creed) fosters structured living through definitive rules and offers absolute beliefs prohibiting personal destructive behaviors. Where personal conservatism may actually pose a risk for morbidity in adolescents is in depriving adherents of resources for coping with infractions of religious creed. In keeping with this notion, Kendler and colleagues (1999) found that whereas personal conservatism protects against ever using substances, it is not associated with prevention against degree of use, and carries a depressogenic effect surrounding social conflict. From this pattern in the findings, the researchers inferred that "rigidity of cultural and/or personal expectations make[s] resolution of these conflicts more problematic and stressful" (p. 142). The lack of protective effect against the degree of substance use and the depressogenic qualities of personal conservatism increase with age in adolescence, potentially suggesting that rigid adherence to creed in adolescence thwarts the questioning process crucial to spiritual individuation and resilience.

The most highly protective dimension of religiousness in adolescence against the most prevalent of adolescent disorders is personal devotion (a direct experience of the Divine). Previous research shows that personal devotion resolves feelings of loneliness (Natale, 1986), fortifies regard for the self and others (Sobson, 1978), and substantiates meaning (Pargament, 1997). Case reports suggest that personal devotion engenders a sense of harmony and enhances spiritual fulfillment. If not fostered through personal devotion, yearnings for transcendence may motivate risk-taking behavior and substance use or devolve into depression. A personal sense of relationship with the Divine is an essential source of the protective qualities of religiousness for adolescents.

> Terrible things have happened. My brother was in a gang and was killed. Sometimes it gets to be so much that I can't take it anymore, I feel like I'm going to explode. So I go in my room, close the door and pray. And, *wow*, it's like *peace*. (Matthew, age 17 years)

Protective qualities of personal devotion are approximately twice as great in adolescents as in adults (Miller et al., 2000, 2001). The greater magnitude of the protective qualities of personal devotion may reflect the strength and centrality of experience in religiousness during adolescence. A search for spiritual relationship with the Creator may be an inherent developmental process in adolescence. Neglect of this quest for personal devotion in adolescence may result in a void, filled instead by pathology.

Gender Differences in Religiousness and Spirituality

Religiosity in adolescence is marked by a primacy of personal religious experience used in the individuation process to reassess and validate belief in religious creed. Within this trajectory of developmental religiosity, gender differences exist in the relative strength and rates of personal religiosity as well as adherence to creed. Each of these two dimensions of religiosity also shows differential protective qualities by gender.

Tamminen (1994) directly assessed gender differences in religiousness among adolescents and found girls, compared with boys, more strongly to endorse dimensions of religiousness that were "personal and based upon their own experience." Adolescent boys, compared with girls, more highly endorsed dimensions of religiousness that were "practical and rule oriented." Among Tamminen's study participants, 78% of girls compared with 61% of boys reported feeling the nearness of the Divine "at least a few times"; 13% of girls compared with 24% of boys reported having never felt the nearness of the Divine. Consistent with Tamminen's findings, other researchers have shown that adolescent boys, compared with girls, tend to report a "legalistic" view of the Divine with an emphasis on ultimate powerfulness (Argyle & Beit-Hallahmi, 1975; Janssen, De Hart, & Gerardts, 1994).

These gender differences in religiousness parallel findings concerning gender differences in moral judgment among adolescents: Compared with boys, girls more strongly base moral reasoning on an internal sense of care or avoidance of harm, whereas boys more strongly adopt a rule-based or institutionalized system of morality (Gilligan, 1994). The simultaneous burgeoning of like gender differences in adolescence within both religiousness and moral judgment (Brown & Gilligan, 1991) may be seen to indicate shared emergent mechanisms or possibly a unified path of moral–religious development.

Beyond gender differences in the rates of religiosity, gender differences exist across development in the association between religiosity and depression, a highly prevalent form of adolescent morbidity. During childhood, exclusively in girls, the development of personal religiousness appears distorted by childhood depression (Miller, Weissman, Gur, & Greenwald, 2002) and by childhood experience of maternal depression (Gur & Miller, 2002). The impact of depression on personal religiousness in girls renders as depressogenic that form of personal religiousness shown to be highly protective against depression in community samples of women (Butler & Nolen-Hoeksema, 1994; Koenig, 1998). A mutagenic path might be that depressive symptoms of guilt, low self-worth, and exaggerated responsibility that frequently occur in female depression distort other centered understandings of service, empathy, or altruism (Zahn-Wexler, Pole, & Barnett, 1991), culminating in a depressogenic interpersonal style. Religious messages to young women, compared with those directed toward young men, might be particularly amenable to this process, as Heggen and Long (1991) argue that some religious traditions discourage self-expression and encourage submissiveness and lack of mastery specifically in women.

From a cognitive perspective, depressed children often demonstrate a scar characterized by self-blame, inwardness, rumination, and lack of efficacy, enduring beyond individual episodes of depression and tending to occur more frequently in girls than in boys (Butler & Nolen-Hoeksema, 1994). Were this self-implicating cognitive style to be integrated into personal religiousness, depressed girls might tend to develop punitive or guilt-inducing forms of religiousness.

From an experiential perspective, a sense of transcendence or personal connection with the Creator often is reported as central to the protective qualities of personal religiousness (Koenig, 1998). If depression occluded a sense of connection with the Creator, then depressed children might struggle with spiritual alienation or an unfulfilled quest for meaning and connection.

Among adolescent girls who have not experienced childhood depression, the protective qualities of personal religiousness against depression are greater than in adolescent boys (Donahue, 1995; Feldman, Fisher, Ranson, & Dimicelli, 1995). The relatively robust protective quality of personal religiousness found in girls appears to augment in magnitude with age and physical maturation, as marked by onset of menstruation and magnitude of secondary sexual characteristics (Miller & Greenwald, 1998; Miller & Gur, 2002a).

Within contemporary research, little is understood of the confluence between the protective strength of personal devotion and onset of menstruation in girls. This notion is consistent, however, with numerous cross-cultural religious traditions surrounding menstruation (Severy, Thapa, Askew, & Jeffrey, 1993) from the Jewish ritual of the Mikvah (Seigel, 1986) to the Native American belief in spiritual powers during menstruation (Atwood, 1991). Psychological anthropologist Lotte Motz (1997) suggests that previous civilizations held knowledge of the confluence between fecundity and spirituality. Motz cites the earliest representation of a human form, the Central European Venus of Willendorf (Upper Paleolithic era, 25,000–20,000 BCE, Central Europe) that forms an almost spherical representation of a fertility goddess, as evidence of knowledge of a confluence between transcendent reality and fertility.

Some correlates of spiritual capacity in women also are correlates of depression in women, including the capacity for absorption, internality, openness to experience, and meaning making (Bateson, Klopher, & Thompson, 1993; Gallemore, Wilson, & Rhoads, 1969; Levin, Wickremesekera, & Hirshberg, 1998). Shared correlates of inversely associated phenomena raise the possibility of a "reservoir effect." To the extent, for instance, that personal devotion is harnessed through prayer or meditation, it serves as a means to deepen spiritual experience and ultimately is a source of resilience. Left to function "willy-nilly," however, the same capacity for absorption might lead to rumination and prompt devolution into depression.

The unified path of spiritual and sexual development in girls may offer preparation for motherhood and procreation. This possibility is supported by previous research showing that (1) the intergenerational transmission of religiosity occurs primarily through mothers (Acock & Bengston, 1978; Okagaki & Bevis, 1999); (2) the intergenerational transmission of religiosity highly protects against depression, as well as other forms of morbidity in offspring (Miller, Warner, Wickramaratne, & Weissman, 1997; Neuman, Quillen, & Chi, 1998); (3) autonomous and responsible sexual practice has been associated with personal religiousness in adolescent girls (Miller & Gur, 2002b); and (4) women in their childbearing years are both at particular risk for depression and tend to derive protective benefit from personal devotion (Miller et al., 1997).

Conclusions

The primacy of personal religiousness in the developmental path of religiousness in adolescence highlights the importance of supporting adolescents in their regard for and understanding of their own personal religious experience. Although the evidence suggests that this holds true for boys and girls, particularly for girls is personal religious experience central to the strength of overall religiosity and to resilience. Youth ministers and youth leaders might consider directly addressing the spiritual path of young girls and be accepting and open to its relationship with the emergence of sexuality, physical maturation, and fecundity. Willingness to explore and support the confluence between physical maturation and spirituality, rather than a blanket prohibitive squashing or shaming of emergent female sexuality, might serve to support the core of spiritual development in adolescent girls.

Acknowledgment

This work was supported by the William T. Grant Faculty Scholars Award for Religion and Resilience in Adolescents.

References

Acock, A., & Bengston, V. (1978). On the relative influence of mothers and fathers: A covariance analysis of political and religious socialization. *Journal of Marriage and the Family, 8*, 519–530.

Argyle, M., & Beit-Hallahmi, B. (1975). *The social psychology of religion*. London: Routledge & Kegan Paul.

Atwood, M. D. (1991). *Spirit healing: Native American magic and medicine*. New York: Sterling.

Bateson, P. P., Klopher, P. H., & Thompson, N. S. (Eds.). (1993). *Perspectives in ethology: Vol. 10. Behavior and evolution*. New York: Plenum.

Brown, L. M., & Gilligan, C. (1991). Listening for voice in narratives of relationship. In M. B. Tappan & M. J. Parker (Eds.), *Narrative and storytelling: Implications for understanding moral development* (pp. 43–62). San Francisco: Jossey-Bass.

Butler, L. C., & Nolen-Hoeksema, S. (1994). Gender differences in responses to depressed mood in a college sample. *Sex Roles, 30*, 331–346.

Donahue, M. (1995). Religion and the well-being of adolescents. *Journal of Social Issues, 51*, 145–160.

Feldman, S., Fisher, L., Ranson, D., & Dimicelli, S. (1995). Is what is good for the goose good for the gander? Sex differences in the relations between adolescent coping and adult adaptation. *Journal of Research on Adolescence, 5*, 333–359.

Fowler, J. (1981). *Stages of faith: The psychology of human development and the quest for meaning.* San Francisco: Harper & Row.

Gallemore, J. L., Wilson, W. P., & Rhoads, J. M. (1969). The religious life of patients with affective disorder. *Diseases of the Nervous System, 30,* 483–487.

Gilligan, C. (1994). In a different voice: Women's conceptions of self and of morality. In B. Puka (ed.), *Moral development: A compendium: Vol. 6. Caring voices and women's moral frames: Gilligan's view* (pp. 1–38). New York: Garland.

Groeschel, B. J. (1983). *Spiritual passages: The psychology of spiritual development.* New York: Crossroad.

Gur, M., Miller, L., Warner, V., Weissman, M. M. (2005). Maternal depression and the intergenerational transmission of religion. *Journal of Nervous and Mental Disease, 193*(5), 338–345.

Heggen, C. H., & Long, V. (1991). Counseling the depressed Christian female client. *Counseling Values, 35,* 128–135.

Janssen, J., De Hart, J., & Gerardts, M. (1994). Images of [G-d] in adolescence. *International Journal of the Psychology of Religion, 4,* 105–121.

Kendler, K. S., Gardner, C. O., & Prescott, C. A. (1997). Religion, psychopathology and substance use and abuse: A multi-measure, genetic-epidemiologic study. *American Journal of Psychiatry, 154,* 322–329.

Kendler, K. S., Gardner, C. O., & Prescott, C. A. (1999). Clarifying the relationship between religiosity and psychiatric illness: The impact of covariates and the specificity of buffering effects. *Twin Research, 2,* 137–144.

Koenig, H. G. (Ed.). (1998). *Handbook of religion and mental health.* San Diego: Academic Press.

Levin, J. S., Wickremesekera, I. E., & Hirshberg, C. (1998). Is religiousness a correlate of absorption? Implications for psychophysiology, coping and morbidity. *Alternative Therapy, 4,* 72–76.

Miller, L., Davies, M., & Greenwald, S. (2000). Religiosity and substance use and abuse among adolescents in the national comorbidity survey. *Journal of the American Academy of Child and Adolescent Psychiatry, 39*(9), 1190–1197.

Miller, L., Greenwald, S. (1998). *Religion and psychopathology among adolescents in the NCS.* Paper presented at the annual convention of the American Psychological Association, New York, NY.

Miller, L., & Gur, M. (2002a). Religiosity, depression and physical maturation in adolescent girls. *Journal of the American Academy of Child and Adolescent Psychiatry, 41*(2), 206–213.

Miller, L., & Gur, M. (2002b). Religiosity and sexual responsibility in adolescent girls. *Journal of Adolescent Health, 31*(5), 401–406.

Miller, L., Warner, V., Wickramaratne, P., & Weissman, M. M. (1997). Religion and depression: Ten-year follow-up of depressed mothers and offspring. *Journal of the American Academy of Child and Adolescent Psychiatry, 36,* 1416–1425.

Miller, L., Weissman, M., Gur, M., & Adams, P. (2001). Religiosity and substance use among children of opiate addicts. *Journal of Substance Abuse, 13,* 323–336.

Miller, L., Weissman, M., Gur, M., & Greenwald, S. (2002). Adult religiousness and history of childhood depression: Eleven-year follow-up study. *Journal of Nervous and Mental Disease, 190*(2), 86–93.

Motz, L. (1997). *The faces of the goddess.* New York: Oxford University Press.

Natale, S. M. (1986). *Loneliness and spiritual growth.* Birmingham, AL: Religious Education Press.

Neumann, J. K., Quillen, J. H., & Chi, D. S. (1998). Physiological stress response and psychological differences as a possible function of perceived paternal religious value similarity and church attendance. *Journal of Psychology and Christianity, 17,* 233–247.

Nolen-Hoeksema, S., Larson, J., & Grayson, C. (1999). Explaining the gender difference in depressive symptoms. *Journal of Personality and Social Psychology, 77,* 1061–1072.

Okagaki, L., & Bevis, C. (1999). Transmission of religious values: Relations between parents' and daughters' beliefs. *Journal of Genetic Psychology, 160,* 303–318.

Pargament, L. I. (1997). *The psychology of religion and coping: Theory, research, and practice.* New York: Guilford.

Park, C. L., Cohen, L. H., & Herb, L. (1990). Intrinsic religiousness and religious coping as life stress moderators for Catholics versus Protestants. *Journal of Personality and Social Psychology, 54,* 551–577.

Seigel, S. J. (1986). The effect of culture on how women experience menstruation: Jewish women and the Mikvah. *Women and Health, 16,* 63–74.

Sethi, S., & Seligman, M. E. P. (1993). Optimism and fundamentalism. *Psychological Science, 4,* 256–259.

Severy, L. J., Thapa, S., Askew, I. G., & Jeffrey, E. (1993). Menstrual experiences and beliefs. *Women and Health, 20,* 1–20.

Sobson, J. G. (1978). Loneliness and faith. *Journal of Psychological Theology, 61,* 104–109.

Tamminen, K. (1994). A viewpoint of religious development between the ages of 7 and 20. *International Journal of Psychology and Religion, 4,* 91–104.

Tix, A. P., & Frazier P. A. (1998). The use of religious coping during stressful life events: Main effects, moderation, and mediation. *Journal of Consulting and Clinical Psychology, 66,* 411–422.

Zahn-Waxler, C., Cole, P. M., & Barrett, K. C. (1991). Guilt and empathy: Sex differences and implications for the development of depression. In J. Garber & K. A. Dodge (Eds.), *The development of emotion regulation and dysregulation* (pp. 243–272). Cambridge: Cambridge University Press.

VI
Connecting to Community

15 Promoting Well-Being Among At-Risk Children: Restoring a Sense of Community and Support for Development

James P. Comer

Yale University

Only 50 to 100 years ago, most Americans grew up and lived out their lives in small towns and rural areas. Indeed, most big cities were collections of small towns. Children were reared within the primary social network of their parents—friends, kin, and organizations in which the family felt acceptance and belonging. Most information came to children from within this primary social network; and those important people were able to censor and sanction— to withhold information that might harm development and sanction children for acting inappropriately in response to information they received. Information from outside a community was minimal and impersonal and thus usually less influential.

The economy of the past absorbed the uneducated and undereducated. Thus, most heads of households could provide for their families without an education, and often at least one parent was at home to supervise child behavior and to promote development. The level of development needed was not high. Most children, without a good education, were in a position to carry out their adult tasks and responsibilities—to work, live in families, rear children if they chose to do so, and participate as citizens of their community and the society.

Housing and material things, health and other services were within a reasonably narrow range throughout the society. Most people walked to work, worship, or recreation; or used slow private or public transportation until about the middle of the 20th century. As a result, authority figures often knew or interacted with each other and were in a position, even expected, to limit the undesirable behavior of children. These interactions were governed by social rules established by the most powerful, but generally accepted and internalized by all, and transmitted to the children.

The chief source of a sense of well-being came probably more from relationships and a sense of belonging than from income and material goods. Neither the private nor public sector was mainly responsible for creating these conditions, particularly in rural areas, where self-sufficiency was possible. Crucially important, conditions of life were in the hands and control of individuals and families more than organizations. All of these factors created a sense of empowerment, place, and belonging, as well as a sense of community. Families that experience these conditions have the best chance of rearing their children in ways that will enable them to be successful.

These life conditions allowed bias and injustices to flourish, particularly against women and minorities. Nonetheless, expectations for children were clear, and support for development was present.

These modest demands and conditions made the American Dream possible—within reach even for marginal groups. This dream is the idea that individuals who work hard, contribute to their community, and support their family will be able to find a sense of purpose in life and feel belonging. From the beginning, an important aspect of the dream was that in time things could get better in America; that there could be free expression, fairness, and greater opportunity for all. Faith in this dream is one of the most powerful driving and unifying forces in our country.

The organizing and direction-giving mindset of the American Dream, coupled with economic and social conditions before the 1960s, made it possible for most families to experience a sense of well-being. Even in difficult economic times, a sense of community, religious faith, and the belief in a better American tomorrow kept hope and well-being alive for most. This sense made reasonably good family functioning and child rearing possible. There was generation-to-generation transmission of a set of attitudes, values, and ways of understanding and managing the world that prepared the young to function adequately as adults.

Nonetheless, throughout American history, there have been families and children at risk—Native Americans, African Americans, certain Latino groups, isolated and poor whites, immigrants, and other exploited and oppressed people. Some families from all of these groups were able to find ways to experience a sense of well-being, function well, and prepare their children to participate in the mainstream culture after major barriers were eroded or broken down (Comer, 1988). But there was a disproportionate number of marginal to dysfunctional families and children from among the groups that experienced the most economic and social stress. These groups were most vulnerable to the ill effects of the rapid pace of change that took place after 1950.

Change

Within the lifetime of many of today's senior citizens, our nation has moved from a horse-and-buggy level of technology through an automobile and jet plane level to an interplanetary rocket level. The changes that are of greatest consequence were created by the emergence of a science- and technology-based economy, high mobility, and mass communications, rapid and visual. As a result of these changes, heads of households now need a high level of development and education to be able to work, take care of themselves and their families, and participate as responsible citizens in an open democratic society (Wilson, 1997). High mobility and communications from outside the primary social network of a child have weakened adult authority and support for development while simultaneously making such support more necessary than ever before.

For the first time in the history of the world, information goes directly to children and not through the important adults in their primary social network who could censor and censure. The information children receive today contains many more models of sexual and aggressive behavior. The information is pervasive—magazines and movies, television, radio, the Internet. Despite the increased amount of information, there are fewer adults to help children learn what to act on and what not to act on, and how to act on the information appropriately.

Working parents, whether single or two parents, are the norm. They are busy and less surrounded by extended family and other network support and are thus under stress (U.S. Census Bureau, 2001b). Teachers and other service providers now usually live a long distance from where they work. They do not know each other or walk through most communities. Thus, the school is no longer a natural part of the community working to support development, as it once did, intentionally or not.

The variety of material things and services needed—housing, health care, education, and others—has grown. The pressure to provide adequately is great and sometimes compromises the time needed to help children grow. Families across the social and economic spectrum are under economic and social stress; the most vulnerable in the past are even more vulnerable today. As a result, too many parents are not able to give their children the preschool experiences that will fully promote their development and prepare them to succeed in school.

Because of these changed conditions, a large number of children are entering school underdeveloped, sometimes simply differently developed. Teachers and administrators are usually not prepared to create school contexts that will reinforce the development of those who previously had good support for development or to help the underdeveloped catch up (U.S. Census Bureau, 2001a). Higher education and the policy makers—in education, government, and business—who influence teacher and administrator pre- and in-service preparation have focused on improving curriculum and instruction rather than helping school staff more effectively support development. Through no fault of their own, school staff view the consequences of underdevelopment as bad behavior and limited ability. This perception leads to control and punishment and low expectations.

Staff expectations are internalized by the students and contribute to low levels of achievement and school failure. Parental hope that the school will make a difference for their children is lost, and a climate of distrust, anger, and alienation often replaces it. Children who see no real chance of succeeding are not motivated to embrace mainstream attitudes about learning and behavior. Because of their universal need to establish identity and belonging, children who are shut out by mainstream society often become a part of countercultures that meet their social and emotional needs but will interfere with their ability to participate in mainstream society—where the legal living-wage jobs are located. This makes it difficult for children to carry out expected adult life tasks.

The growth of behavior problems among middle- and upper-income children over the past 25 years strongly suggests that inadequate support for development is not limited to the poor and non-mainstream. We must consider the effects of social and economic change on family and community, and, in turn, on support for child development. Our society has been slow to do so. We have often blamed families for not being able to prepare, or not being interested in preparing, their children for school. We do not give sufficient attention to the need of societal institutions, public and private, to adjust adequately to the new conditions of life. To address the root of the problem, we must focus on understanding the child development process and on understanding how to adjust all our institutions to better support child development, as well as teaching and learning of a kind necessary to help the young meet all adult tasks and responsibilities.

Before considering how our institutions can better support child and adolescent behavior, particularly for non-mainstream children, I would like to share my personal experience, as it has been an important source of insight in my work in schools.

A Personal Perspective

I am an African American from a low-income family. My mother was the daughter of sharecropping parents in rural Mississippi. Her father was a good man who worked hard to provide for the family. But when my mother was 6 years old, he was killed by lightning. Because there were no family support programs at that time, and the seven children were too young to work, a cruel stepfather came into their lives. The family lived under extreme conditions of abuse and deprivation, and the stepfather would not allow them to go to school. At about 8 years of age, my mother decided that education was the only way to a better life. At age 16 she ran away to her sister in East Chicago, Indiana, with the hope that she could go to school. But my aunt did not support my mother's dream, and she had to leave school and go to work as a domestic.

When my mother left school, she declared that if she ever had children she would make certain that every one of them got a good education. Over time, my mother, with less than 2 years of education, and my father, a steel mill laborer with a rural Alabama 6th grade education, sent all five of their children to college for a total of 13 degrees.

Three neighborhood friends attended elementary school with me. It was my impression that they were just as intelligent and able as myself and my siblings—or anyone else in our predominately white, middle- and upper-income school—but all three of them went on a downhill life course. One died early from alcoholism; another was frequently incarcerated; and the third was perpetually battling mental illness.

When I returned home to do my internship in medicine, my friends' lives were already in decline. What happened to them? We had similar intelligence and potential. We attended the same school, and our parents were similarly employed. Why did we have such very different outcomes? Answering these questions became a driving force in my life and led me to change my intended career path from becoming a general practitioner in my hometown to training in public health and child psychiatry and then work in schools. My concern was not only for my friends and children like them; it also occurred to me that a society like ours could not afford the loss of so many able people on an ongoing basis and expect to survive and thrive.

Eventually, I realized that the difference in life outcomes was due largely to the quality of our developmental experiences. My family was enmeshed in an African American church culture with values and styles very close to those of the larger society. In her work as a domestic, my mother was able to observe and acquire mainstream success skills and contacts by interacting with her employers and was able to translate that knowledge into lessons for us. Those networks, and the chance to work, even at low-income levels, made it possible for my parents to give us a good developmental experience. Work and belonging gave them a sense of adequacy and worth. It allowed them to believe in the American Dream. All of this encouraged them to provide us with everything they could to help us grow and achieve in school and as adults.

They provided us with nurturance, knowledge, guidance, and skills. We received many warm, memorable experiences with them in our earliest years: popcorn and malted milk on the porch on warm summer evenings; play at the Lake Front Park; discussions around the dinner table in which we learned the rules of conversation, with informal after-dinner debates in which we learned to express our ideas as well as how to control our emotions and angry impulses; protection of our aspirations from the "naysayers"; and much more. They exposed us to and discussed all things they believed educational—museums, political activities, books and newspapers, and so on; and they provided us with all the social skills necessary to engage in these activities.

The lessons, skills, and connections my parents taught and made enabled us to take advantage of educational and social opportunities that were unavailable to my friends. Indeed, many of the jobs we received that helped us pay for our education grew out of our family connection to more powerful people and networks. Thus, our primary family social network and people and institutions in the larger community supported our family functioning and child development. My friends and their families did not have such ties and experiences, and these bonds and support from the community are much weaker today.

The realization that meaningful connections within the family and community promote good youth development has driven my work all these years (Bowlby, 1988). I now understand that it takes a coalition of resources, including the family, schools, local and state policy, and civic institutions like the local recreation center, or a family's place of worship, to ensure optimum child development. Through my academic work over the past four decades, carried out through the School Development Program (SDP), I have investigated the impact of this loss of social network on a child's success in school. Indeed, our SDP training program helped to popularize the proverb, "It takes a whole village to raise a child."

My work in schools began in the mid-1960s, when I began to examine the disconnect between children's experiences at home and at school. I wanted to know how the contrasting experiences affected their psychosocial development, which in turn shaped their academic achievement and future success in life. This contrast was especially sharp for non-mainstream, poor, minority children and families. I speculated, and over time have demonstrated, that underdevelopment and the resultant failure to bridge the social, cultural, and academic learning preparation gap between the home and larger institutions, such as schools, are at the root of the poor academic and social performance of these children (Comer, 2004).

Our clinical intervention in failing schools required an understanding of child and adolescent development and how to promote it in school. Changing the culture or social context of schools so that they could support development required a public health and/or ecological (interactive) perspective. These perspectives can help us change our institutions in ways that will enable them to help all adults better help all young people grow.

The Child Development Contexts and Process

Children are born into three networks of people and organizations, and the policies and practices they generate. Again, the first is a primary network of immediate family, extended family, friends, communal and faith organizations (such as synagogues, temples, mosques, and churches), and others. The family receives services needed for survival and functioning in the secondary social network, including job or work opportunities. In modern society, education or the school is an important part of the secondary network. Policy makers at every level who make decisions that affect services and family life constitute the tertiary network.

In this age, unlike in the past, many critically important life conditions are greatly influenced by private- and government-sector policies and programs of the secondary and tertiary networks—education, work, housing, and so on. The decisions made are guided as much or more by ideology, self-interest, and quest for personal power as they are by the need to empower families to function and to rear their children well.

Regardless of societal structure and function, caretakers must be able to provide children with food, clothing, shelter, and protection from physical and psychological harm. Children must be able to feel trust and receive affection from one or more adults from whom they can learn. And caretakers must be able to help them control their aggressive and impulsive energy in order to learn, work, and play in continually more mature ways. This provides children with the competence, confidence, and comfort needed to begin to make their way in personal and larger worlds that will continually grow more complex.

Fortunately, whereas heads of households have little control over the secondary and tertiary networks, they have great power to influence the quality of family and primary social network life. It is in the home and school that society can best make adjustments that will help today's young people develop in ways that improve their chances for school and life success. And because of their need to provide their children with a good education, parents have an interest in and the potential to influence schooling. I will return to a discussion of school change. But first, I would like briefly to discuss the basic principles of child development that parents, community organizations, and schools must know to be better prepared to help children grow.

Brain and behavioral research has confirmed that an interaction of nature and nurture (biological and social environment), not fixed intelligence or talent, brings about the full expression of human intelligence and other potentials (Bransford, Brown, & Cocking, 2002). Without good caretaking interactions between adults and children, children can lose the intellectual potential with which they were born, as well as the potential for desirable behavior with which they are born. It is important to remember that children are not passive recipients of input. They are born exploring their world and trying to make sense of and cope with it. But they are profoundly immature at birth and therefore dependent. When healthy, they are born with the capacity, even the need, to form relationships. This is what makes caretaking interactions necessary and possible and is what positions the caretaker to help children develop.

With reasonably well-functioning parents in a reasonably well-functioning family, a child can make an emotional attachment and bond that enables the parent(s), and other important caretakers, to protect and promote desirable or positive development. Initial learning and growth take place largely through child identification, imitation, and internalization of the attitudes, values, and ways of important caretakers. Good interactions help children channel their life-sustaining, but potentially harmful, aggressive energy and impulses into the energy of learning, work, and play. Attachment, bonding, development, and learning take place in all life activities—commonplace and random, planned and systematic.

The activities are so commonplace that few pay attention to the development and learning involved. The knowledgeable parent names parts of a child's body, clothing, and household furniture they use. As they play, parents often name where they are in space—up, down, under, over. They warn that the stove is hot, the water cold. They identify relatives and friends and help children learn protective stranger etiquette. Parents help toddlers work things out rather than fight over possessions. Children learn the rituals of worship by observing their parents. Parents help children learn to wait their turn rather than go to the front of the buffet line; and much more, every day.

Parents read to their children—both for pleasure and to promote growth. Reading is the critical skill of the new age and is perhaps the best exemplar of how adults help children grow. Children often cuddle up close to their parents, receiving intimate special attention. Books can be intriguing, stimulating, and exciting. The stories often help them manage their own anxiety and fears. For these reasons, they often want to hear the story, or a favorite part, again and again. They often internalize reading behavior and recite by memory along with the reader. If their memory reading is greeted with support and approval, they are further motivated to learn to read. All of this makes reading a warm, emotionally charged learning experience.

Reading, then, the most primary of academic skills and an important social skill, is largely the product of a positive relationship with an important adult. The relationship motivates and facilitates academic learning. For example, the symbol "A" has no more tangible meaning for a young child than does scribble. Why learn about it? The symbol becomes significant because an important caregiver helps to make it so. Children want to please and win the approval of adults; and displaying their competence is a way of doing so, and is also self-satisfying. Thus, they learn to recognize the symbol, how to pronounce and eventually how to use it, and combine it with other symbols to form more complex sentences and thoughts.

Higher-order thinking is equally important and can be promoted by an activity as commonplace as a visit to the gas station. The mother of a 5-year-old was filling up the gas tank of her car, and her son asked her what she was doing. She went beyond the obvious and stated that she was giving the car its breakfast, as he had just had. She went on to discuss other similarities and differences between living and inanimate things, including the danger of ingesting fuel. The youngster was fascinated by the discussion and raised one question after another.

I have given examples of but a few of the many interactions of children and their caretakers. And again, they appear commonplace and random. But these, and many others, indeed all, are promoting or interfering with growth along several pathways—physical, linguistic, psychological, social, cognitive, and ethical. Although there are other pathways, a high level of development along these six is needed for school and life success.

Growth along the pathways from conception and birth to maturity until death is interactive and simultaneous. And growth is uneven to varying degrees, for example, well-developed social skills, but less well-developed cognitive skills, or any combination thereof. But to facilitate observation and to be able to point to the various determinants of behavior at given times, we speak about them separately.

The pathway concept is well established in child and adolescent development and the social and behavioral sciences. But in our earliest work in schools in 1968, we discovered that most educators viewed child behaviors through a moral–cultural lens (good or bad) or as a reflection of intelligence. This approach usually led to punishment or external control rather than a focus on helping a child develop the capacity and desire to function appropriately and to take personal or inner responsibility for doing so. We introduced the lens of developmental pathways in schools to help teachers understand that much undesirable child behavior and performance, both social and academic, is due to underdevelopment or poor preparation for school; that a focus on development would enable teacher and child to be more successful (Comer, Haynes, Joyner, & Ben-Avie, 1996).

For example, if children do not begin to learn to negotiate as toddlers, and do not have adequate impulse control, they are more prone to fight in school. Help with reflection, negotiation, making good choices, and more, is more useful to teacher and child than simple punishment. Knowledge of the fact that young children can't sit still very long should enable school staff to plan activities that will not require them to do so. Frequent changes of adult staff make it difficult for young children to gain and maintain the level of trust that makes it possible for them to take the chances necessary to explore and learn. Thus, a school should make its best effort to provide continuity, or support when change is necessary.

There are multiple and different developmental opportunities and issues at each age that knowledge of can help the caretaker be more helpful to the child. The 5- or 6-year-old still likes to imitate adult work. Curriculum activities can take this tendency into account. It helps to understand that cliques are a way 10- or 11-year-olds become part of a "new family" while maintaining their base in their own. At the same time, cliques can be harmful in the absence of a school climate that helps everybody value and feel belonging and ownership. And early adolescents without a future orientation, but in search of an identity, can drift or lose interest in schoolwork. School staff who "think development" can not only prevent problems but also tap into what is going on with students developmentally to promote interest in the academic program.

We discovered, however, that we could not expect school personnel to change lifelong personal and professional beliefs and ways of working simply by explaining child development. It is difficult for school staff to think and work differently in a difficult staff–parent–student relationship climate. To get adults to work together in a way that would establish conditions that promoted development and learning, we had to create a conceptual and operational framework based on development and public health and/or ecological principles. This framework enabled them to give up self-defeating behaviors and to focus on supporting student development. The pathway lens helped to made this shift possible.

Figure 1 illustrates child growth across the six developmental pathways toward life goals.

Again, children from well-functioning, mainstream families have the best chance of receiving the kind of support for development that leads to success in school and life. A child from a poor, marginalized family is more likely to enter school without adequate preparation in all six of these developmental areas.

The usual "bad and dumb" assessment, and the punishment, control, and low expectation response, can be replaced with support for development in schools where all the adults—administrators, teachers, parents, support staff— are using the developmental pathways lens.

A school working in this way can help. But it is important to remember that the family has primary responsibility for providing a quality of rearing and development that prepares children for learning in school. The dilemma of the modern age is that so much of what families need to function well comes

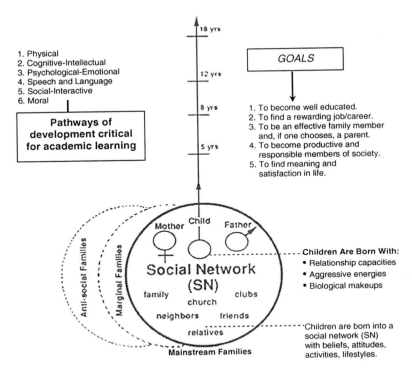

© 1991, Yale Child Study Center School Development Program

Figure 1. Child growth and development

from government and private institutions over which they have little control. Policies and practices established by opinion and institutional leaders, public and private, must make it possible for most families to function well, to rear their children well, so that schools can adequately prepare today's children to work, live in, and rear families in an open, democratic, and much more complex society.

Toward a School for the 21st Century

In the preceding sections, I described how our society has changed and placed new challenges on individuals, families, and institutions, pointing out that today, public and private institutions beyond the control of families must be involved in making it possible for most children to function well in school and in life. The involvement must be focused as much on development as on academic learning, must be inside and outside of school, and must be reasonably well coordinated (Epstein & Salinas, 2004; Henderson & Mapp, 2002). These needs are reasonably new and have important implications, but they are difficult to accept.

Our School Development Program work in New Haven, Connecticut, now in many places across the country, is still short of the fully coordinated school and community interaction that is needed. But even as a work in progress, it suggests what is possible and the elements and processes that are necessary to meet the needs of children and families in the 21st century.

Before describing our past, present, and future SDP work, I want to respond to the question sometimes asked, often by educators: Why the school? Several parts of the "old natural community" are still around and involved in support for child and youth development. There are other civic institutions like the Boys and Girls Clubs, YMCA, and YWCA, other community programs and recreation centers, faith-based programs, and others that help families. Some educators argue that the school has too much to do already.

All our institutions can be helpful, but none is in the position to be as effective and efficient as the school. It was the continuous immersion, linked and interacting relationships with meaningful people aspect of the natural community that made it so effective in supporting development. School is the only institution remaining that retains all of these essential elements. It provides an opportunity for adults to be in contact with children, adolescents, and young adults almost from birth to young adulthood. During this period, relationships can be created that permit interactions enabling the young to gain the attitudes, values, skills, and ways needed to be successful in school and in adulthood. And almost everybody goes to school.

There is no stigma attached to the work of the school. School staff are in the position to call on the resources of the family, community, and larger society to carry out its mission. There are scattered programs that make good education and life opportunities possible for "at risk" children. For example, "Prep for Prep" prepares underprivileged students to attend elite private schools, and

"A Better Chance" places urban young people in good suburban and rural schools. However, such programs do not serve the large masses of able young people, like my childhood friends, who are lost at a young age.

Again, even "good schools," from an academic learning standpoint, generally do very little to prepare students to live in an open democratic society. And only the public school was created to do so, with supervision and oversight responsibility. A citizenry so prepared has been the key to American social and economic progress and well-being. These, and others, were the reasons I decided to focus on public schools as the site for re-creating the critical elements of community needed to adequately support development.

The New Haven School-Community Model

In 1968, my colleagues and I began the Yale Child Study Center's involvement in the two most troubled and underachieving inner-city elementary schools in New Haven, Connecticut. Our project was eventually called the School Development Program. We did not try to impose preconceived notions, research findings, or action theory on the schools. Our five-member behavioral science team lived in the schools, experienced the difficulties, and with parents and staff began to create a change model that addressed authentic problems.

We recognized that the major reason the schools were failing was because of difficult interactions between home and school. The students were underdeveloped or differently developed, and the staff was unprepared to help them. The resultant school environment was one of conflict, defensiveness, and defeat of everybody—parents, students, and staff. However, everybody wanted to be successful. We gradually created a nine-element change process made possible by three mechanisms, three operations, and three guidelines (Comer, Joyner, & Ben-Avie, 2004). This framework is both conceptual and operational, and it transformed the two project schools (Figure 2).

Again, our observations and the design of the clinical intervention were informed by our life experiences, our social and behavioral science knowledge and skills, and my public health and child and adolescent development knowledge and experience. Thus, the focus was not on the individual and not on pathology. We recognized that factors in all three networks were operating to create dysfunctional conditions but that we could not influence issues beyond the school. Thus, our focus was on parents, staff, and students in school. Our goal was to gradually decrease interactions that created difficult conditions and to replace them with interactions that promoted student development, good teaching, and learning.

The School Planning and Management Team (SPMT), or the governance mechanism, is the "engine" and steering wheel of the model. It provides direction, drive, energy, and coordination to the system. It is representative of all the adult stakeholders in the school—administrators, teachers, parents, and professional and nonprofessional support staff. Students serve on this body, or

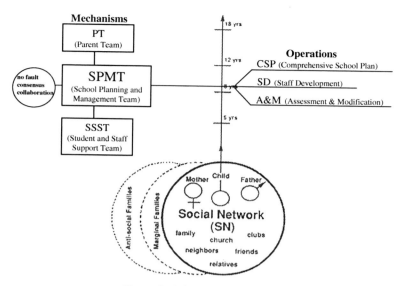

Figure 2. School transformation

otherwise advise it, in middle and high schools. In this way, everybody owns the program implementation, outcomes, challenges, and successes. Ownership promotes belonging and the motivation for success among parents, staff, and students.

The SPMT carries out the three traditional tasks and/or operations of organization leadership. It develops a Comprehensive School Plan that has both a social and an academic focus; oversees Staff Development based on district expectations and building needs; and oversees Assessment and Modification of its work on a periodic and ongoing basis.

Mutual trust and respect are needed to work in these interactive ways. Schools serving children from families under economic and social stress are least likely to produce these conditions. This led to the creation of guidelines to live by—no-fault problem solving (i.e., fixing, not blaming); consensus decision making based on what is in the best interest of children; and collaboration. These approaches are generated and reinforced first in the SPMT, and then in all the activities in the school.

The Parent Team, or the second mechanism, selects its representatives to serve on the SPMT, and its members inform and work in support of all the activities of the Comprehensive School Plan, both social and academic.

The third mechanism, the Student and Staff Support Team, focuses first and foremost on prevention and secondarily on the problems of individual or small groups of children. All the helping professionals in a school serve on this team—psychologist, social worker, nurse, and so on. Outside professionals working with particular children or families sometimes serve temporarily.

These nine elements working simultaneously and in a coordinated way decrease overlap, fragmentation, and communication problems. They promote efficient problem solving and make it possible for all involved to create and exploit learning opportunities on an ongoing basis. This coordination creates a school culture that makes it possible for children to attach to and bond with school people and program and be motivated to learn. It greatly reduces behavior problems among students, staff, and parents; or creates a learning community. Indeed, it re-creates in school the essential elements of community that have been lost or greatly reduced in the larger community by the effects of science- and technology-driven change.

This approach does not lock school staff into the rigid implementation of any particular math, reading, or other academic approach. It empowers staff to grow and be creative. It permits organic school change and improvement. Organic change led us to a program designed to help school people provide underdeveloped students with the experiences they need to develop adequately and to succeed in school and, in time, in life.

In 1977, we developed a program called the Social Skills Curriculum for Inner City Children (SSCICC). Based on parent input about what they wanted for their children as adults, we designed a program that pointed school activities toward the venues in which students will need skills to be successful as adults—politics and government, business and economics, health and nutrition, spiritual and expressive recreation time. Basic academic skills, social skills, and appreciation of the arts were integrated into these four activity areas.

There was a 7-month gain in academic achievement the first year after this program began, and it continued over the next 2 to 4 years until the students were more than a year above grade level in one school and 7 months above in the other. The attendance was the best in the city, and there were no serious behavior problems. Importantly, there was no teacher turnover for 13 years.

Dissemination

Implementation of the SSCICC requires a well-functioning school. Thus, when we began to disseminate our work in 1983, we had to use our nine essential elements model. Using a trainer of trainers method, eventually in collaboration with several colleges and a social service agency, we were in almost 700 schools across the country by 1996. But we noted that buildings could not sustain the changes without the sponsorship and support of their districts. We now work at the district level in most places and ask them to develop a steering committee that acts at the district level very much like an SPMT acts at the building level.

Districts expressed concern about the limited supply of staff able to work in today's schools. It is our observation that this is the case largely because preservice staff are not prepared to work in a way that will create a school context enabling them to help children grow. This led us to a focus on teacher and administrator preparation in several schools of education. The schools work with us in supporting districts while simultaneously changing their university programs to better prepare their students. We also have done some preliminary work with education, business, and government policy makers.

Note that our work has moved us from a focus on the classroom and building, including work with parents (the first and second networks), to work with policy makers in the third network, where decisions are made that affect school practices. Our intent is to encourage coherent child- and adolescent-oriented policies and practices from the state house to the classroom. All that is done should make attachment and bonding, good development, teaching, and learning more possible.

The School of the 21st Century

Again, until the middle of the 21st century, the family and its primary social network did a reasonably good job in preparing the young to meet their adult tasks and responsibilities. As the society changed, the family needed more coordinated, coherent support from public and private organizations in the society—health care, sometimes housing and income, schools, and so on. These helping organizations and programs developed separately, in a fragmented way. A silo mentality emerged, with school and community programs operating independently.

Also, a frontier, self-sufficiency mentality persists among many in our society. As a result, income, housing, and other family support programs have experienced significant societal ambivalence and opposition. Thus, the notion that these programs are needed, valued, and must be adequately supported in order to make it possible for most modern families to function well is not a deeply held and pervasive sentiment in the society. For these reasons, it has not been apparent that these programs must be interactive and well coordinated. Only recently has it become clear that the silo mentality and organization are inefficient and ineffective.

A focus on schooling would help us to begin to understand the need and to establish the interactivity among agencies and programs required to help 21st-century families function adequately. Community organizations can be organized around a focus on helping families support the development of their children at home *so that they will be ready for school*, and around *the development of children in school* in a way that will prepare them to become successful family members, workers, and citizens of an open democratic society. But schools and districts must be functioning reasonably well before they can successfully engage community organizations and programs.

In New Haven, we are simultaneously working to create schools capable of ongoing self-improvement and on creating a structure that will enable community organizations and programs to interact with each other and with schools in a way that will have a positive, if not a synergistic, effect. We saw the potential for this when our Social Skills Curriculum for Inner City Children was at its highest level of implementation. The SSCICC related the children and their families to the larger community in a natural and personal way and brought the people and programs of the community into the schools in ways that motivated parents, students, staff, and service providers.

We currently have school-based health clinics and other important family empowerment services operating, but without adequate interaction with the academic program and without ties to larger community services. Nor are the latter services as coordinated and focused on family functioning for child development as they must become. *Importantly, school people and other human services workers cannot be asked to do more without more help and time, better preparation, and rewards.*

In 2001, New Haven mayor John DeStefano established a study group to think through how all community organizations can best serve schools. Simultaneously, our School Development Program again began to work on an in-school pre-K–12 coordinated curriculum that integrates personal development and academic and social learning. The intent is to restore the essential elements of community that once supported families and to provide the students with experiences that truly prepare them for the complex world of today and tomorrow. Again, this is a work in progress, but we believe it is an important start in the right direction. Such a program could go a very long way toward promoting well-being among at-risk children and, indeed, among all children.

References

Bowlby, J. (1988). *A secure base: Parent-child attachment and healthy human development.* New York: Basic Books.

Bransford, J. D., Brown, A. L., & Cocking, R. R. (Eds.). (2002). *How people learn: Brain, mind, experience, and school.* Washington, DC: National Academies Press.

Comer, J. P. (1988). Educating poor minority children. *Scientific American, 259*(5), 42–49.

Comer, J. P. (2004). *Leave no child behind: Preparing today's youth for tomorrow's world.* New Haven, CT: Yale University Press.

Comer, J. P., Haynes, N. M., Joyner, E. T., & Ben-Avie, M. (Eds.). (1996). *Rallying the whole village: The Comer process for reforming education.* New York: Teachers College Press.

Comer, J. P., Joyner, E. T., & Ben-Avie, M. (Eds.). (2004). *The field guide to Comer schools in action: When children develop well, they learn well.* Thousand Oaks, CA: Corwin Press.

Epstein, J. L., & Salinas, K. C. (2004). Partnering with families and communities. *Educational Leadership, 61* (8), 12–18.

Henderson, A. T., & Mapp, K. L. (2002). *A new wave of evidence: The impact of family, school, and community connections on student achievement.* Austin, TX: Southwest Educational Development Laboratory.

U.S. Census Bureau. (2001a). *Historical living arrangements of children.* Available at http://www.census.gov/population/www/socdemo/hh-fam.html.

U.S. Census Bureau. (2001b). *Married couples by labor force status of spouses: 1986 to present.* Available at http://www.census.gov/population/socdemo/hh-fam/tabMC-1.txt.

Wilson, W. J. (1997). *When work disappears: The world of the new urban poor.* New York: Random House.

Additional Sources

Boykin, W. (1994). Comparing outcomes from differential cooperation and individualistic learning methods. *Social Behavioral & Personality, 22*(1), 91–103.

Comer, J. P. (1987). New Haven's school-community connection. *Educational Leadership, 44*(6), 13–16.

Comer, J. P. (1997). *Waiting for a miracle: Why schools can't solve our problems—and how we can.* New York: Dutton.

Comer, J. P. (2001). Schools that develop children. *American Prospect, 12*(7), 30–35.

Comer, J. P. (2002). The place of education. *Boston Review, 27*(1), 17–18.

Darling-Hammond, L. (1998). Teacher learning that supports student learning. *Educational Leadership, 55*(5), 6–11.

Goleman, D. (1995). *Emotional intelligence.* New York: Bantam.

Mowery, D. C., & Rosenberg, N. (1998). *Paths of innovation: Technological change in 20th-century America.* Cambridge: Cambridge University Press.

16 Sex, Guns, and Rock 'n' Roll: The Influence of Media in Children's Lives

Leonard A. Jason and Kerri L. Kim

DePaul University

This chapter is intended to educate readers about the influence of media in children's lives, both good and ill, as well as explore ideas of how to empower parents and those who work with youth in appropriately guiding and/or limiting media exposure. As influential as the media may be, real individuals who have significant relationships with children are even more influential in their lives.

The explosion of electronic entertainment over the past two decades is not necessarily a negative development; indeed, most of these innovations represent an amazing leap forward in the realms of entertainment, education, communication, and everyday fun. The Internet is frequently used for school-related tasks (LaFerle, Edwards, & Lee, 2000), and high-quality programs, games, software, and Web sites can serve as entertaining, informative parts of a child's day. As an example of constructive uses of media, exposure to educational television programs (e.g., *Sesame Street, Mr. Rogers' Neighborhood*) during early childhood is associated with later academic success and imaginative behavior during adolescence (Anderson, Huston, Schmitt, Linebarger, & Wright, 2001). An analysis of strong educational programs offered by commercial broadcasters documented little violence (Jordan, Schmitt, & Woodard, 2001). In addition, these media influences frequently represent just one part of a child's day, balanced with a mix of social, physical, and imaginative pursuits (Jason, Hanaway, & Brackshaw, 1999). Modern theories of cognition support the notion that children are active viewers of television or other media. In other words, viewing even television is not a completely passive experience. Calvert (1999) suggests that the media can challenge stereotypes, foster nonviolent forms of dispute resolution, and educate and inform.

For all the promise of the electronic frontier, however, many parents, educators, researchers, and child advocates have legitimate reservations about the wholesale adoption of electronic entertainment on the part of American children and youth. Of the two chief concerns, one is a problem of time, the other a problem of content. American children spend an average of 6 hours 32 minutes each day involved with various forms of media (i.e., television, movies, video games, computer, and the Internet) (Roberts, Foehr, Rideout, & Brodie, 1999), during which time they are exposed to 8.5 hours of media messages, a result of a portion of children using two or more media simultaneously (Roberts, Foehr, & Rideout, 2005). Parents and educators around the country are increasingly concerned over this amount of time. Part of this concern stems from the fact that a considerable amount of violence and sexuality is regularly portrayed on television and other media technologies. In addition, excessive use of electronic entertainment can interfere with the development of crucial social skills and meaningful family interaction. Excessive viewers also sacrifice both physical and imaginative play as well as reading time, all of which can affect cognitive development and academic achievement (Jason & Hanaway, 1997).

Many parents feel at a loss to control the tide of information rushing toward their children. A parent's natural reaction might be to blame the media industry, and although the industry does bear much of the responsibility, solutions are going to have to come from all quarters, including parents. The industry remains responsible for its content, but as a business, television and its related industries will do as much as they can to remain profitable, even at the expense of children.

Because of exploding technology, parents must step in if enduring, meaningful change is to come about—the kind that touches individual children in individual homes—and no one can achieve such change better than parents. Parents and educators need to become familiar with the power of media and the solutions, and their respective limitations, offered by social scientists and various arms of the industry (ratings, V-chip, etc.). This chapter will provide a review of what can be done to guide and limit media exposure.

Consequences of Viewing Violent and Sexual Images

According to the American Academy of Pediatrics, exposure to violence in television, movies, video games, and the Internet is a significant risk to the health of children and adolescents (American Academy of Pediatrics, 2001). Research findings over the past 40 years indicate that viewing media violence is an important contributing factor to the development of aggressive behavior (Huesmann, Moise-Titus, Podolski, & Eron, 2003). The average child in the United States has watched 100,000 acts of violence and 8,000 murders by the time he or she leaves elementary school, and by the end of high school has been exposed to 200,000 acts of violence (Huston et al., 1992; Villani, 2001). Eighty percent of parents are concerned that their children are exposed to excessive violence and sex on television (Henry J. Kaiser Family Foundation, 2001b).

More than 75% of surveyed parents are also concerned that their children view sexually explicit images on the Internet (Wartella & Jennings, 2000). In the following section, we will review the nature of violent and sexual materials found in media and parental concerns associated with children's exposure to such images.

Defining Violence

According to Gerbner, Gross, Morgan, and Signorielli (1980), violence is "the overt expression of physical force (with or without a weapon, against self or others) compelling action against one's will on pain of being hurt and/or killed or threatened to be so victimized as a part of the plot" (p. 11). The broad scope of this definition allows the incorporation of varying types of violent media, including the cartoon antics of Wile E. Coyote, the reports of shootings and murder on the local news, and the graphically advanced, violent Tekken 3 video game. In other words, there are many ways in which children can become exposed to inappropriate violent messages, and the availability of hundreds of cable channels, video games, and the Internet contributes to children's exposure to violent and sexual materials (Jason et al., 1999). Moreover, the boundaries between violence and sexuality have increasingly been blurred; the result has been media violence that is inherently sexually oriented (Levine, 1996).

Level of Comprehension

Over the years, the portrayal of media violence has become more realistic and cruel (Jason et al., 1999), and this type of violence is more likely to have a negative effect on children (Levine, 1996). Eron (1980) claims that vulnerability to television violence begins as early as age 3, and young viewers rarely understand the motives and consequences behind violent and sexual images. Children may fail to understand or misinterpret program content if they lack the essential background knowledge, and they may accept program content as accurate "information" while more knowledgeable viewers know it to be otherwise (Dorr, 1986). Television's brilliant colors, sound effects, and sharp graphics hold children's attention effortlessly (Singer, 1980). As children get older and begin to understand the media better, they view the violence as less realistic, and they are less frightened by it (Surgeon General's Scientific Advisory Committee on Television and Social Behavior, 1972). But exposure to media violence can still have a lasting effect, as we shall see here.

Modeling

According to Albert Bandura's social learning theory, modeling plays a fundamental role in a child's social development. Bandura (1965) set out to test the relationship between a child's viewing of aggressive behavior and the child's own subsequent aggressiveness. Repeatedly, children who observed aggressive models were seen to display comparable behaviors. Since Bandura's classic work in the 1960s, research has consistently found a positive relationship between excessive television viewing, with its high level of violence, and subsequent aggressive behavior among children (Singer, Singer, & Rapacynski, 1984). Unfortunately, media violence teaches children how to behave aggressively toward others and use violence as a means to resolve their problems (American Academy of Pediatrics, 2003). Habitual early childhood exposure to television violence is predictive of more aggression by children later in life, independent of their own initial childhood aggression, intellectual capabilities, social status, parents' aggressiveness, and parents' viewing habits (Huesmann et al., 2003). Further, children who achieve less tend to watch television more often and identify more strongly with aggressive television characters, and these children are more apt to believe that aggressive television content is real.

Children prefer to model the characters they like and identify with, and children are more likely to model behaviors if they see the perpetrator as being rewarded for performing violence (Levine, 1996). Regrettably, negative consequences rarely follow the violence that is glamorized by media. As an example, the majority of child-oriented cartoons include violence, but pain and suffering rarely accompany the violence (Jason & Hanaway, 1997). In addition, nearly half of violent perpetrators in media suffer no consequences for their acts. There are more than twice as many violent acts per hour on children's programs as on prime-time television. Additionally, 70% of all prime-time television programs contain violence, with men typically depicted as the perpetrators and women as the victims, and this programming teaches males to be aggressive toward females. Even more alarming is the statistic that more than 90% of programs on children's weekend and daytime television contain violence (Jason et al., 1999). Children are repeatedly observing their television heroes solving problems by employing violence, and this encourages them to act aggressively.

In today's advanced technological world, media exposure includes acts of violence that are witnessed in the form of video games (Roberts, 2000). Approximately 85% of video games examined in one study required players to act violently (Bowman & Rotter, 1983). Practicing violent acts may contribute more to aggressive behavior than passive television watching (National Institute on Media and the Family, 2002b. Of the games analyzed, 89% contained some kind of violence, and 9 out of 10 player-controlled killings were justified in the games. More than 75% of the games rated "E" (meaning appropriate for "everyone") contained violence (Children Now, n.d.). Studies have established that young children become more aggressive and show less prosocial behavior when they are observed after playing an aggressive game (Silvern & Williamson, 1987; Subrahmanyam, Greenfield, Kraut, & Gross, 2001). Video games place a child in the role of the aggressor and reward the child for violent behavior. Griffiths and Hunt (1998) maintain that video games allow players to rehearse an entire behavioral script and that they could produce a dependence in children and adolescents because children want to play them for long periods of time in order to advance to higher levels. Even the Surgeon General has warned that the addictive nature of video games can increase violent behavior in children (Sneed & Runco, 1992).

Children with constant access to violent images can become easily frightened by media content (American Academy of Pediatrics, 2003) or desensitized to real-life violence (Huesmann et al., 2003; Jason et al., 1999; Linzer-Schwartz, 1999). The U.S. military uses computer games for combat training to influence military recruits to be more willing to kill (Children Now, 2003; Subrahmanyam et al., 2001). If such games are capable of making recruits more inclined to use violence, similar images can increase children's propensity to engage in aggressive actions.

Television and music videos glamorize the carrying and use of weapons, and children in grades 4 through 8 prefer video games that award points for violence against other people (Funk & Buchman, 1996). Interactive media are relatively new, and consequently there has been less time to assess their influence, but several studies indicate that these types of media may be even more harmful than those of passive media, such as television (Anderson & Dill, 2000; Irwin & Gross, 1995). After playing violent video games, children exhibit measurable decreases in prosocial behaviors and increases in violent retaliation to provocation. In fact, playing violent video games has been found to account for a 13% to 22% increase in adolescents' violent behavior (Anderson, 2000). Whereas viewing television is a fairly passive experience, playing video games and surfing the Internet are highly interactive, and these new electronic media sources can promote violence and hate (Sher, 2000). More research is needed on the possible negative consequences of involvement with these newer, more interactive forms of media.

Sexual Content

Today, sexual dialogue and behavior are prominent on television, videos, and DVDs, video game systems, 100-plus cable channels, and countless Web sites and chat rooms. Greater exposure to sexual content has been associated with a stronger endorsement of recreational attitudes toward sex (Ward & Rivadeneyra, 1999). This is unfortunate given that more than half of teenagers aged 15 to 19 have had sex, and AIDS has become the sixth leading cause of death among those ages 25 to 44 (Brown, Steele, & Walsh-Childers, 2002). Of a sample of 45 television programs, 82% contained some talk about sex or sexual behavior (Brown et al., 2002). In addition, 56.6% of music video programming contains violence, and of these violent videos, a full 81% also depict forms of sexual intimacy (Sherman & Dominick, 1986). When teenagers have been asked about their primary sources of sex information, entertainment television ranked fourth (behind friends, parents, and courses at school). More than half of the respondents believed that topics such as pregnancy, personal consequences of sex, and the likelihood of contracting a sexually transmitted disease were presented on television in a realistic manner (Harris & Associates, 1986). In a study by Browne and colleagues, 75% of characters did not experience any clear consequences associated with their sexual behavior. Further, of the 80 scenes examined that contained sex, only 11 had an emphasis on risk or responsibility (Brown et al., 2002)

With a few notable exceptions, television, computer games, and the Internet still largely fail to address the issues of teen pregnancy and sexually transmitted diseases, including AIDS, among teenagers. At a time when young people are being urged to abstain from sex for their own personal safety, television, computer games, and the Internet continue to emphasize the glamour of sex. The excess of sexual images available in the media, which do not address the realistic potential consequences of sexual behavior, encourage children to adhere to notions that favor recreational attitudes toward their sexual life.

School Performance and Health

Researchers report that excessive television viewing and video game, VCR, computer, and Internet use negatively affect school performance because viewing replaces time that might otherwise be spent reading or pursuing other school activities (Jason & Hanaway, 1997). Practice time is lost, and, as a result, children (particularly those with learning disabilities and other difficulties who are in need of the practice) lose fluency and automaticity in skills such as reading (Corteen & Williams, 1986). Researchers have also found that children's writing is often similar in style to television show scripts—fragmented and disconnected without regard to logic (Doerken, 1983).

One study reported that 39% of children stated they would prefer to surf the Internet than to engage in their favorite after-school activity (Henke, 1999). Greenfield (1999) found that 6% met criteria for compulsive Internet use, and more than 30% reported using the Internet to escape from negative feelings. The vast majority admitted to feelings of time distortion, accelerated intimacy, and feeling uninhibited when online. Clearly, some youngsters are spending excessive amounts of time with these types of media.

In addition, eating snacks and drinking regularly accompany viewing television (Van den Bulck, 2000), and children who watch more television are less likely to participate in vigorous activity (Anderson, Crespo, Bartlett, Cheskin, & Pratt, 1998). Findings indicate that reducing media use might be an effective way to prevent childhood obesity (Robinson, 1999), which is reaching epidemic proportions in the United States.

Stereotypes

The typical media character is a physically fit, male, successful European American. Clearly, the entertainment industry habitually hides society's physical and demographic diversity. Characters who fall outside this mold are portrayed in stereotypical ways, and this pattern is both harmful and limiting (Jason & Hanaway, 1997). As an example, men are more often than not depicted as intelligent, work-oriented, and independent, whereas women are shown as emotional and family-oriented (Morgan, 1987). It should not be surprising that greater sex typing occurs among children who spend more time watching television (Freuh & McGhee, 1975). Although people of color (African American, Asian American, Latin American, and others) represent one-third of the U.S. population (Blaine, 1999), they are greatly underrepresented in media sources, and when portrayed they are frequently in comic roles, service workers, or associated with criminal activity (Jason & Hanaway, 1997). Although individuals over the age of 65 represent 11% of the actual U.S. population, they represent only 2.3% of the characters in media (Jason & Hanaway, 1997). Finally, although 15% to 20% of the population has a disability, people with disabilities represent less than 0.5% of television characters (Linzer-Schwartz, 1999). The media need to do a better job representing the many groups and cultures within our country, and in this way, children and adolescents will better recognize and appreciate the rich diversity that exists within our society (Wroblewski & Huston, 1987).

Strategies for Dealing with Media

The media are ever-present in modern-day society, and as technology continues to advance, there is a clear need to investigate strategies that will help parents and those who work with youth deal more effectively with the influence that media play in children's lives. Concerned parents and educators should adopt a realistic view about the role the electronic entertainment industry can or will have in creating a safer media environment for children. For example, parents should recognize that the television industry (with the obvious exception of cable channels like Nickelodeon and the Disney Channel) is not particularly interested in attracting an unprofitable child audience. By limiting child- and family-friendly programming during the traditional family hour, by promoting sensationalistic afternoon talk shows and reality programming, and by offering children's programs that are product-merchandising efforts, network television has very clearly indicated its priorities. Inadequate governmental compliance with efforts such as the Children's Television Act of 1990 has failed to increase educational programming for children. In the following section, we will discuss ways in which parents and educators can guide and limit children's media viewing.

Parental Supervision

To ensure a more balanced use of time spent on media and non–media-related activities, parents need to play an active role in monitoring the amount of time children devote to this electronic entertainment (Jason & Fries, 2004). Many articles have been written describing the actions parents can take to help their children use the media appropriately, and one common feature is active parental supervision (American Academy of Pediatrics, 2003; Jason et al., 1999; Jason & Hanaway, 1997; National Institute on Media and the Family, 2002a). Observing media-viewing patterns is a necessary preliminary step in understanding the nature of a child's media use. Unfortunately, Levine's (1996) review of the literature indicates that the majority of parents are *not* making the effort to monitor what their children are viewing. Clearly, parents need to spend the time becoming better acquainted with their children's media-viewing patterns (Levine, 1996).

No doubt, the task of monitoring children's media habits is made more difficult by the prospect of working parents and single-parent homes. Those parents who find themselves unable to monitor their children's television, video, and computer consumption might consider finding quality after-school programs, instituting certain homework or chore requirements, developing a level of trust that television privileges will not be abused, or investigating the available products that are aimed at limiting and monitoring children's media consumption in the absence of parental supervision.

Promoting Comprehension

One of the best ways parents can monitor media's content is simply by watching with their children, serving as clarifiers, translators, and even censors when necessary. Studies show that when parents watch television with their children, and actively discuss media content, children's understanding of the messages improves (Levine, 1996). Educating children to be critical, active consumers of media can minimize and counteract the negative ideas and stereotypes media present (Gorham, 1999). Not only does this approach keep media on the level of a family activity, but it also provides a great forum for teaching valuable information. Demeaning stereotypes can be countered, positive messages can be applauded, consequence-free violence can be challenged, and delicate conversations on difficult topics like sex and racism can be broached. Parental involvement is the ideal, but in the real world parents cannot always be on hand to monitor media viewing. To help them learn to make appropriate decisions on their own, children need clear guidelines regarding acceptable and unacceptable programs and material.

Developing Media Rules

Parents need to determine content limits and, no less important, explain their reasoning to their children. Not only will an explanation make content limits seem more logical and less punitive, it also will provide children a solid model for their own decision-making processes. Moreover, when children understand a parent's reasoning, they may be less likely to push the boundaries when they are on their own.

There are several simple actions that parents can take to help develop media rules. First, by limiting the amount of time a child is allowed to view or interact with media, the amount of inappropriate materials reaching the child is also limited (Jason et al., 1999; Villani, 2001). The American Academy of Pediatrics (2003) suggests limiting total viewing time to no more than 1 to 2 hours per day; however, parents might need to consider personal circumstances and conditions when establishing such guidelines (Jason & Fries, 2004).

In addition to taking a more active role in a child's media life, parents also need to model appropriate media use patterns. In other words, parents should lead by example (Jason & Hanaway, 1997). If parents excessively view media, their children are likely to adopt similar media use styles (Levine, 1996). Moreover, parents need to place less emphasis on the use of media as a solitary endeavor (American Academy of Pediatrics, 2003), and this can be done through parents' more actively supervising their children's media use and engaging in conversation about the media content.

Finally, parents can also establish ground rules that would limit a child's media viewing. For example, parents could place time limits on media use, determine that use is not permitted one day per week or on school nights, and allow only certain types of contents to be viewed (Jason & Hanaway, 1997). Parents could also allow media use as contingent upon completion of certain other activities, including homework. Additionally, rules can be developed to limit media exposure by requiring that homework not be completed when the television is on, as doing so interferes with the retention of information. While remaining firm and consistent with enforcing these types of media rules, parents need to be flexible when unexpected situations arise—for example, when a child wants to watch a special program that might require several hours of television viewing.

Although establishing clear rules and expectations is a natural start, the better and more enduring part of monitoring involves the use of diversionary tactics—that is, introducing children to pleasures beyond media to make electronic media less attractive in the first place. Homes that heartily encourage art, music, storytelling, reading, imaginative play, sports, and nature will find that television and other electronic entertainment naturally play less central roles in their children's lives. This approach to family life is easiest to institute when children are very young, but even families with older, dedicated viewers will see positive changes if new interests and opportunities are introduced.

Creating Knowledgeable Consumers

Schools are a natural setting for media literacy programs, and a benefit of presenting these programs within the school environment is that underserved populations will have greater access to this information (Jason et al., 2002). Media education should begin early on, when children are most impressionable to the materials being presented. Lessons should promote critical thinking, encourage students to pay close attention to details, describe what they see, and discuss what aspects they like and dislike (Linzer-Schwartz, 1999; Media Awareness Network, 2003). Media education can equip students with the tools they need to think, respond, and act critically in regard to media content (Media Awareness Network, 2003). And finally, media literacy programs can teach children to recognize their ability to affect the media industry as consumers (Center for Media Literacy, 2003).

In addition to developing rules concerning media use, parents can help their children become knowledgeable consumers of media (Wartella & Jennings, 2000). Parents and children can voice their opinions about damaging messages and portrayals that are being relayed to the public (Knight & Giuliano, 2001) by writing short, well-thought-out letters to producers of programs as well as advertisers. Large corporations, such as Johnson & Johnson and General Motors, have canceled their sponsorship of certain shows because of pressure from the public (Levine, 1996).

Behavior Modification

Parents can use behavioral techniques to aid in monitoring and reducing their children's media use. The simplest of such methods is self-monitoring, which involves recording the amount of media use a child engages in daily. This method has been reported to be effective with some families in reducing children's excessive levels of television viewing (Jason et al., 1999). Self-monitoring can highlight excessive media patterns and help motivate parents to actively limit children's inappropriate media use (Jason & Fries, 2004).

Behavior modification generally involves record keeping and the reinforcement of desired positive behaviors. In the case of media use, children might be required to engage in particular prosocial behaviors, such as completing homework, performing chores, or playing outside with friends. The completion of these alternate activities would earn the children media time. This simple behavior modification system has been used to develop new behaviors as opposed to simply extinguishing media use. For example, Faith et al. (2001) used contingent television to significantly increase physical activity and reduce television viewing among a group of overweight participants. The key to implementing this type of behavior modification system is to keep it enjoyable for the involved children and family members (Jason & Fries, 2004).

Parents who do not have the time to consistently monitor their children's media involvement have found electronic devices helpful in lessening media use (Jason, 1987). As an example, Jason (1985) had a parent provide her child tokens that were earned for participation in certain positive activities such as reading, doing chores, or playing with friends. The tokens could be used to turn on the television set for a half hour. The child's daily average TV viewing was decreased from 7 hours at baseline to 1 hour at a 9-month follow-up. At the conclusion of the study, the mother reported: "It geared her into other areas that she wouldn't have gone into without the program (swimming, musical instruments, interviewer at church). Her grade in science increased from D to A and she recently won the second prize in a science fair." Other devices have been used that require a child to ride a bicycle in exchange for television-viewing time (Jason & Brackshaw, 1999). Tools of this kind can be applied to reduce media use time, particularly with children who are excessive media users. However, once lower levels of media use are achieved, it is best to gradually phase out the use of these external devices.

One of the reasons these behavior modification systems have been successful is that they provide structured opportunities for parents and children to dialogue with each other. Through regular discussions, the families learn better ways to work cooperatively and resolve issues. In several studies, after 1 or 2 weeks of involvement in a behavioral program, important changes in the children's viewing occurred, and after about 8 weeks, the children had shifted their interests into more productive activities. It is possible that both parents and children learn important new communication skills in these types of behavioral interventions.

Ratings, the V-Chip, and Other Blocking Technologies

Other mechanisms are geared toward helping parents monitor media use for their children. For example, networks have created and implemented rating systems for programs, but these ratings can be ambiguous and misleading. Four out of 10 parents *do not believe* the ratings are accurate (Henry J. Kaiser Family Foundation, 2001b). In addition, the rating systems are premised on the idea that children are being exposed to media in a supervised environment, and clearly this often does not occur.

The V-chip (violence chip) is an electronic device that is built into television sets and is used to read the ratings of programs provided by networks. It adds to parents' ability to control what the television set is allowed to play and, therefore, what their children are permitted to view (Huesmann et al., 2003). However, only 40% of parents now have television sets with V-chips, and of those individuals who do have access to a V-chip, 53% do not know they have it, while only 17% use it to block shows (Henry J. Kaiser Family Foundation, 2001b). In addition, network producers have been allowed to rate their own shows, and there is a clear need for an independent and less biased source for these ratings.

Cable companies offer blocking options for those channels that subscribers deem undesirable. Programs like "SurfWatch" have been developed to aid parents in limiting what their children are able to access online (Bremer & Rauch, 1998). An electronic computer can be attached to a television and allocates to children a designated amount of time that television can be watched each day (Johnson & Jason, 1996). In general, these solutions only seek to regulate or restrict the flow of material, rather than improve the material in the first place. Despite video game ratings, many retail outlets sell or rent games to anyone regardless of age. As for the Internet, a source of serious concern for many parents, recent efforts at creating a child-friendly cyberspace have proved inevitably weak, as there are now millions of Web pages, and many have not been rated by the Recreational Software Advisory Council or SafeSurf. Meanwhile, software products have been developed to block objectionable material and limit the times of day when kids can surf the Internet. Regrettably, most of these products can be defeated, and those that cannot are fairly to extremely restrictive, preventing children from getting the most out of their online experience.

Conclusions

Increasing disengagement among adolescents from family and community is due to multiple factors, but, clearly, inappropriate media content is an important contributing factor (Schwartz & Greenfield, 1999). Decades of psychological research have shown that violence in media may influence children to be less sensitive to the pain and suffering of others, more fearful of the world around them, and more likely to behave in aggressive and harmful ways toward others (Jason et al., 1999). Children themselves have reported that television makes them think people are dishonest, selfish, and care more about money than other people. Video game manufacturers specialize in violence, and Web site creators invite children to view pornography and violent scenes. To deal with these ubiquitous problems, parents must play an active role in talking with their children and monitoring their use of media. Television ratings and the V-chip will not replace the need for parents to supervise the content and overall amount of media exposure.

Many experts suggest limiting overall media use to no more than 2 hours a day, but families individually need to consider their own goals and develop expectations and strategies accordingly. Even with 2 hours of viewing a day, parents have cause for concern as media content includes violence, sex, and stereotyping that can negatively affect impressionable children. The average child views 6.5 hours of media daily, and each hour spent viewing media reduces the valuable time that children could otherwise be engaged in simple yet somehow essential childhood pursuits such as riding bikes and playing with friends. Heavy viewing beyond this 6.5 hours per day is a clear sign that a problem needs to be addressed as there is mounting evidence that excessive viewing can seriously challenge a child's social, emotional, mental, and physical well-being (Jason & Hanaway, 1997).

Parents need to commit to the hard work of monitoring how much time is spent watching television and playing computer games, surfing the Internet, and interacting with other electronic entertainment. The issue of content will have been mitigated in part simply by limiting the time of children's overall exposure. Even with time rules in place, however, content issues will continue to require monitoring.

Parents and public policy officials need to become more involved in the content debate by actively voicing their disapproval (or support, as the case may be) to local stations and national networks. Parents have a legitimate basis on which to continue arguing for increasing high-quality programming for children. Parents have an absolute right and responsibility to express their opinions and to follow up with boycotts and letter-writing campaigns if necessary. Networks will be more responsive when ratings and profits are at stake.

To develop into healthy, independent adults, children need to participate in the real world and develop hobbies and lifelong interests (Jason, 1997). Television, video games, and Internet surfing are simply too passive, impersonal, and limiting to wholly serve the developing needs of children. No matter what obligations the electronic entertainment industry has toward children and families, no producer or network president will provide the environment that will ensure a healthy, balanced childhood. This is a job for parents and educators.

Acknowledgment.

The authors thank Amber Jurgens for her editorial help on this manuscript.

References

American Academy of Pediatrics. (2001). Media violence. *Pediatrics, 108*, 1222–1226.
American Academy of Pediatrics. (2003). *Understanding the impact of media on children and teens.* Available at http://www.apa.org/family/mediaimpact.htm. Retrieved April 4, 2003.
Anderson, C. (2000). The impact of interactive violence on children. *Hearing before the Senate Committee on Commerce, Science, and Transportation.* 106th Congress, 1st session.
Anderson, C. A., & Dill, K. E. (2000). Video games and aggressive thoughts, feelings and behavior in the laboratory and in life. *Journal of Personality and Social Psychology, 78*, 772–790.
Anderson, D. R., Huston, A. C., Schmitt, L., Linebarger, D. L., & Wright, J. C. (2001). Early childhood television viewing and adolescent behavior. *Monographs of the Society for Research in Child Development, 66* (1, Serial No. 264).
Anderson, R. E., Crespo, C. J., Bartlett, S. J., Cheskin, L. J., & Pratt, M. (1998). Relationship of physical activity and television watching with body weight and level of fatness among children: Results from the third National Health and Nutrition Examination Survey. *Journal of the American Medical Association, 279*, 938–942.
Bandura, A. (1965). Influence of models' reinforcement contingencies on the acquisition of imitative responses. *Journal of Personality and Social Psychology, 1*, 589–595.
Bowman, R. P., & Rotter, J. C. (1983). Computer games: Friend or foe? *Elementary School Guidance and Counseling, 18*, 25–34.
Bremer, J., & Rauch, P. K. (1998). Children and computers: Risks and benefits. *Journal of the American Academy of Child and Adolescent Psychiatry, 37*(5), 559–560.
Brown, J. D., Steele, J. R., & Walsh-Childers, K. (Eds.). (2002). *Sexual teens, sexual media: Investigating media's influence on adolescent sexuality.* Mahwah, NJ: Erlbaum.
Calvert, S. (1999). *Children's journeys through the information age.* New York: McGraw-Hill
Center for Media Literacy. (2003). *Assignment media literacy—Maryland Project.* Available at http://www.medialit.org. Retrieved April 2, 2003.

Children Now. (n.d.). *Fair play? Violence, gender and race in video games.* Available at http://www.childrennow.org. Retrieved March 30, 2003.

Corteen, R. S., & Williams, T. M. (1986). Television and reading skills. In T. M. Williams (Ed.), *The impact of television: A natural experiment in three communities* (pp. 39–86). Orlando, FL: Academic Press.

Doerken, M. (1983). *Classroom combat: Teaching and television.* Englewood Cliffs, NJ: Educational Technology Productions.

Dorr, A. (1986). *Children and television: A special medium for a special audience.* Beverly Hills, CA: Sage.

Eron, L. D. (1980). Prescription for reduction of aggression. *American Psychologist, 35,* 244–252.

Faith, M. S., Berman, N., Heo., M., Pietrobelli, A., Gallagher, D., Epstein, L. H., et al. (2001). Effects of contingent television on physical activity and television viewing in obese children. *Pediatrics, 107*(5), 1043–1048.

Freuh, T., & McGhee, P. (1975). Traditional sex-role development and amount of time spent watching television. *Child Development, 11,* 109.

Funk, J. B., & Buchman, D. D. (1996). Playing violent video and computer games and adolescent self-concept. *Journal of Communications, 46,* 19–32.

Gerbner, G., Gross, L., Morgan, M., & Signorielli, N. (1980). The "mainstreaming" of America: Violence profile no. 11. *Journal of Communication, 30*(3), 10–29.

Gorham, B. W. (1999). Stereotypes in the media: So what? *Howard Journal of Communications, 10,* 229–247.

Greenfield, D. N. (1999, August). *The nature of Internet addiction: Psychological factors in compulsive Internet use.* Paper presented at the meeting of the American Psychological Association, Boston, MA.

Griffiths, M. D., & Hunt, N. (1998). Dependence on computer games by adolescents. *Psychological Reports, 82,* 475–480.

Harris, L., & Associates. (1986). *American teens speak: Sex, myths, TV, and birth control.* New York: Planned Parenthood Federation of America.

Henke, L. L. (1999). Children, advertising, and the Internet: An exploratory study. In D. W. Schumann & E. Thorson (Eds.), *Advertising and the World Wide Web: Advertising and consumer psychology* (pp. 73–80). Mahwah, NJ: Erlbaum.

Henry J. Kaiser Family Foundation. (1994). *Kids and media at the new millennium: A Kaiser Family Foundation Report.* Menlo Park, CA: Author.

Henry J. Kaiser Family Foundation. (2001a). *Fact sheet: Kids and media.* Available at http://www.mediaandthefamily.org. Retrieved March 26, 2003.

Henry J. Kaiser Family Foundation. (2001b). *How parents feel about TV, the TV ratings system, and the V-chip.* Available at http://www.mediaandthefamily.org. Retrieved March 26, 2003.

Huesmann, L. R., Moise-Titus, J., Podolski, C., & Eron, L. D. (2003). Longitudinal relations between children's exposure to TV violence and their aggressive and violent behavior in young adulthood: 1977–1992. *Developmental Psychology, 39*(2), 201–221.

Huston, A. C., Donnerstein, E., Fairchild, H., Feshbach, N. D., Katz, P. A., Murray, J. P., et al. (1992). *Big world, small screen: The role of television in American society.* Lincoln: University of Nebraska Press.

Irwin, A. R., & Gross, A. M. (1995). Cognitive tempo, violent video games, and aggressive behavior in young boys. *Journal of Family Violence, 10,* 337–350.

Jason, L. A. (1985). Using a token-actuated timer to reduce television viewing. *Journal of Applied Behavior Analysis, 18,* 269–272.

Jason, L. A. (1987). Reducing children's television viewing and assessing secondary changes. *Journal of Clinical Child Psychology, 16,* 245–250.

Jason, L. A. (1997). *Community building: Values for a sustainable future.* Westport, CT: Praeger.

Jason, L. A., & Brackshaw, E. (1999). Case study: Reducing TV viewing and corresponding increases in physical activity and subsequent weight loss. *Journal of Behavior Therapy and Experimental Psychiatry, 30,* 145–151.

Jason, L. A., Curie, C. J., Townsend, S. M., Pokorny, S. B., Katz, R. B., & Sherk, J. L. (2002). Health promotion interventions. *Child and Family Behavior Therapy, 24*(1–2), 67–82.

Jason, L. A., & Fries, M. (2004). Helping parents reduce children's TV viewing. *Research on Social Work Practice, 14,* 121–131.

Jason, L. A., & Hanaway, L. K. (1997). *Remote control: A sensible approach to kids, TV, and the new electronic media.* Sarasota, FL: Professional Resource Press.

Jason, L. A., Hanaway, L. K., & Brackshaw, E. A. (1999). Television violence and children: Problems and solutions. In T. P. Gullotta & S. J. McElhaney (Eds.), *Issues in children's and families' lives: Vol. 11. Violence in homes and communities: Prevention, intervention, and treatment* (pp. 133–156). Washington, DC: National Mental Health Association.

Johnson, S. Z., & Jason, L. A. (1996). Evaluation of a device aimed at reducing children's television viewing. *Child and Family Behavior Therapy, 18,* 59–61.

Jordan, A. B., Schmitt, K. L., & Woodard, E. H. (2001). Developmental implications of commercial broadcasters' educational offerings. *Journal of Applied Developmental Psychology, 22,* 87–101.

Knight, J. L., & Giuliano, T. A. (2001). He's a Laker; she's a "looker": The consequences of gender-stereotypical portrayals of male and female athletes by the print media. *Sex Roles, 45*(3–4), 217–229.

LaFerle, C., Edwards, S. M., & Lee, W.-N. (2000). Teens' use of traditional media and the Internet. *Journal of Advertising Research, 40,* 55–65.

Levine, M. (1996). *Viewing violence: How media violence affects your child's and adolescent's development.* New York: Doubleday.

Linzer-Schwartz, L. (Ed.). (1999). *Psychology and the media: A second look.* Washington, DC: American Psychological Association.

Media Awareness Network. (2003). *Media education and media violence.* Available at http://www. reseaumedias.ce/english/issues/violence/role_media_ education.cfm. Retrieved April 1, 2003.

Morgan, M. (1987). Television, sex-role attitudes, and sex-role behavior. *Journal of Early Adolescence, 7*(3), 269–282.

National Institute on Media and the Family. (2002a). *Fact sheet.* Available at http:// www.mediaandthefamily.org. Retrieved March 26, 2003.

National Institute on Media and the Family. (2002b). *What goes in must come out: Children's media violence consumption at home and aggressive behaviors at school.* Available at http:// www.mediaandthefamily.org. Retrieved March 26, 2003.

Roberts, D. F. (2000). Media and youth: Access, exposure, and privatization. *Journal of Adolescent Health, 27*(suppl.), 8–14.

Roberts, D. F., Foehr, U. G., & Rideout, V. J. (2005). *Generation M: Media in the lives of 8–18 year-olds.* Menlo Park, CA: Kaiser Family Foundation.

Roberts, D. F., Foehr, U. G., Rideout, V. J., & Brodie, M. (1999). *Kids and media @ the new millennium.* Menlo Park, CA: Kaiser Family Foundation.

Robinson, T. N. (1999). Reducing children's television viewing to prevent obesity: A randomized controlled trial. *Journal of the American Medical Association, 282,* 1561–1567.

Schwartz, L. L., & Greenfield, M. R. (1999). Tuning into the media: Youth, violence, and incivility. In L. L. Schwartz (Ed.), *Psychology and the media: Vol. 2. Psychology and the media: A second look* (pp. 173–214). Washington, DC: American Psychological Association.

Sher, L. (2000). The Internet, suicide, and human mental functions. *Canadian Journal of Psychiatry, 45,* 297.

Sherman, B. L., & Dominick, J. R. (1986). Violence and sex in music videos: TV and rock 'n' roll. *Journal of Communication, 36,* 79–83.

Silvern, S. B., & Williamson, P. A. The effects of video game play on young children's aggression, fantasy, and prosocial behavior. *Journal of Applied Developmental Psychology, 8*(4), 453–462.

Singer, J. L. (1980). The power and limitations of television: A cognitive-affective analysis. In P. H. Tannenbaum (Ed.), *The entertainment functions of television* (pp. 31–65). Hillsdale, NJ: Erlbaum.

Singer, J. L., Singer, D. G., & Rapacynski, W. S. (1984). Family patterns and television viewing as predictors of children's beliefs and aggression. *Journal of Communication, 34,* 274–278.

Sneed, C., & Runco, M. A. (1992). The beliefs adults and children hold about television and video games. *Journal of Psychology, 126*(3), 273–284.

Subrahmanyam, K., Greenfield, P., Kraut, R., & Gross, E. (2001). The impact of computer use on children's and adolescents' development. *Applied Developmental Psychology, 22*, 7–30.

Surgeon General's Scientific Advisory Committee on Television and Social Behavior. (1972). *Television and growing up: The impact of televised violence.* Washington, DC: U.S. Government Printing Office.

Van den Bulck, J. (2000). Is television bad for your health? Behavior and body image of the adolescent "couch potato." *Journal of Youth and Adolescence, 29*, 273–288.

Villani, S. (2001). Impact of media on children and adolescents: A 10-year review of the research. *Journal of the American Academy of Child and Adolescent Psychiatry, 40*(4), 392–401.

Ward, L. M., & Rivadeneyra, R. (1999). Contributions of entertainment television to adolescents' sexual attitudes and expectations: The role of viewing amount versus viewer involvement. *Journal of Sex Research, 36*, 237–249.

Wartella, E. A., & Jennings, N. (2000). Children and computers: New technology—old concerns. *Future of Children, 10*(2), 31–43.

Wroblewski, R., & Huston, A. C. (1987). Televised occupational stereotypes and their effects on early adolescents: Are they changing? *Journal of Early Adolescence, 7*(3), 283–297.

17 The Civil Society Model: The Organic Approach to Building Character, Competence, and Conscience in Our Young People

Bill Stanczykiewicz

Indiana Youth Institute

> The question for our time is not whether all men are brothers. That question has been answered by God who placed us on this earth together. The question is whether we have the strength and the will to make the brotherhood of man the guiding principle of our daily lives. (President John F. Kennedy, quoted in Federer, 1994)

The time for reading had arrived in the second-grade classroom, and an ambitious boy climbed onto the lap of the volunteer teaching assistant. As the volunteer prepared to read to the assembled circle of eager students, the curious boy on his lap studied the man's face, touching the tips of his fingers against end-of-afternoon whiskers.

"What are those?" the boy asked, his amazement surpassed only by the volunteer's astonishment. The child was truly dumbfounded by the little stubs growing out of the man's cheeks. "Do they hurt?" the boy inquired further.

The teaching assistant could not believe it. This boy and many of his classmates had never been close to an adult male, let alone close enough to observe a man shaving in the morning (Terry West, personal communication, September 1992).

Whereas the second-grade boy was searching for an explanation, children at the Lifeline Community Center are finding their way. Lifeline was launched in inner-city Indianapolis in 1997 by Ermil Thompson, a retired federal worker who grew weary of watching young children roaming the rough streets with nothing to do. Thompson responded by raising $30,000, mostly by cooking lunches at $5 a head for area businesses. She used the funds to purchase and renovate an abandoned house where prostitutes and drug addicts congregated.

Midway through the renovation, the criminal element struck back by setting the building on fire. The blaze was stopped, but Thompson was not. She simply cooked more lunches, raised more money, and opened the Lifeline Community Center to 25 low-income children in a crime-infested neighborhood.

Tutoring, arts and crafts, and other fun learning activities fill summer days and school-year afternoons. Donations—from food to computers—provide needed supplies. And thanks to Thompson's remarkable resourcefulness, there is always enough money left at the end of the summer to take the kids on field trips to places like Washington, D.C., and the University of Notre Dame.

Providing a safe haven in the midst of danger and despair would be enough for most folks interested in the well-being of children, but not for Ermil Thompson. Growing up in a household of 17 children prepared her for instilling dignity and respect in the youngsters at Lifeline. Rules for proper behavior are strictly enforced. Striving for excellence is consistently encouraged. Achievement is an expectation, not a surprise. One result: All of the children arrived as struggling students; 10 are now on the honor roll.

The activities at Lifeline Community Center display the basic truth of healthy youth development: What all kids need most are positive relationships with caring adults who are passionately committed to their very existence— first and foremost in their family, ideally with two married parents, and also in their surrounding community. Yes, these relationships can ensure the fulfillment of basic needs such as food, shelter, and safety, and caring adults also can provide interventions for children suffering from physical or emotional health problems. More important, however, these relationships reach deeper into the very human essence of the child.

Although the process is intangible, the outcomes are not. Research supports common sense. When children have those positive and caring relationships—in their families and in their communities—they tend to do better in life, regardless of how that is measured. They tend to do better in school, delay parenthood until marriage, avoid crime, and stay away from cigarettes, drugs, and alcohol. Civil society indeed is decisive in the healthy development of children and youth.

Out of the Mouths of Babes

Like the curious second grader who was shocked by whiskers, none of the children at Lifeline have fathers in their homes. One summer, as Father's Day approached, Thompson asked the kids what they would like to do with their dads if they were around. The replies ranged from playing basketball to riding bikes to taking a walk around the block. Incredibly, not one of these poverty-stricken children said, "Go to the store and buy me things." Instead, their responses were both simple and profound: "Just be with me. Please!" (personal communication, July 1999).

The same message was delivered by more than 100,000 teens surveyed or interviewed in a national longitudinal study commissioned by Congress through the National Institutes of Health. Conducting the National Longitudinal Study of Adolescent Health (Add Health), researchers provided anonymous questionnaires to nearly 90,000 students, grades 7 through 12, in 145 American schools. An additional 35,000 students provided information during in-home interviews. Although a thorough analysis of the data will not be available for several years, an initial overview provides important learnings.

Looking at the data, researchers Robert Blum and Peggy Mann Rinehart (1998) find that most kids are physically healthy. "Threats to their health," Blum and Rinehart warn, "stem primarily from their behavior. Drinking and driving, involvement in violence, early and unprotected sex, and drug abuse create immediate threats; use of tobacco, poor nutrition, and sedentary lifestyles can lead to health problems in later years" (p. 5).

Through the questionnaires and interviews, one fourth of adolescents said they smoke cigarettes, about half that number reported smoking marijuana in the previous month, and just under 18% reported drinking alcohol more than once a month. More than 10% of boys and more than 5% of girls reported committing a violent act in the past year. Nine percent of young people reported having suicidal thoughts, dropping to 4% who have actually attempted suicide. Nearly half of the teens said they have experienced sexual intercourse (pp. 10–14).

But the adolescents also described the connections that help them avoid those dangerous behaviors. Not surprisingly, family matters most. As Blum and Mann Rinehart summarize, "Across all of the health outcomes examined, the results point to the importance of family and the home environment for protecting adolescents from harm. What emerges most consistently as protective is the teenager's feeling of connectedness with parents and family" (p. 31).

Whether low-income youngsters are talking with Ermil Thompson, or a cross section of American teens are talking with trained researchers, a basic conclusion can be reached: Kids are hardwired to connect, first in family, and then in their local communities.

Not Rocket Science

The circuit board for this internal hardwiring has been the subject of constant scientific study. In examining more than 100 of those studies, Dr. Peter Benson gleaned 40 common attributes—which he terms *assets*—that all kids need to thrive. Now published as Search Institute's 40 Developmental Assets, the list translates dense data into simple science (Benson, 1997).

Three of the first six assets depict the same connections described by the Add Health teens—connections such as "Family life provides high levels of love and support," and "Young person and her or his parent(s) communicate positively, and young person is willing to seek advice and counsel from parents." Also near the top of Benson's list are affirming relationships with nonfamily adults, including, "Young person receives support from three or more nonparent adults," and "Young person experiences caring neighbors." Other assets emphasize positive activities such as community service, reading for pleasure at least three or more hours a week, and spending one or more hours per week in activities in a religious institution. Safety, honesty, and integrity also make the list (Benson, 1997, pp. 32–33).

The assets are not complicated, but that is exactly Benson's point. All adults can become engaged in meaningful ways—through family and community—in the lives of young people. As Benson often says, when it comes to youth development, "If you breathe, you're on the team."

In important and intuitive ways, Benson's research demonstrates that the more assets a child possesses, the more likely that child will be to avoid negative behaviors and display thriving behaviors. For example, a survey in Minneapolis of more than 5,000 students in grades 6 through 12 revealed that 63% of adolescents who reported having 0 to 10 assets consumed alcohol three or more times in the previous month, compared with just 12% of young people who reported having more than 30 assets. Other survey results demonstrated that 75% of kids who said they had at least 26 assets are involved in volunteer community service (Benson, 1997).

Benson concludes: "Developmental assets are powerful predictors of behavior. They serve as protective factors: they inhibit, for example, alcohol and other drug abuse, violence, sexual intercourse, and school failure. They serve as enhancement factors: they promote positive developmental outcomes. And they also serve as resiliency factors: they help youth weather adversity. For each important function (protection, enhancement, resiliency), the key dynamic is this: the more assets, the better" (Benson, 1997, p. 55).

Peter Benson is not alone in deducing understandable patterns from complex studies on human development. James Q. Wilson conducted a similar review and is convinced that people are hardwired with what he terms the *moral sense*. "Most of us do not break the law most of the time," Wilson writes, "not simply because we worry about taking even a small chance of getting caught, but also because our conscience forbids our doing what is wrong" (Wilson, 1993, p. 13).

Wilson contends that the moral sense is something we are born with, as infants exhibit moral behavior before they develop the language skills needed to be taught the difference between right and wrong. "The rudiments of moral action—a regard for the well-being of others and anxiety at having failed to perform according to a standard—are present well before anything like moral reasoning could occur. If morality had to be written on a blank slate wholly by means of instruction, then it would not emerge until well after language had been acquired so that concepts could be understood, and by that time it would probably be too late" (Wilson, 1993, p. 130)."

Wilson's notion of the moral sense is consistent with America's religious heritage. For example, Christians cite the Apostle Paul, who wrote, "Indeed, when Gentiles, who do not have the [Jewish] law, do by nature things required by the law, they are a law for themselves, even though they do not have the law, since they show that the requirements of the law are written on their hearts, their consciences also bearing witness, and their thoughts now accusing, now even defending them" (Romans 2:14–15, New International Version). Similarly, the Jewish prophet Jeremiah recorded, " 'This is the covenant I will make with the house of Israel after that time,' declares the Lord. 'I will put my law in their minds and write it on their hearts. I will be their God, and they will be my people" (Jeremiah 31:33, NIV).

The influence of religion cannot be discounted. A summary of studies on the impact of religious belief on personal behavior reported that states with higher levels of religious belief have lower rates of teen pregnancy; teens who regularly attend religious services are less likely to consume drugs or alcohol; and religiously active teens experience less anxiety and depression (Fagan, 1996).

But, according to Wilson, positive consequences such as these do not just happen on their own. The implanted *moral sense* needs careful cultivation. "Children do not learn morality by learning maxims or clarifying values. They enhance their natural sentiments by being regularly induced by families, friends, and institutions to behave in accord with the most obvious standards of right conduct—fair dealing, reasonable self-control, and personal honesty. A moral life is perfected by practice more than by precept; children are not taught so much as habituated" (Wilson, 1993, p. 249).

In short, a child's natural hardwiring still is in need of a good electrician, or as Wilson underscores, electricians—plural: "families, friends, and institutions." Benson's 40 Developmental Assets also begin with the family, followed by nonfamily adults and other community factors. The sociologist David Popenoe (1995) ties together these vital influences of family and community into a civil society package of healthy youth development: "For the moral development of children, no aspect of community support is more important than the community's ability to reinforce the social expectations of parents; that is, to express a consensus of shared values. Young people need to hear a consistent message about what is right and wrong from all the important adults in their lives; they need not only a social community but a moral community" (p. 73).

In effect agreeing with Wilson, Popenoe adds: "The central significance of the community for moral development is this: moral development in children takes place in part through repetition and reinforcement, and through adapting fundamental moral values to a variety of social circumstances beyond the family. As the child moves into the outside world, the moral lessons taught by the parents must be sustained by others" (1995, p. 82).

The engagement of "others" is described by the sociologist Robert Putnam (2000) through the lens of *social capital*, most often demonstrated by neighbors who interact with each other on a frequent basis and who participate in civic and voluntary organizations. In the context of child well-being, Putnam confidently states, "Child development is powerfully shaped by social capital" (p. 296).

Putnam has developed a state-by-state national measurement of social capital—the Social Capital Index—and he compares the index against data on child well-being from the Kids Count indexes published and supported by the Annie E. Casey Foundation. He concludes: "States that score high on the Social Capital Index—that is, states whose residents trust other people, join organizations, volunteer, vote, and socialize with friends—are the same states where children flourish: where babies are born healthy and where teenagers tend not to become parents, drop out of school, get involved in violent crime, or die prematurely due to suicide or homicide. Statistically, the correlation between high social capital and positive child development is as close to perfect as social scientists ever find in data analyses of this sort" (Putnam, 2000, pp. 296–297).

The value of social capital also is realized in the classroom. "States with high social capital have measurably better educational outcomes than do less civic states," Putnam writes. "The beneficial effects of social capital persist even after accounting for a host of other factors that might affect state educational success—racial composition, affluence, economic inequality, adult educational levels, poverty rates, educational spending, teachers' salaries, class size, family structure, and religious affiliation, as well as the size of the private-school sector. Social capital—not poverty or demographic characteristics per se—drives test scores" (Putnam, 2000, pp. 299–300).

The author James Traub (2000) agrees, arguing that academic achievement is dependent upon the human touch—Putnam's *social capital* interacting with Wilson's *moral sense*. In a review of public spending on a wide range of education reforms, Traub writes, "It turns out that almost anything can work when instituted by a dedicated principal supported by committed teachers. Jaime Escalante, the teacher celebrated in the movie *Stand and Deliver*, prodded his impoverished Chicano students to extraordinary achievements on their Advanced Placement math tests, but any method that depends on a Jaime Escalante is no method at all." And since "whom you hang out with, both during and after school, can matter more than what happens in the classroom," Traub contends that "there's a strong argument for universally available after-school activities. No less important would be the restoration of the web of church, community and police-sponsored programs that once flourished in big cities. The breakdown of families means that we have to ask more of social institutions—and not just schools—than we used to. Of course we also have to ask more of the families themselves."

Community Youth Organizations

Traub's "web" of out-of-school youth programs can include nationally affiliated nonprofits like the YMCA, Boys and Girls Clubs, 4-H, Boy Scouts and Girls Scouts; local agencies such as community centers; and the diverse range of faith-based youth ministries. Summarizing the extensive research on the positive impacts of youth groups such as these, the University of Chicago's Chapin Hall Center for Children reports, "Youth-serving organizations share the aims of contributing to the positive development of young people. In fact, many programs for young people function as engaging and rigorous settings for cognitive and social development. They provide opportunities to participate in activities and issues of importance, involving participants in environments of high expectations and sustained support. These opportunities can contribute to developing competencies critical for individual achievement in both education and employment and for participation in civic life" (Wynn, 2000, p. 9).

The National Research Council (NRC), reviewing two decades of studies, finds that the most successful community youth organizations enjoy the following eight characteristics:

Physical and Psychological Safety: At the most basic level, safety is essential for positive development....

Clear and Consistent Structure and Appropriate Adult Supervision: Development requires that a child experience a stable, predictable reality.... A critical element of structure is consistent monitoring and enforcement of rules and expectations....

Supportive Relationships: The quality of relationships with adults comes up again and again as a critical feature of any developmental setting....

Opportunities to Belong: One of the first issues for an adolescent walking through the door or even thinking about trying a community program is whether he or she can belong to this group of people: "Will I fit in, will I be comfortable?"...

Positive Social Norms: Community programs have an internal culture of social norms that shapes youths' perception of appropriate behavior for good or ill, depending on the social norms that emerge....

Support for Efficacy and Mattering: If adolescents do not experience personal engagement and a sense of mattering, they are not likely to grow personally....

Opportunities for Skill Building: Good settings provide opportunities to acquire knowledge and learn both new skills and new habits of mind....

Integration of Family, School, and Community Efforts: There is every reason to believe that community programs will be more effective when they coordinate their activities with parents, schools, and communities. (Eccles & Gootman, 2002, pp. 129–138)

The NRC emphasizes that "the more of the eight positive features described that a community program has, the greater the contribution it will make to the positive development of youth" (Eccles & Gootman, 2002, p. 112). This statement adds further weight to the conclusion that kids are hardwired to connect, and that civil society—in this context expressed through community-based youth agencies—energizes that wiring. Revisiting the list reveals that at least six of the eight characteristics permeate into a child's internal dynamics: a stable and structured setting with enforced guidelines and expectations; quality relationships with adults; a sense of belonging; social norms that shape appropriate behavior; personal engagement and mattering; and learning new skills and new habits of mind. Each of these qualities carries positive current into the hardwired child.

The NRC also highlights the healthy influences of religious faith: "Research on faith-based institutions and the role of religious organizations, such as churches and synagogues, suggests that they can contribute to community-wide efforts to promote youth development in several key areas, helping to reduce risky behaviors, building a value base from which young people make decisions, and involving a variety of people across the life span. While schools and social service agencies reach only targeted populations, congregations often touch a cross-section of the population" (Eccles & Gootman, 2002, p. 142).

The reason, according to a study released by Public/Private Ventures, is that youth workers in faith-based ministries are responding to hardwiring of their own: "Faith-motivated volunteers draw strength from their sense of mission, even when program goals do not press for youth to find faith themselves. They see faith as that which enables them to do the difficult work of ministering to underserved youth, to take the time necessary to develop relationships of trust and accountability, and to endure the struggles and setbacks that inevitably come when youth 'fall away' or become recidivists. Faith becomes the motivation for being involved in the lives of high-risk youth, the impetus for caring" (Trulear, 2000, p. 17).

Taking It to the Streets

One of the nation's most compelling examples of faith-based motivation is found in the Dorchester neighborhood of Boston. Over an 8-year stretch, a church-based initiative named the Ten Point Coalition worked closely with teens, law enforcement, and social service providers to reduce the neighborhood's annual number of juvenile homicides from 60 to zero.

This remarkable effort was born out of crisis. During the funeral for a teenager in the Morning Star Baptist Church, another teen was chased into the sanctuary and stabbed in front of the congregation by rival gang members. Instead of throwing up his hands, the Rev. Eugene Rivers led with his feet, encouraging 43 other ministers to join him on Dorchester's meanest streets to persuade teens to leave their lives of gang warfare and prostitution.

In addition to the tragic stabbing inside his church, Rivers was inspired by his relationship with a neighborhood drug dealer. "Selvin [the drug dealer] explained to us, 'I'm there when Johnny goes out for a loaf of bread for Mama. I'm there, you're not. I win, you lose,'" Rivers said. "It's all about being there" (Leland, 1998, p. 20).

That's why Rivers became active in the life of a 10-year-old boy he describes as "America's worst nightmare," a boy living in dire poverty—both materially and emotionally—his father dead and his mother addicted to drugs. Rivers would visit the boy in school and at home, and then spend additional time with him at the church youth center. After one encounter at school, Rivers remarks, "You see that smile? You see the way he lit up? See, he's doable. We can get him. But you got to do an intensive thing with him. He'll go for the love thing, 'cause he's never seen it from a black male before." And revealing a confidence in the inner desire of kids to connect with caring adults, Rivers adds, "He's almost wishing someone would care enough to spank him" (Klein, 1997, p. 41).

Olgen Williams (2001) has seen the same story himself. Responding to the murder of two arson investigators in his inner-city Indianapolis neighborhood of Haughville, Williams used a neighborhood community center—Christamore House—as a centralizing force. Williams pulled together neighborhood associations, churches, business and labor, law enforcement, residents, and local government into a collaboration with dramatic results. For example, when Indianapolis experienced a record homicide rate in 1997, the murder rate in formerly rough-and-tumble Haughville went down by 70%. Dozens of kids have received computers in recognition of their academic success, with one teen rising to the position of Governor of Boys State (the American Legion program for high school seniors)—an achievement that would have been unthinkable in Haughville a decade before.

"Real solutions are found when common people work together to create results. In order to bring health to our communities, there must be cooperation among government agencies, churches, synagogues, mosques, neighborhood organizations, schools, labor unions, charities, businesses, and citizens" (Williams, 2001, p. 149).

And those citizens include the young people themselves. That's the lesson from Columbus, Indiana, where adult leaders stepped aside and let a group of ambitious teenagers renew their local community. Joe Nierman, at the time a high school sophomore, was weary of receiving public nuisance tickets for skateboarding in public places. Nierman finally told park department director Chuck Wilt, "You build basketball and tennis courts on park property, and people can play for free. So you should do the same for kids who want to skateboard."

Wilt agreed, on one condition. "You build it, Joe, and adults will help." So Nierman responded by organizing nearly two dozen of his skateboarding buddies, and they raised about $100,000 in donations—almost all of it in cash, quite remarkable in a town of roughly 30,000 residents. After he and his friends reviewed existing park space for the perfect site, Nierman drew up the blueprints for Columbus's forthcoming attraction. The talented teen then persuaded construction professionals from the cable network ESPN—which features skateboarding competitions as part of its "X Games" broadcasts—to travel to Columbus and turn a dream into reality.

Three years later, graffiti and criminal activity are nonexistent at the skateboard park, which is filled daily with young people who otherwise would be on the streets or loitering in public places. More important, parks director Chuck Wilt notes, "We need to listen to kids and give them a chance to be involved. This gives young people a chance to build confidence and important skills that will last them the rest of their lives" (personal communication, February 1999).

Building confidence also explains what happened to a South Bend, Indiana, second grader—Derrick—who was matched with a high school senior through the School-Based Mentoring Program of Big Brothers Big Sisters of St. Joseph County. "Derrick is very bright," explains program director Deborah Burrow. "But he was behind in his school work and withdrawn from his peers due to some personal issues. When we matched him with a high school senior who volunteered as a Big Brother, Derrick really changed, telling his teacher, 'Finally. You finally found someone who understands me.'"

Burrow also tells of the small child who was picked on by classmates before being matched with a local high school football star. "Boy, have his confidence and status been elevated now that he's been matched with his new friend," Burrow exclaims. In 2001, all 173 children in the mentoring program advanced to the next grade level, 67% improved at least one letter grade, 69% improved their attitude toward school, and 93% gained in self-confidence (personal communication, February 2002).

Similar outcomes were delivered in small-town Goshen, Indiana, where the Boys and Girls Club worked with Chamberlain Elementary School on an extensive tutoring program called "Power Hour." A staff member from the club consulted with the school's principal and teachers on third-grade curriculum and then trained more than a dozen volunteers to work with students with failing grades. Nearly 100 students received this added in-school instruction, which continued after school at the Boys and Girls Club. The results? In the 2000–2001 school year, 71% of Chamberlain's third graders passed the math portion of a statewide proficiency exam, up from 47% the year before. In language arts, 60% passed, up from 42% the previous year (State of Indiana, 2000–2001). Encouraged by this remarkable success, club director Kevin Deary is now expanding Power Hour into two more elementary schools (personal communication, January 2002).

Transformations such as these are not just for young people in dire straits. In 2002, the *Indianapolis Star* named its statewide Academic All-Stars—40 high school seniors from around the Hoosier state who have been selected as best in class. You would think brilliant high school scholars would have no hangs-ups and thus no need for the caring relationships necessary for healthy youth development. And you would be wrong. Each Academic All-Star named at least one teacher who had made a vital difference in her or his success.

According to Mary R. W. Dicken of Floyd Central High School, "I did not value my musical abilities or believe music was a worthy field of study." That changed forever after Mary met choral director Angela Hampton. "She showed me the musician inside," Mary wrote, "inspiring me to share music with others. I now believe music educators are among the most valuable of people" (Fleming, 2002, p. D1).

At surface level these several examples, along with Lifeline Community Center, seem to have more differences than similarities—the big cities of Boston and Indianapolis compared with the little towns of Columbus and Goshen; nationally affiliated Big Brothers Big Sisters and Boys and Girls Club versus the radically independent Christamore House and Lifeline Community Center; faith-based and secular; urban, suburban, and rural; hundreds of children served compared with just a small number.

Despite these differences, the core principles and stellar performances are the same. Each of these youth organizations—working within civil society—is promoting healthy development of children and youth who are hardwired to connect.

Jail and Java

She actually wanted to stay on probation.

The teenage girl had committed a serious crime, and her sentence included probation. For the first time in her life, she had to report to a probation officer. And for the first time in her life, she found someone who cared.

Along with ensuring that the terms of probation were being met, the officer asked her about school, talked with her about her favorite music, and challenged her to think about what she could do when she became an adult.

That's why when her probation was drawing to a close, the young offender did not want to leave. "Once I'm off probation," she said, "there will be no one in my life who cares about what I do." Not in her family. Not in her community. Not anyone at all.

Her story is instructive, demonstrating that all kids are yearning for positive relationships with caring adults who are passionately committed to their very existence. Kids need parents who are involved and neighbors who care, and they need consistent moral messages about right and wrong. Research supports common sense. Young people who have those healthy relationships and who absorb those moral messages tend to do better in life, no matter how or what we measure.

This will only happen if we commit to one another and commit to connections with children and youth. As we do so, we can draw inspiration through an astonishing story from across the border.

Of Mexico's 31 states, Chiapas by far is the poorest. This southernmost state, bordering on Guatemala, is a centerpiece of the once-mighty Mayan culture. The terrain is rich in terms of lush mountains, fertile fields, and other natural resources, but the region's residents remain poor in terms of money, housing, and vital social services. This poverty is exacerbated by the native belief that history has not treated them kindly. Outsiders moved into the area centuries ago seeking European and religious conquest. Today's "conquistadors," in the eyes of the locals, are found in a national government and an international business sector that residents believe will exploit their land.

Midway up the mountain range sits San Cristobal, truly a paradox. In the courtyards of centuries-old church buildings, folks come from the fields to sell their homegrown produce and their homemade garments. Down the street, a smoke-filled rock-and-roll bar offers Internet access for the equivalent of just 1 dollar an hour.

The top of the mountain range, 12,000 feet high, seems close enough to touch yet in reality is a 2-hour car ride away. Along the battered two-lane highway that winds its way to the top, one-room homes with dirt floors exist alongside small plots of corn, beans, and tomatoes. Without running water, women wash clothes in streams. Without electricity, modern miracles such as cell phones and e-mail, and not-so-modern miracles such as fans and light bulbs, are nonexistent. The only sign of modern life is seen in armed soldiers, sent by the national government in response to the presence of Zapatista rebels.

If you think these poor, downtrodden residents of Chiapas have surrendered to their plight, think again. For on these mountain tops, hundreds of farmers have formed a cooperative to grow organic coffee. These farmers do not have America's latest agriculture technology. They don't even share the same language, with some speaking Spanish and others speaking two different dialects of Maya (Tzotzil and Tzeltal).

Yet by working together, these resourceful farmers have figured out how to combine their efforts to grow enough organic coffee each year to satisfy the entire United States of America for 1 full week. Even better, the coffee co-op formed by these farmers has negotiated a premium price for their product in European markets.

No floors in their houses. No electricity. No running water. No common language. And no excuses. Just hard work and cooperation on behalf of the greater good. These farmers are a living testament to the adage that working together works.

This remarkable method of growing coffee is not too different from how we should grow our children—by working together to build on our strengths and conquer our challenges. Whereas those farmers in Chiapas overcame historical scars and contemporary obstacles without the tools of modern life, we of course have countless resources at our disposal. Which leaves just one question: What's our excuse?

The juvenile offender who wants to stay on probation just to find someone who cares needs an answer, just as she needs someone to walk alongside her on her journey to adulthood.

Will Allen Dromgoole's memorable poem, *The Bride Builder*, shows the way. An old man encounters "a chasm, vast, and deep, and wide, / through which was flowing a sullen tide." Thanks to his wisdom and experience, the old man is able to cross the chasm without fear. Once safe on the other side, he looks back and realizes that the crossing might not be as easy for future generations. So he builds "a bridge to span the tide."

Another traveler comes along and criticizes the old man for his laborious efforts. The traveler notes that the old man himself will never use the bridge, as the old man already has found safety on the other side. The old man's reply is an encouragement for us all:

"'There followeth after me today, / a youth, whose feet must pass this way. / This chasm, that has been naught to me, / To that fair-haired youth may a pitfall be. / He, too, must cross in the twilight dim; / Good friend, I am building the bridge for *him*' " (Dromgoole, 1993, p. 223).

References

Armour, S. (2001, October 4). American workers rethink priorities. *USA Today*, B1.

Benson, P. L. (1997). *All kids are our kids: What communities must do to raise caring and responsible children and adolescents*. San Francisco: Jossey-Bass.

Benson, P. L. (1999, November). Plenary speech presented at the KIDS COUNT Conference. Indianapolis, IN.

Blum, R. W., & Rinehart, P. M. (1998). *Reducing the risk: Connections that make a difference in the lives of youth*. Minneapolis: University of Minnesota, Division of General Pediatrics and Adolescent Health.

Dromgoole, W. A. (1993). The bridge builder. In W. J. Bennett (Ed.), *The book of virtues: A treasury of great moral stories*. New York: Simon & Schuster.

Eccles, J., & Gootman, J. A. (Eds.). (2002). *Community programs to promote youth development*. Washington, DC: National Academy Press.

Fagan, P. F. (1996). *Why religion matters: The impact of religious practice on social stability*. Washington, DC: Heritage Foundation.

Federer, W. J. (Ed.). (1994). *America's God and country*. Coppell, TX: FAME Publishing.

Fleming, M. (2002, April 21). These mentors more than made the grade. *Indianapolis Star*, p. D1.

Klein, J. (1997, June 16). In God they trust. *New Yorker*, pp. 40–48.

Leland, J. (1998, June 1). Savior of the streets. *Newsweek*, pp. 20–29.

Popenoe, D. (1995). The declining social virtue: Family, community, and the need for a natural communities policy. In M. A. Glendon & D. Blankenhorn (Eds.), *Seedbeds of virtue: Sources of competence, character, and citizenship in American society* (pp. 71–104). Lanham, MD: Madison Books.

Putnam, R. D. (2000). *Bowling alone: The collapse and revival of American community*. New York: Simon & Schuster.

State of Indiana, Department of Education. (2000–2001). School snapshot, Chamberlain Elementary School, 1829, Benchmarks. Available at http://mustang.doe.state.in.us/search/benchmark.cfm?subnum=303&hidden=1829&ip95=checked&istavg=checked& colobg=FFFFFF; and http://mustang.doe.state.in.us/search/benchmark.cfm?subnum=203&hidden=1829&ip95=checked&istavg=checked&colobg=FFFFFF. Retrieved July 10, 2006.

Traub, J. (2000, January 16). What no school can do. *New York Times Magazine*.

Trulear, H. D. (2000). *Faith-based institutions and high-risk youth*. Philadelphia: Public/Private Ventures.

Williams, O. (2001). *Healing the heart, healing the hood*. Indianapolis: Martin University Press.

Wilson, J. Q. (1993). *The moral sense*. New York: Free Press.

Wynn, J. R. (2000). *The role of local intermediary organizations in the youth development field*. Chicago: University of Chicago Chapin Hall Center for Children.

VII
Commentaries

18 Caring and Character: How Close Parental Bonds Foster Character Development in Children

Elizabeth Berger

Good Character Is Fundamental to Families

An upright character is our fundamental American value. Its image is everywhere—the men and women most admired in our nation's history are the very embodiment of strong character qualities: courage, ingenuity, loyalty, responsibility, and altruism. These values emerge in our greatest documents—for example, the speeches of Abraham Lincoln and Dr. Martin Luther King Jr. Popular books, movies, and TV shows are unified by these themes: the good guy displays these virtues and battles the bad guy. The underdog defeats the larger villain through his pluck, common sense, and determination. On a more sophisticated level, the good guy battles within himself and becomes a better guy. The Hollywood movies and human interest stories in the newspapers that illustrate these dramas may not be great works of art, but they are great works of cultural self-definition. The American consensus of who we want our children to be is beyond controversy—it can be exploited, stereotyped, and satirized, but it continues to unite and inspire us. We are one people because we value this—the steadfast heart of the noble Everyman.

What parents are after perhaps foremost is the capacity to know right from wrong; the growth of the child's conscience. Character also involves courage, realism, and the ability to accept loss squarely. It involves creativity, empathy, and the capacity to love. And character involves a respect for the human condition, a commitment to other human beings, and a love of justice both private and public. These qualities are what prepare a young person for the eventual demands of adulthood, for being a good parent and a fine citizen. For Americans, part of the meaning of character lies in its individuality. This acknowledges that each person is irreplaceable and precious in his or her own singular way, and unlike every other person. A person's character is in this sense related to his or her soul or spirit, intangible and absolute. Character involves the fundamentals of living. It is the sum of a person's responses to the profound polarities of human existence: love and hate, man and woman, life and death.

It would seem like a tall order for ordinary families to accomplish "character education" if it were a separate discipline like gem cutting or understanding particle physics or hitting home runs, and sometimes parents worry that they lack familiarity with the proper curriculum or skills. Fortunately, however, character development is not the result of special lessons. It is embedded in and is the product of the child's growth. Parenting involves a great deal of teaching—pots are hot, the street is dangerous, and hitting isn't allowed—and as the child matures, families may hold valuable discussions with their children on abstract subjects like truth, commitment, and ideals. But the child's inner capacity for these things has taken shape long before his ability to discuss them. It is through the intimacy of the ordinary day that the child's character—the capacity for morality, devotion, and ideals—is shaped and enhanced.

Good Character Begins with Reliable Parental Love

Understanding child development from the perspective of human relationships illuminates how character qualities emerge from everyday interactions in loving families. Naturally, the value the parents place on the child is the child's first "value" and helps define the child's image of himself and of other people from the very beginning. Scientists who study infants now acknowledge what parents have known all along: that infants even in the very first days and weeks of life are quite complicated in their capacity to love and be loved and to interact on a unique, intimate level. Very early—around 8 months of age—babies begin to comprehend that other people understand their ideas and emotions. At this time, babies begin to show powerful loyalty for certain loved persons and may display worry or outrage at the approach of strangers.

From the age of 1½ years, the child begins to use symbols for ideas and speak in two- or three-word phrases. Complex social emotions, such as embarrassment, envy, and empathy, are expressed nonverbally. The age of 2 years heralds the emergence of pride, shame, and guilt. The child has entered the social environment as a separate entity, aware that the meeting ground between the wishes of others and his own needs must be negotiated. He already has a considerable repertoire of intimate interpersonal skills.

This remarkable personal growth is grounded in brain development, but it is equally dependent upon the participation of loving adults who respond to the child and care for his body and spirit. Parents do not do this because they have mastered a text of intellectual material. They do it because they love their infant, and because of the intense pleasure that getting to know, feeding, caring for, and playing with their infant gives them. The experience is personal, emotional, and deeply intimate for both parent and child. For many families, it is the most profound fulfillment of all. Any ordinary parent would gladly give his life for his child. This emotional reality, although not often explicit, is the very core of a child's psychological life. It is out of this fundamental experience of having received devotion that the child begins to achieve the capacity to be devoted. Herein lies the foundation of character.

The love relationship between parent and child is not all roses, of course, as in any ordinary day an infant is hungry or too hot or too cold or suffers some other trouble. The baby knows only his need of the moment, and his ideas of love for the parents are temporarily lost. In the regularity of the satisfaction of the need, and the human magic that goes with it, however, the baby begins to form more complex and durable concepts of satisfactions that are anticipated, and of the trustworthy people who bring these satisfactions. Here we find the origins of joy, of optimism, of faith, and of friendliness. They grow in the child as a consequence of his being alive and loved, and because his needs were met reliably.

Forgiveness and Tolerance Grow from Devotion

Small children have the tendency to see all sensation, both good and bad, as coming from the powerful parents. Gradually, an awareness grows within the child that the loved person who often relieves desires and the hated person who sometimes frustrates desires are indeed the very same person. Wrestling with the emotional attachment to someone who is alternately loved and hated, and transforming it into a more realistic image of someone who contains both good and bad qualities simultaneously, is part of the work of early childhood— a task that often persists incomplete throughout life. From this complicated inner realization comes the capacity for toleration of human faults and for forgiveness. Likewise, well before the age of 3, the child begins to understand that he himself can be both good and bad—that the same little self who so brilliantly mastered the use of a fork in the morning, to everyone's admiration, went on at lunch to pull the cat's tail, strictly for spite. At some point, probably before 2 years of age and certainly before the child's language can express the sentiment, the child begins to be sorry, to regret his own destructiveness. Being sorry is part of love and can develop only in the context of devotion.

All of this happens at the same time that the toddler is attaining the capacities—walking, talking, feeding himself—that allow for increased physical independence. In that independence, however, the child is thrown back upon his inner resources to draw upon the self-esteem, the courage, and the friendliness that have grown there, laid down in memories of receiving care. The memory of parental warmth and imagination animates the child's inner life as he begins to experience himself as a separate being. The 2-year-old gains confidence by leaning on the parent's greater capacities and expertise, but also by pushing the parent away, as if to say, "I'm in charge here!" We notice that there is a certain paradox involved: The parent who is pushed away already has been taken in. The child has absorbed the parents' guidance—he's become a little expert himself.

Children Absorb the Values of Those They Love

It is hard to overemphasize the strength of a small child's desire to *be like* his parents, the power of the child's ambition to inhabit the parents' values and habits of mind just as he aims to inhabit Daddy's shoes and eyeglasses. The small child takes in like a sponge the qualities of those he loves. He mirrors in his human relationships the respect and trust and commitment that he experiences from his parents' relationships with him and with each other. A small child nurtures his teddy bear with tender guidance, identifying with the nurturing he has received. The rhythm of living and the music the family brings to it are themselves aspects of the parents' soothing and caring. To the degree that children are little and dependent, they need to feel that parents are structuring and supervising daily life, and making decisions for them in their best interest. In time, the parents' leadership guides the child in learning to manage himself—to slowly take over the functions of the parents. The child needs both inspiration and information. This is perhaps the greatest challenge of parenthood, because it draws heavily upon the parents' own strength of character—patience, forbearance, self-discipline, energy, and wisdom.

First and foremost, parents keep the child safe, and only gradually can they actively enlighten the youngster about the outside world. When the parent crosses the street, he holds the small child's hand and explains how traffic may be dangerous. He does so tenderly because the child is precious to him. Next week, we see the child muttering under his breath, "Now look both ways and hold my hand." As a child matures, staying out of the way of cars is a means of preserving forever within himself the relationship with his parents; he manages himself in relation to dangers as the parent once did, with respect for his own body and for the reality of danger. In this way, the bond with the parents, and the rules that govern the world, slowly become a durable part of the child's inner life. The child respects the parents' authority, first because it has kept the child safe when he was too little to do so himself, and second because the parents' wisdom has been useful and imparted to the child in a way that respects the child's feelings and developmental level.

A child's eventual outlook on all forms of authority depends upon the positive quality of his relationship with the adults upon which he depends. There are many moments, of course, during any child's day when the child is fussy or whining or otherwise at the end of his rope, and at those moments the child's personality has temporarily moved backward into a kind of babyish collapse. A wise parent understands that it is not possible to teach anything to a person, child or adult, who is in this temporary collapse and that all one can do is attempt to survive this awful moment without disaster and get on with the next thing. But apart from these many moments of collapse and backsliding, the growing child struggles within himself to be a better person because of his ardent desire to be like those he loves.

Wise Parents Communicate the Universality of Rules

The wise parent recognizes that the child's struggle is to be his best self, a struggle within himself so to speak, and approaches rules as features of an outer reality that we must all accept, rather than the parent's own invention. This is the magnificence of rules—they apply to everyone equally; the child can see that they are designed to protect everyone, including the child. Thus it is that the mature parent avoids power struggles by explaining the way the world works. Of course, parents do whatever is needed to preserve safety—so that the child does not fall out the window, throw books at his grandmother, or run into the street. These matters are not subject to negotiation. But beyond the arena of safety, parents acknowledge that only the child can *want* to be respectful, generous, fair minded, or hardworking. The parent cannot "make" a child be any of these things. The child aspires to these qualities through his admiration of people close to him, encouraged by the parents' leadership and example.

It is an error to suppose that children begin as wholly selfish beings and come to acknowledge the needs of others through disapproval. We observe that a baby in arms makes efforts to feed his mother, and to comfort other babies who are distressed, long before he learns to speak. This fundamental and innate human responsiveness, a capacity for empathy, is the basis for all mature forms of love and loving-kindness. Naturally, an infant's kindness doesn't go very far in the real world—the next moment he needs something for himself and starts to fuss. Only very slowly does the child begin to understand that other people are truly entitled to feel things, to believe things, and to want things that are different from his own feelings, beliefs, and desires. To grow up to be truly responsible, generous, and concerned, the child needs to feel that his parents respect human beings and put human priorities first. This begins with a respect for the child and his needs, but is balanced by the laws of reality—including, of course, moral laws—and the claims of other individuals' needs. Parents may structure these priorities with rules, but the child can only learn to respect other people's thoughts and feelings if he can observe the genuine ongoing interest in people's thoughts and feelings that lies behind the rules.

All small children grapple with the deep disappointment of their magical wishes—to fly, to own an elephant, to grow up and marry Daddy because he is the most handsome and powerful man in all the world. Parents need not teach children that they cannot have everything they want; daily reality teaches this lesson on its own. Childhood involves many frustrations; the most fundamental of these is to be weak and small in a big world where the grown-ups are in charge. From the infant's very primitive identification with his parents, "I am the King of the Mountain!" comes the 3- or 4-year-old's bittersweet awareness: "I cannot be Mommy. I cannot marry Mommy— she's already married to Daddy." This disappointment paves the way for the promise that "I'll be a mommy one day and do an even better job! I'll have 50 children!" The child's ambition first to engulf and to *be* the parent is transformed into the ambition to be *like* the parent in time, introducing the capacity to yearn for a future self and to work toward its accomplishment. Through this process, the child at the close of the nursery era learns to wait not just for a cookie but for rewards that are far away and require an ongoing self-discipline. He learns to apply himself. The child comes to terms with his relative smallness in order to discover a personal future, to begin the lifelong process of dedicating himself to the effort involved in achieving his ideals. The resolution of this psychological task, which depends upon the child's ambition not just to *be* in the here and now but to *become* somebody in time, signals his growing readiness for school.

Schools Build on the Family's Foundation

Public education in America is the child's first sustained experience with social systems that are impersonal, disciplined, and oriented around public values rather than oriented around intimate personal relationships. The school experience builds on the youngster's eagerness to *become* somebody—and almost every child in America knows that to become somebody you need to master in school both the academic subjects known as the three R's and a second domain called citizenship. Some of the magic of parents rubs off on the teacher as a beloved figure, but in addition to this the teacher is beloved in a new way—as the guardian angel of the child's ambitions to work, to apply himself, and to fulfill his dreams, not just in Mommy's and Daddy's heart, where you are loved passionately no matter what, but in the eyes of the larger world, where you are assessed dispassionately for what you can accomplish.

Success in school not only depends on the child's character but also contributes to the child's character. The capacity for work is always related to one's conscience; it means giving up something that is more fun. It requires an inner struggle. Giving up fun in order to do schoolwork is something the child owes himself because of the importance the child places on his future. These attitudes come from within the child, and a good school will encourage the consolidation of these attitudes. The discipline of school provides a deep sense of meaningfulness. School measures in small steps his sense of getting somewhere on the road of his own life. Loving school reflects the part of a child's sense of well-being that comes from applying himself diligently and being successful. Working hard in school is the cardinal sign of a child's self-respect, and often a good indicator of his respect for other people. Of course, working hard in school contributes to success in school, which reinforces the youngster's self-respect.

It is a wonderful thing if a child is so interested in a subject that he pursues it for its own sake, and this happens sometimes. But by and large, children are not deeply interested in irregular verbs or the exports of Spain. They are interested in class work because they know that doing a good job in the fourth grade will prepare them to do a good job in the fifth grade, and that this process will enable them eventually to make use of their potential and what society has to offer in a satisfying way. The child focuses on the stuff on the blackboard and what the teacher has to say because he is motivated from within. This is not primarily because he is being entertained, or because he loves the past participle, or because he wants to avoid getting in trouble. It is because he sees his own self-interest in learning and the teacher's interest in teaching as progressing in the same direction. The teacher is concerned with each child in a relatively impersonal way. The teacher aims to be fair, but the bond between the teacher and student is not necessarily intimate. This is another aspect of the discipline of education.

The maintenance of firm classroom discipline is a manifestation of our American values of free speech, fairness, and justice for all. This doesn't mean that everyone shouts at once—on the contrary, it means that everyone listens quietly with respect and open-mindedness to the opinions of others. Schools are concerned not only with communicating ideas that are beyond debate but also with communicating the important concept that many significant ideas are and always have been subject to vigorous debate. School opens a child's mind to the ways in which human beings in different times and places have had views both remarkably like and remarkably unlike those held by the child's family and community. The teacher emphasizes the importance of trying to understand the real meaning of views that seem at face value to be foreign or ridiculous. This moves the child forward from the natural reaction of intellectual immaturity—laughing at unfamiliar customs and ideas—to the reaction of intellectual discipline and curiosity, a respectful wish to understand things that seem new and confusing. A teacher stimulates students to adopt a posture of thoughtfulness and considered judgment, and to mistrust shallow emotionality, whether in schoolyard gossip, the nightly news report, or the pronouncement of nations.

Good Teacher–Child Relationships Promote Good Citizenship

A teacher stands for the value of process in all things: the process of critical thinking on an individual level and the process of group discourse, upon which civic devotion to due process depends. To carry forth their responsibilities in our democracy successfully, our children must be able not only to read but also to respond critically to what they read—to see things not just superficially but in their wider implications for the individual and for the group.

The relationship between the child and the teacher, and the child and the youngster sitting next to him, is the perfect laboratory for these issues. These are the building blocks of participatory citizenship. A capable teacher controls the class so that all students have a fair opportunity to express their viewpoints. The teacher structures the discussion so that children learn to disagree with each other and with the teacher in an energetic and constructive spirit. This makes it plain that toleration of another's ideas and choices does not necessarily imply agreement. One may attack an idea without attacking the person who holds it. The teacher enhances the student's self-regard by insisting that each voice be heard with respect. In this way, the classroom becomes safe from the bullying, ridiculing tendencies of the mob mentality that occur so readily among children. At the same time, when the teacher calls for a consensus, the fundamental mechanism of democracy is put into action.

Through all of these activities, school teaches American civic values—both as facts (for example, the Bill of Rights) and as principles of personal consideration and intellectual freedom. This approach builds character in each student by interrelating the child's intellectual growth, the dynamics of classroom decorum, and the history and ideals of our country. It prepares the child to approach any decision with a certain gravity and to weigh his wishful impulses against realistic pros and cons. The implications for the child in all spheres of living—as an educated citizen, and as a potential spouse and parent, are profound.

School-Age Children Emulate Parents

Despite his exposure to a broader world, the school-age child of 6 through 12 years continues to be an admiring apprentice to his parents' values and worldview—because of the powerful high esteem in which the parents are held. School-age children will argue bitterly and mightily among themselves whether a Ford or a Chevrolet is the best sort of automobile to have, because "my dad said so." Only gradually does the school-age child come to see that his parents, far from being the majestic god and goddess of his early childhood, are indeed quite ordinary people, rather like the folks next door. But with this process, the passionate ideal that the parent once represented is transferred to other people, to other things—to teachers and coaches and admired older friends, and later to transcendent yearnings expressed in art, in religion, and in efforts to better the world through social justice.

Children who come from homes in which people really are interested in other people—how others think and what they feel, how they got to be who they are, their goals and values and dreams—are nice to be with. They have learned that intimate communication is a two-way street; they are great talkers, but they are also respectful and attentive listeners. They become shrewd observers of human nature and keen judges of character. Nice children come from the richest kind of homes, where what is valued is the human spirit, its needs for love and respect, for solitude, for beauty, for transcendence, and for challenge and accomplishment.

The lively involvement of other family members creates a situation where one may air one's troubles and upsets in an atmosphere of trust, and may appeal to others for advice, support, and encouragement. It takes parents' vigorous presence within the home to set the stage for this kind of family life, which brings out sharing, a concern for others, and real thoughtfulness. Such parents provide their children with the most valuable thing of all—a sense of meaning.

It is the home's orientation toward human beings that stimulates the child to acknowledge his authentic and vivid emotions, including love and hate, concern, jealousy, triumph, and despair. His feelings are not given the brush-off as inconvenient or unattractive. Home provides the constant presence of living models who demonstrate how more mature personalities deal with emotions in a way that is expressive, productive, and responsible. The fact that the home functions with each member's best interest at heart, with an emphasis on consideration and respect, leads toward resolution of the inevitable conflicts that family life involves. The values of loyalty, commitment, and generosity may not be preached, but they are embedded in behavior. This is the home that supports with interest and pride the achievements and activities of the young child and cheers on the adolescent's steps toward real independence.

One can imagine that a young person of 12 or 13 years emerging from a home and a school that foster the development of character is already an individual of some mettle. He has already consolidated into his personality the values and outlook of his family and his nation. By junior high, such a youngster doesn't need constant adult supervision. Of course, he still needs his parents to "be there" for him, but by now this has largely come to mean that he knows they have trust and confidence in his good judgment, rather than that they are perpetually physically present. We recognize this trust when we let a youngster of 12 or 13 babysit for an infant or toddler. We are saying that the young teen is responsible enough to be the sole authority for a little person who is entirely dependent upon him, at least for several hours at a stretch. The babysitter role is an excellent example of something that demands ordinary authentic maturity of character—the kind every preteen should have. It is a benchmark for what needs to be in place well before he undergoes the personal transformation of puberty and the physical, intellectual, and social changes that go with it.

The Troubled Teen

It is clear that a great many young people in America enter adolescence without this necessary backbone of firm character, and that this is the common denominator that underlies a vast spectrum of adolescent problems that will become dramatic only in time. Such a youngster is Jell-O inside. He has no powers of resistance to the impulses coming from within, or to peer pressures coming from without. Disaster is always just around the corner because he lacks the judgment, self-protectiveness, and respect for others that would help him navigate around peril. These are the young teenagers that one would not put in charge of an infant—one would not put them in charge of a potted plant.

It is predictable that every aspect of the adult world that is suddenly spread out in front of this young adolescent can be the focus of serious problems: drugs, alcohol, sexuality, weapons, crime, and all manner of rebellion, risk taking, and personal failure. This sad state of affairs is so commonplace that many people think it is normal. Onlookers are in a quandary, constantly waiting for disaster to strike, yet unable to provide supervision of every moment. The piece of the picture that often does not come into focus is that the youngster has never been able to manage his own life adequately from the inside. Something that should have been consolidated by the time childhood was drawing to a close was never achieved. The youngster's body has become large and strong, but his character hasn't.

The reason many teenage problems do not respond to a quick fix is that the development of the problem was not quick. The problem teen is often the result of a long process in which the stability of the youngster's inner world failed to become anchored through strong positive relationships. These are adolescents who do not feel invested in their own futures, who feel empty and hopeless and angry. They are disinclined to master their impulses because they see no point in doing so; achieving relief in the moment seems to them a more reliable satisfaction than aiming for some distant and abstract goal. They feel they have been betrayed by the world of adults and thus owe it no loyalty. The voice inside that reassures each individual that he is good and loved and worthy of protection speaks rarely to these teens and only in a whisper; their memories of childhood are full of bitterness and hostility and a sense of loss.

Circumstances Undermine Families

At this time, the number of unstable, unhappy, and unreliable young people has reached the level of national crisis. How can we understand this situation? How are we to make sense of this threat to our national well-being that has already established a beachhead in our communities?

The answer is not that American parents do not love their children, or that they are bad people. The answer is the totality of our circumstances—both material and intangible—that so often undermines the integrity and depth of the bond between parents and children. What children need is a home with vigorous, optimistic, self-reliant parents—grown-ups who are more or less fulfilled with regard to their own lives, who demonstrate trustworthiness, patience, humor, loving respect for others, commitment, and self-discipline as parents and human beings. What children need is a home that makes the enrichment of human relationships its greatest priority. Distressed homes that do not embody these values produce distressed young people.

Parents who struggle with material hardship are often compromised in these areas because the pressures of surviving rob them of the integrity, peace, and presence of mind so fundamental to parenting. Poorer and poorer outcomes on every measurement, such as domestic violence or perinatal mortality, are obtained as one travels down the socioeconomic gradient—a gulf that is growing steeper and deeper every decade. The crucial entity of "stress" is related both to poverty and to the ill health that often accompanies poverty. Poverty is itself perhaps our main source of stress, not only for the 20% of Americans surviving below the poverty line but also for a huge number of overworked families just over the poverty line—parents who work two jobs and leave children substantially unsupervised or in inadequate day care, parents who come home to a welter of unmet needs, tension, and anxiety about survival. The patience and forbearance that parenting demands are just what the stressed parent is least likely to be able to give. In situations of inadequate housing, nutrition, safety, and supervision, the stressed parent is likely to look for a quick solution—corporal punishment or threats that prevent disaster in the moment but undermine the child's emotional growth in the long term. It doesn't take riches to give a child optimism and security, but it does take serenity and hope. Parents must have not only strong values inside but also a strong situation outside to support those values.

But materially impoverished parents often manage to communicate, despite all, that the child is their greatest joy and fulfillment, the apple of their eye. In contrast, many families who are not financially pressed nevertheless place such great value on material success that intimate relationships become yet one more commodity. These are the parents who confuse giving of themselves with giving of their wallets and spoil the child with things when the child needs communication and trust. The child's yearning for closeness is given the brush-off; his room is full of stuff, but his heart is empty. Parents need not only to mean well in general but also to deliver in the moment. When the toddler's button won't go through the buttonhole, when the cup of juice spills, when the child's or adolescent's vulnerability calls for the steadying presence of a loving adult—these are the simple moments where parenting takes place, where courage and strength and self-discipline are transmitted from one generation to the next. Parents whose spirits are preoccupied elsewhere—with personal aggrandizement or pressing professional demands—may give short shrift to the child's need for intimacy.

Why Families Need Access to Good Health Care and Good Schools

A child's need is for closeness—so simple and yet so hard for us as a nation to provide. And why? Around us we may take inventory of our national disaster areas, social as well as personal, that appear as an aggregate both interrelated and overpowering: foremost, of course, poverty, followed by decaying infrastructure of neighborhoods, addictions, joblessness, divorce, violence, crime, untreated mental illness, bigotry, the trend toward the commercialization of all human relationships, the greed and materialism that saturate popular culture, the loss of regard for human dignity and its needs for transcendence. This list of social ills is all too familiar and self-perpetuating.

What we must recognize is that all of these ills take their greatest toll in the coherence of the moment between parent and child. From the child's point of view, the point of impact of any social problem is on the ability of the parent to meet the needs of the child's body and spirit. From the perspective of a child's character growth, the health of his family is ground zero. We cannot directly provide families with "happiness" and "love" through public policy, but we can speak intelligently about concrete impediments to family integrity and stability.

Any comprehensive plan to address our hopes for our country's youth must start with the goal of supporting families and shoring up their capacity to function. The most fundamental of these supports are good basic medical care and good basic education for our children. Families can achieve remarkable things for themselves in a breadth of other domains if good basic services in these areas are available to them and their children.

Good basic medical care is accessible, comprehensive, team oriented, integrated, and family based. Such services are focused upon prevention, upon a public health model, upon long-term management of chronic disease, and upon outcomes-based interventions. Medical care based on these principles is cost effective; moreover, by emphasizing early recognition of emotional and behavioral distress, good basic medical care can capture and treat early on the parental depression, alcohol problems, sexual abuse of children, drug dependency, domestic conflict, malnutrition, end-of life issues, parent–child difficulties, and child-developmental disorders that are everywhere apparent in their dismal consequences and rarely appropriately managed. A flexible team of physicians, nurses, social workers, psychologists, and learning specialists can respond to "multiproblem" families in such a way that upfront costs would be more than balanced by downstream savings in public expenditures in such areas as the court and penal system, preventable hospital stays, emergency room visits, time lost from the workplace, disability, suicide, and the detention of children and youth languishing in lockup facilities or foster care arrangements. Of course poverty, divorce, and joblessness are not medical illnesses. Yet the appropriate medical interventions—including psychological interventions—for families on the brink of poverty, divorce, or joblessness can often avert or ameliorate their worst outcomes in spectacular and surprising ways.

The fundamental treatment for poverty is education; understandably, American families place their faith in our schools as the second public institution that promises all of our children a better life. But the disrepair of thousands of schools in every state is a scandal, and all the more because poor schools dash the hopes of many youngsters who enter them with high hopes. For millions of small students, the unchallenged bullying, the threats and examples of school violence, the overcrowding of classes, the burnout among their teachers, the decay and filth and sheer dangerousness of the school building itself powerfully convey to them the low value that society places on their worth and well-being.

But even in middle-class neighborhoods, most schools are not prepared to respond adequately to the large numbers of troubled youngsters at their doorsteps. A lack of personal commitment to what is happening in the classroom is often a youngster's initial cry for help, the first sign of a breakdown in his trust and optimism. Floundering in school is a sensitive predictor of complex problems that emerge down the line—family distress, substance use, emotional disorders, or crime—and thus signals an opportunity for intervention. It is one thing to identify children at risk. It is quite another to have somewhere to send the family to get appropriate services.

Along with good basic medical care, good basic schooling is a fundamental building block for parents aiming to provide their children with a fair start in life—an even playing field. But poor families live in poor communities, and poor communities cannot fund good schools for their children because they cannot raise the revenues to build, maintain, and staff them. The absence of good schools perpetuates the impoverishment of any community because such communities cannot attract or even hold on to families with the resources and aspirations to provide good education for their children. Poor schools both create and are created by poor communities.

Common National Goals Can Unite Us in Supporting Families

Health and education have been traditionally public domains in America—we believe as a nation that every child and every family has an equal right to good basic services in these areas. Yet the immense chasm between rich and poor families is the silent presence in child-rearing throughout America. Not enough material wealth and an overabundance of material wealth share at least one thing in common—a deep fixed preoccupation with what money can buy. If we as a nation are to raise our children with values beyond the scramble for material things, we need to actively address the gulf between rich and poor, and the toll this discrepancy takes on our spiritual wholeness.

These public institutions of health care and education hold the key to stabilizing a host of problems—variably social, psychological, educational, economic, and medical—that are at this time conceptualized and addressed in exceedingly inadequate, fragmented, and wasteful ways. We must devote ourselves to an intense, preoccupying national effort to design, build, and staff the infrastructure of health care and education for all of our children.

Ordinary human goodness is hard to extinguish in parents. Given a reasonable chance, parents raise children with the capacity for hard work, commitment, responsibility, and devotion—and they accomplish this not through any special agenda but through the workshop of the everyday. What protects children from risk and harm are their parents' good faith and confidence in them and in the meaningfulness of daily life lived in very ordinary ways. America was founded on these sunny and simple principles. We can return to these principles and restore them as a legacy for our children, but only if we leave our children a nation that lives up to its promise.

Author's Note

Portions of this chapter have been excerpted and modified from my book, *Raising Kids with Character: Developing Trust and Personal Integrity in Children* (Lanham, MD: Rowman & Littlefield Publishers, Inc., 2006). The book was originally published under the title *Raising Children with Character: Parents, Trust, and the Development of Personal Integrity* (Northvale, NJ: Jason Aronson, 1999).

19 Gather Around the Children

Enola Aird and the Mothers' Council Task Force on the Needs of Children

The latest research in the neurosciences confirms what many mothers have long known. Children are born to bond. They develop through intense emotional relationships with the beloved people around them. Children have an innate need to connect deeply with other people, and they long for a sense of moral and spiritual purpose. These are human imperatives. When they are not met, a child's potential is stifled.

Children's needs are best met through nurturing communities in which mothers, fathers, and other adult caregivers spend ample time with children, telling stories and sharing traditions—communities that articulate a clear and inspiring vision of a good and meaningful life and then lovingly help children bring that vision to pass in their own lives.

Children in Crisis

Why is it that, in a nation of unprecedented material abundance, growing numbers of children are suffering from depression, addiction, anxiety, suicidal thoughts, and other grave mental health and behavioral problems? Why, in spite of our unmatched scientific, technological, and economic progress, are so many children in the United States hurting themselves and others?

The Commission on Children at Risk, a group of distinguished physicians, scholars, scientists, and youth service professionals, has sought to answer these questions by amassing and integrating the most recent neuroscientific and social science evidence. In the *Hardwired to Connect* report, the commission makes a compelling case that the problems facing young people are due in large part to our cultural failure to meet children's most basic human need for connectedness—connectedness with other people and to a sense of meaning and purpose.

A number of studies over the years have warned of growing threats to the well-being of children in the United States and called for action to address the needs of children at risk. These studies have been largely ignored. Our nation has so far been unable to muster the will to take the steps necessary to dramatically improve conditions for children.

With its remarkable report, the Commission on Children at Risk presents a new and powerful scientific case, and offers us yet another opportunity, to change course for the sake of our children.

The commission urges all sectors of American society to take action to meet children's needs. As members of the Mothers' Council Task Force on the Needs of Children, we hope that every individual and institution will respond to this groundbreaking work.

We hope that mothers, fathers, and other primary caregivers will draw on the report to reaffirm their commitment to the work of raising their children, deepen their connections with other young people within their spheres of influence, and strengthen their advocacy and activism on behalf of all children.

We call on fathers to assess the report's implications for fathering and to respond.

Initial Reflections on the Commission's Report

In 2002, in *Call to a Motherhood Movement* (available at www.watchoutforchildren.org), the Mothers' Council urged mothers to "refuse to accept the continuing decline in the quality of our children's lives." It called upon mothers across the United States to "move boldly to change the conditions under which we mother and under which our children are living."

In keeping with that mothers' statement, we joined with the Commission on Children at Risk in calling for a national mobilization to change the conditions of childhood in the United States. We are committed to doing all we can to engage, energize, and empower mothers to play a leading role in that mobilization.

The Commission on Children at Risk is calling adults to attention. It is telling us that too many of our children are running on empty—they are empty of love, parental time and attention, empty of stories, of traditions, of relationships, of guidance, of purpose, and meaning.

The stakes are high. If we lose our ability to connect, we lose our humanity. We must gather around our children and change the direction in which our culture is heading. Regarding the commission's recommendations, we offer the following general observations.

1. *We prefer the term* connected communities.

We agree that the commission's 10 characteristics are the minimum necessary to create communities in which children have opportunities to flourish. We commit ourselves to using our best efforts through the Mothers' Council to spread the word and contribute to the revitalization and creation of such communities across the nation.

But we think *connected communities* is a better term than *authoritative communities*. It is, in our view, a more user-friendly term and fully consistent with the spirit of the commission's findings on the importance for children of sustained bonds with parents and communities.

2. *There is important news here for mothers.*

If, as the commission demonstrates, a child is born to connect with people, the most important person at the beginning of a child's life is his or her mother.

According to the commission, a child's brain actually develops as a result of the emotional communication and growing relationships she has, first with her mother, then with her father or other caregivers, and later on with others.

Mothers, it seems, are also primed to attach, even if they are not biologically related to their children. As the commission puts it, "Oxytocin is … released during birth and lactation and appears to strengthen the mother's attachment to the baby." And, "caretaking, among other things, boosts some of the very neurotransmitters that appear to facilitate caregiving." This points to the central role of birth mothers and adoptive mothers in the lives of children. It also points to the fact that when mothers are not able to provide care, other loving and consistent primary caregivers can successfully step in to provide the nurturing and sense of connectedness that children require.

Nevertheless, in most cases, a child's first relationship is with his or her mother. Mothers therefore play a foundational role in the process of connectedness—the process that sets the stage for children's gene transcription, the development of their brain circuitry, their emotional and mental health, their morality, and their spirituality. This primary relationship influences the capacity to respond to stress, and the development of personality, self-worth, the capacity for intimacy, and conscience.

In the *Call to a Motherhood Movement*, the Mothers' Council urged an end to the culture's devaluing of mothers and mothers' work. The council noted that "whether mothers are employed in the workforce or not, the work that we do as mothers is of paramount importance, but profoundly undervalued and demeaned."

The findings of the Commission on Children at Risk show how important mothers are and how valuable mothering is. They show that we give short shrift to the work of mothering at great risk to our children and to our society.

The commission's findings should give mothers the strength to say that mothers are central to children's development; we are not easily inter-changeable with other people. These findings should give us the courage to declare that bonding is a feminist issue and a human rights issue. They should embolden us to assert that efforts to improve the quality of life for children must also include efforts to improve the quality of life for mothers. They should give us courage to insist that our nation value and support all mothers, whether they are also employed in the workforce or not.

Viewed through the lens of the commission's deliberations, the work of a mother—work that is often sentimentalized, trivialized, and devalued—can be seen for what it is: foundational to the health and well-being of human beings as well as to the vitality of the communities human beings create.

The commission's report gives mothers reason to celebrate. And, it gives us reason to work together to ensure that all mothers—in the paid and unpaid workforce—receive the emotional, practical, and economic support they need in order to do the vital work of mothering.

3. *Missing from* Hardwired to Connect: *A prominent role for parents.*

The commission does not say enough about the important part parents play in creating the connectedness that children need. In identifying next steps, the commission calls on "youth service professionals and civic leaders" to guide the national conversation about solutions to the crisis facing our children.

Children are born to parents, not to institutions. In the first instance, children connect with people, not communities.

If we are to overcome the problem of disconnectedness in our culture, we must include mothers and fathers as leaders in this societal transformation. Our efforts must be more bottom-up than top-down. Specialists and civic leaders must be recognized and valued as resources and partners, but not as substitute leaders for parents themselves.

We must reach out to parent support groups across the country, such as La Leche League, a global leader in promoting connectedness. It has been working for years in neighborhoods across the nation and the world to empower mothers and create communities of mothers to support one another in breast-feeding, a vital part of biology's design for securing children's first relationship—the relationship with their mothers.

We cannot help children without addressing directly the needs of mothers and fathers. They, too, must be valued and supported. (For an overview of leading mothers' organizations, please see "Gathering the Mothers," by Peggy O'Mara, in *Mothering* magazine, July–August 2003.)

4. *The commission underestimates the magnitude of the challenge we will face in changing the ecology for our children.*

The most powerful forces in the United States promote a value system that is diametrically opposed to the value system necessary to foster connectedness.

The commission is asking a great deal of us. It is asking that we assess and, in many cases, work to change the tenor of our relationships with our spouses or partners and with our children, that we assess and change the way we run our homes, the way we relate to our neighbors, the way we run our early childhood centers, schools, and all other institutions that touch our nation's children.

Changing course will mean that we will have to put our children ahead of materialism and radical individualism; that we will have to dust off that long-derided word: sacrifice. To change the ecology for our children, we must offer ourselves and be prepared, as Gandhi taught, to be the change we seek.

The commission recognizes our crisis of values but offers no specific recommendations for dealing with this most potent challenge to the realization of its goals. It asserts that we must deepen our societal commitment to the values that "build and sustain authoritative communities and reconsider our commitment to those values that often replace and undermine them." We agree. But fundamental change will require a great deal more than a simple "reconsideration" of the values that undermine our quest for connectedness. We must work aggressively to make changes wherever we can to improve conditions for our children. But to transform the ecology of childhood, we will need to work on a fundamental reordering of the values and priorities of our society.

The commission admits that fundamental social change will "require something from almost all of us." We believe that it will require a lot from all of us. Curiously, the commission fails to ask very much of our corporate community. It does not speak directly to the corporations that create and support the media environment that contributes in largely negative ways to our cultural ecology.

Unless we squarely confront and overcome our crisis of values, we will be condemned to tinkering around the margins of what our children need; we will not be able to effect fundamental social change.

A Call for Mothers' Voices and Activism

We believe that mothers can play a critical role at this moment. We can be powerful and irresistible advocates in this cause. Our work as mothers helps us see and understand in the most concrete ways what it takes to help our children grow and flourish. In this culture that is rapidly forgetting what it takes to nourish the human spirit, we mothers have our own urgent message to deliver. Because of our work, we know something of what it takes to love actively—to offer love that listens, observes, values, and empathizes. We know that it takes sacrifice to enable another human being to grow. We know that it takes a spirit of interdependence for human beings to be nourished. We know that raising a child often requires humility, a willingness to admit what we do not know and reach out to others for help and support. These and related qualities—qualities of the "mother world"—are precisely the qualities our culture will need to cultivate to be able to make the changes the commission proposes.

We call for the passion of the lionesses for their cubs. We call on mothers to be relentless in making the case for, and working to build, a more caring culture—from the inside out: from our relationships to our homes, our neighborhoods, communities, organizations, media institutions, workplaces, and government.

Conclusions

Let us be bold. Let us set our sights high—intent on creating something entirely new. Let us build on the gains of the women's movement to propel us forward to a newfound leadership for mothers in the public and the private spheres. Let us create healthy, nurturing families—families founded on principles of equal dignity and equal regard. Let us build a place of joy for children.

About Enola Aird and the Mothers' Council

The Mothers' Council was convened in 2001 by the Motherhood Project of the Institute for American Values to examine—and spark public debate and mobilization on—matters affecting mothers, children, and the work of mothering. The Council's Task Force on the Needs of Children is charged with developing and implementing strategies for deepening the public debate on children's needs.

The members of the Task Force on the Needs of Children are Heidi Brennan, board of directors and public policy adviser, Family and Home Network; Brenda Hunter, psychologist and author; Loretta Pleasant-Jones, mother; Lysa Parker, executive director, Attachment Parenting International; Barbara Nicholson, president, Attachment Parenting International; and Enola Aird, director, the Motherhood Project, Institute for American Values. The full text of this statement and the complete list of Mothers' Council members is available at www.watchoutforchildren.org.

Index

ABC (Attention Behavioral Cognitive) Relaxation Therapy, 257
Absolute Unitary Being (AUB), 168–74
Add Health. *See* National Longitudinal Study of Adolescent Health
Adler, Alfred, 152–54, 156, 159, 160
adolescence
  defined, 263–64
  eating and sleeping, 265–66
  evolutionary context, 264
  motivational stimuli and positive affects, 266
  psychobiology of, 263–75
  social behavior and interactions, 264–64
  universality vs. individual differences, 267–68
  See also child and youth development; puberty
Adolescent Medicine: State of the Art Reviews (Resnick), 146
advocacy and activism, 145, 373
African American youth, and community, sense of, restoring, x, 305–20
aggression, 17, 88, 90, 93–97, 99
Ainsworth, Mary, 106, 109–15, 155, 160
Aird, Enola, xi, 374
alcohol abuse, 14, 87–89, 93–95, 96, 98–99, 193. *See also* drug abuse
American Academy of Pediatrics, 324, 326, 327, 330–31
American Psychological Association (APA), 167
American Society of Democratic Brothers, 293
amphetamines, 76
anger, and healing, 254
animal studies, 48n42. *See also* specific animals
Annie E. Casey Foundation, 4, 33–34, 37, 343–44
anxiety disorders, 4, 257
APA. *See* American Psychological Association
arginine vasopressin (AVP), 75–77
Aristotle, 56–57n117
assets, developmental. *See* developmental assets

Association for the Advancement of Mental Health Research and Education (Indianapolis, Ind.), 135
at-risk, term, use and prevalence of, 7
at-risk model, inadequacies of, 7–9
at-risk youth
  programs for, xiii, 34
  resilience and social competence among, 142
  well-being, promoting among, x, 305–20
attachment
  biochemistry of, 72–77
  as biological, 10–12
  through emotional communication, 10
  vs. love, 248–49
  and morality, 19, 20–21, 123–24
  and parenting, 11
  and place preference, 76
  quality of, 109–13
research, viii, xxiv, 19, 103–19
and resiliency, 112
secure, 89–90, 95, 110–11, 115, 232
social environment, supports by and for, 115–19
  spiritualization of, 21–22
  See also bonding; connectedness; mothers and mothering; nurturing
Attachment Parenting International, 374
attributes, developmental. *See* developmental assets
authoritative communities
  building and renewing, xviii, 34–35
  common commitment to, xv
  concept introduced, xvii
  vs. connected communities, 370–71
  core proposition, 26
  core rationale, 26
  defined, 26–27
  families as, 32
  framework for, embraced, xi
  immediate next steps, 42
  as long-term focus, 29
  in low-income neighborhoods, 35–37
  main characteristics, 26–31, 43

authoritative communities (*Continued*)
  main propositions, 10–25, 42
  as multigenerational, 29
  primary value of, 27
  real-world vs. ideal examples, 57n123,
    59n145
  scientific case for, vii, 3–43, 9–25
  and social connectedness, 65n171
  weakening of, results, 31–34
  See also connectedness
authority, 127–28, 358
autonomy, 111, 124, 125, 175, 178, 285

Bakwin, Harry, 107
Bandura, Albert, 325–26
Barkley, Charles, 20
Baumrind, Diana, 27, 227–28, 233–34
Beck, Aaron, 158
behavior modification, media use, to aid in
    monitoring, 332–33
behavior therapy, 256
behaviorism, 158, 256
*Bell Curve, The: Intelligence and Class Structure
    in American Life* (Murray & Herrnstein), 15
Bellah, Robert N., 27
belonging, 143, 144
Bender, Loretta, 107
Bennett, A. J., 97–98
Benson, Peter L., 341–43,
Berger, Elizabeth, x, xxiii, 368
Berger, Peter L., v–vi, 27
best practices, 141–42, 145
Better Chance, A, school program, 315–16
Big Brothers Big Sisters, 348
bio-psycho-social-cultural model, of child
    development, xiv
biochemistry
  of attachment, 72–77
  of connection, 10–12
  of family and youth competence, vii, 71–83
  of parental commitment, 77–83
  and resilience, vii, 71–85
  See also biology
biology, of attachment, 10–12. *See also*
    biochemistry; neurobiology;
    psychobiology
blame and blaming, 254
Blankenhorn, David, xiii–xv, 290
blood pressure, high, 191
Blum, Robert, 341
Boeme, Jacob, 171
bonding
  biochemistry of, 11, 73–76, 371
  disposition to, 155
  as feminist and human rights issue, 371
  See also attachment

Borysenko, J., 255–56
Bowlby, John, 92, 104–9, 112, 115, 155, 160
*Bowling Alone: The Collapse and Revival of
    American Community* (Putnam), 32–34
Boy Scouts, 344
Boyce, W. T., 15
Boyden, Stephen, 143
boys, male elders and role models for, ix–x,
    281–93
Boys and Girls Clubs, 315, 344, 348
brain development, 15–17, 263, 268–75. *See also*
    child and youth development
Brain-Heart conscience, 126
breast-feeding, importance of, 372
Brennan, Heidi, 374
Bronfenbrenner, Urie, 117
Brookings Institution, 41
Brown, David, 282
Bucke, R. M., 171
Buddhism
  basic tenants, 245–46
  Buddha, defined, 246
  Buddha nature, 246
  Bodhi, defined, 246
  Bodhichitta (transformation), 246–55
  bodhisattvas, 247–48, 250
  Chitta, defined, 246
  compassion vs. burnout, 249–50
  counseling behaviors, 259
  empirical research of concepts, 255–59
  equanimity (*upeksha*), 251
  Four Nobel Truths, 246
  healing difficult emotions, 253–54
  impermanence, 252
  interdependence, 252, 253
  joy and rejoicing, 250–51
  love vs. attachment, 248–49
  mindfulness, 245–59
  non-self or egolessness, 252–53
  and parenting, 56n109
  and spiritual development, 168, 171
  and well-being, 245–59, ix
  See also meditation; religion; spirituality
Burlingham, Dorothy, 108
burnout, vs. passion, 249–50
Burrow, Deborah, 348
Burt, Martha, 145
Burton, Linda M., 37

Call to a Motherhood Movement, 370–71
Calvert, S., 323
Capps, Donald, 227
caregiving and caretaking, biochemistry of,
    11, 371

caring, 156
Carnegie Council on Adolescent Development, 145
cartoons. *See* media and technology
Casey (Annie E.) Foundation. *See* Annie E. Casey Foundation
causation, 23
CDC. *See* Centers for Disease Control and Prevention
Census Bureau (U.S.), 60–61n151, 307
Center for Media Literacy, 332
Centers for Disease Control and Prevention (CDC), 4, 190
character
    civil society model for building, x, 339–51
    families, fundamental to, 355–56
    parental bonds for fostering, x, 356–57
    and teenagers, 363–64
    See also conscience; values and value system
chemistry. *See* biochemistry
child and youth development, 137–46, 310–15. *See also* adolescence; brain development
child psychiatry, 46n29, 104
Child, Irving, 288–89
Children at Risk: State Trends 1990–2000, 4
Children Now, 326
Children of the Great Depression (Elder), 117
Chödrön, P, 246–48, 249–51
Christianity, 168
citizenship, 143, 360–62
civic engagement, 32–33, 37, 67–68n189
civic values, 362. *See also* values and value system
civil society, x, 27, 31–32, 36, 59n141, 339–50
cocaine, 76
Coleman, James, 23–24, 228–31
Columbine High School, 130
Comer, James P., x, xxiii, 27, 36–37
Commission on Children at Risk (Washington, D.C.), vii, xi, xvii, 3–43, 369–73
    membership, 43
    name, reasons for, 7
communication, emotional, and attachment, 10
community, well-being, promoting, x, 305–20. *See also* authoritative communities; neighborhoods
compassion, 31, 249–50
competence
    academic, 141
    biochemistry of, vii, 71–83
    civil society model for building, x, 339–51
    developmental influences, 79–83
    sense of, 140, 142, 156, 311, 312
    social, viii, 79, 142, 231
computers. *See* media and technology

comradeship, 143
confidence, 111–12, 114, 117, 124, 142, 143, 311, 347–48, 357, 363, 367. *See also* self-confidence
connected communities, 370–71
connectedness
    and civil society, 341
    meeting basic needs for, 26, 369, 371
    and parenting, 372
    of social institutions, 32–33
    social, 33
    and value system, 372–73
    See also attachment; authoritative communities
connection, biochemistry of, 10–12
conscience
    in adolescence, 126–33
    Brain-Heart, 126
    civil society model for building, x, 339–51
    conceptualization of, 126–33
    and developmental process, vii, viii, 19, 123, 124–34
    external stage, 131
    fostered by parents, 35
    integrated stage, 131–33
    during mid-adolescence, 127–31
    moral-emotional responsiveness, 124–25
    and morality, vii, 19, 123–26, 127
    during older adolescence, 131–33
    personified, 126–27
    and pluralism, 30
    and success, 360
    during young adolescence, 126–27
    youth organizations, policies for improving, 134
    See also character; values and value system
consciousness, 159, 167, 169, 171
conservatism, personal, 297
cooperation, 31
coping and coping mechanisms, 23
corporations and corporate communities, and cultural ecology, changes in, 373
Cortés, Ernesto (Ernie), Jr., 36
critical thinking, 361
Crouter, Anne C., 37
culture, and myth, 289

danger zone emotions, 125
d'Aquili, Eugene, 25
Dare to Discipline (Dobson), 227
Darwin, Charles, 87
day care, 113–15
DBT. *See* Dialectical Behavior Therapy
deafferentation, 169, 176, 182
Deary, Kevin, 348

death and dying
  decreased rates among youth, 5
  religion, impact on longevity, 190–91
  See also homicide; suicide
deculturation, 293
delinquency, 193–95, 197. *See also* risk taking
  and novelty seeking
Democracy in America (Tocqueville), 59n141
depression
  prevalence and statistics, 3–4
  and spirituality/religion, 192, 298, 299–300
DeStefano, John, 320
detachment, 251
developmental assets, 140, 341–43
devotion, parental, 357–58
devotion (spiritual), personal, 24, 297, 299, 300
Dialectical Behavior Therapy (DBT), 257–58
Dicken, Mary R. W., 348
dignity, equal human, 31
discipline. *See* education and schooling; rules
  and rulemaking
Disney Channel (cable television channel), 329
Dobson, James, 227, 233–34
Doherty, William J., 67–68n189
dopamine, and brain development, 269–71
Dromgoole, Will Allen, 350
drug use, 76, 266, 274. *See also* alcohol abuse;
  specific drug(s)

Eberly, Don, 27
ecology, cultural, and social change, 372–73
education and schooling
  academic competence, 141
  attainment, and religion, 197
  and character development, 360–62
  and child development, 319
  classroom discipline, 360–61
  need for access to, 365–67
  troubled youth, responding to, 366–67
  for 21st century, 315–16
  See also teachers
efficacy, and mattering, 345
efficiency, technocratic, 28–29
ego, defined, 252. See also self
ego psychologists, 154
ego strength, 156
egolessness, 252–53
Elder, Glen, 117
Ellis, Albert, 158
emotional communication, and attachment, 10
emotions, 124–25, 253–54
empathy, 51–52n74
enjoyment, of life, 144
Enlightenment project, 151–52

environment (nurture), vs. heredity (nature),
  13–15
environmental conditions, and deteriorating
  health of youth, xiii
Epstein-Fenz Manifest Anxiety Scale, 257
equal human dignity, 31
equal moral regard, 300–31
equanimity or nonattachment, 251
Erikson, Erik, 32, 156, 159, 284, 285, 293
Escalante, Jaime, 344
ethology, 88
Etzioni, Amitai, 27
Evans, T. David, 194
expectations, establishing, 28. *See also* rules
  and rulemaking

Fahlke, C., 93
Fairbairn, W. R. D., 154–55
faith, 166–67, 175, 182–83. *See also* religion;
  spirituality
families, 63n161, 63–64n166, 63n167
  as authoritative communities, 32
  biochemistry and youth competence, vii,
    71–83
  and character development, 355–56
  and civic engagement, 67–68n189
  and developmental assets, 341–42
  recommendations, 39
  stability, and religion, 239–40
  structure, importance of, 231–32
  supported by common national goals, 367
  undermined by circumstances, 32, 344,
    364–65
  See also marriage; parents and parenting
Family and Home Network, 374
fantasy, and imagination, 177–78
fathers and fatherhood, role models for
  boys/sons, ix–x, 281–93. *See also* parents
  and parenting; paternal care; patriarchy
fear, individual differences in regulation,
  89–90, 91–93, 95–97, 99
Ferree, Myra Max, 227
fight or flight response, 174
Floyd Central High School, 348
Focus on the Family, 233
forgiveness, 357–58
foster care, 118
4-H, 344
Fowler, James, 167, 174–79, 181–83
Francis, Darlene D., vii, xxiii
Frankl, Viktor, 157
Franklin, Robert Michael, 37
free will, 159
friends and peers, 129–31, 132
Freud, Anna, 108

Freud, Sigmund, 53n83, 151–54
Fromm, Erich, 157
Fukuyama, Francis, 27

Gandhi, Mohandas, 372
"Gathering the Mothers" (O'Mara), 372
Gehlek, Nawang, 254
gender, 17–18, 298–300
gene-environment interactions, 97–98
generativity, 156
genetics, vs. social contexts (environment),
   13–15. See also heredity (nature); nature
Girl Scouts, 344
girls, spirituality and resilience in, x, 295–302
Glasser, William, 158
goals and goal setting, 132–33
Golden Rule ethic, 30–31, 130–31
Goldfarb, William, 107
Gottman, John, 242
grandparents, 29
gratitude, 23
Gutmann, David, ix–x, xxiii, 20, 51n70
Gyatso, Tenzin, 250

hardwired, defined, 46n32
Hardwired to Connect, v, vii, xi, xvii, 3–43,
   369–73
Harris, Eric, 130
Hartmann, Heinz, 154
Harvard University, 30, 82
healing emotions, 253–54
health care
   and environmental conditions, xiii
   need for access to, 365–67
   religion, organic, impact of, 187, 189–95, 198,
      202–18
Health, Education, and Welfare Dept.
   (U.S.), 143
helplessness, learned, 158
Henry J. Kaiser Family Foundation, 324
heredity (nature), vs. environment (nurture),
   13–15. See also genetics; nature
Herrnstein, Richard, 15
Hinduism, 168, 169, 171
homicide death rates, among youth,
   prevalence and statistics, 5
honesty, 31, 64n168, 342, 343
hope, and religion, 195–96
hormones, 11, 266–67
HPA. See hypothalmic-pituitary-adrenal
   activity
Hrdy, Sarah Blaffer, 19, 51–52n74
humility, 373
Humphreys, Christmas, 245

Hunter, Brenda, 374
Hunter, James Davison, 230
hypertension, 191
hypothalmic-pituitary-adrenal activity,
   89–90, 92

ideals and idealizations, 20–21, 57n123, 59n145
identity, 17–18, 144, 160
imagination, and fantasy, 177–78
immigrants, health status for children of, 5–6
impermanence, 252
independence, 160, 363
Indiana Youth Institute, 9
individual differences, vs. universality, 129,
   267–68
individualism, radical, 372
individuation, 131, 153, 160
infancy, 79–80, 175–77
infotainment, 130
innateness, 155
Institute for American Values, xvii, 374
Institute of Medicine. See National Research
   Council and Institute of Medicine
institutional actors, types of, 228
integrity, 342
intellectual models, inadequacy of, 6–9
intelligence, 15
interconnectedness, 182–83
interdependence, 250, 252, 253, 373
intergenerational participation
   elders and sons, 281–300
   and needs for human development, 143–44
   and parenting, 231, 232, 240
   See also multigenerational communities
involvement, personal, 143
IQ tests, 15
Ironson, Gail, 21–22
Izard, Carroll, 124

Jason, Leonard A., x, xxiii
jealousy, 250–51
Jerry Springer Show, The (television talk
   show), 230
Johns Hopkins University, 110
Johnson, Byron R., ix, xxiv, 22–23
joy and rejoicing, 250–51
Jung, Carl, 152–54, 158, 159

Kabat-Zinn, Myla and Jon, 248, 251, 252, 253
Kagan, Jerome, 30
Kaiser (Henry J.) Family Foundation. See
   Henry J. Kaiser Family Foundation
Karen, Robert, viii, xxiv, 19
Katz, Steven, 168

Kendler, K. S., 296
Kennedy, John F., 339
Kids Count, 343–44
Kiecolt-Glaser, Janice K., 11–12
Kim, Kerri L., x, xxiv
King, Martin Luther, Dr., 289, 355
Klebold, Dylan, 130
Klein, Melanie, 154–55
Kline, Kathleen Kovner, v, vi, xxiv
Kohlberg, Lawrence, 126
Konopka, Gisela, 143–44
Ku Klux Klan, 31

La Leche League, 372
learning, and nurturing, 28
Leung, P., 259
Levy, David, 107
Lieberman, Alicia, 112–13, 116
Lifeline (Stenson), 233
Lifeline Community Center (Indianapolis, Ind.), 339–40, 348
limits. *See* expectations
Linehan, Marsha, 257–58
List of Human Universals (Brown)
love, 143, 248–49
low-income neighborhoods, authoritative communities, building, 35–37
loyalty, 31

Main, Mary, 111
Making Connections, program, 37
Mana (power), 282, 290
manhood, male elders and role models for, ix–x, 281–93
Mann Rinehart, Peggy, 341
marijuana use, prevalence and statistics, 5
marriage, 32, 37, 60–61n151, 62n152, 66–67n182. *See also* families
masculine development, paradox of, 285
Maslow, Abraham, 157–58, 159
materialism, 4, 369, 372
Maternal Care and Mental Health (Bowlby), 107–8
maternal responsiveness
  biochemistry of, 77–83
  nongenomic transmission across generations, 80–81
  See also mothers and mothering
mattering, and efficacy, 345
May, Rollo, 157
McCullough, M. E., 190
McQuillan, Julie, 227
Meaney, Michael, 80

meaning, search for, 24–25, 56–57n117, 17–173, 195–96
media and technology
  behavioral modification, to aid in monitoring use, 332–33
  blocking mechanisms, to aid in monitoring use, 333–34
  and childhood obesity, 328
  comprehension, 325, 330
  and cultural ecology changes, 373
  education and literacy regarding use, 331–32
  influence in children's lives, x, 323–35
  modeling behaviors and social development, 325–27
  parental supervision, 329–31
  rules and limits for use, 330–31, 332
  school performance, affect on, 328
  sexual content, 327–28
  stereotypes portrayed in, 328–29
  strategies for dealing with, 329–34
  violence, defined, 325
  violent and sexual images, consequences of viewing, 324–29
Media Awareness Network, 332
mediating structures, 27
medical care. *See* health care
meditation, 167, 169–72, 247–48, 253, 257–59
memory, 29, 126
menstruation, 299
midlife crisis, in men, 292
Mikulas, W. L., 256–57
Miller, Lisa, x, xxiv, 24
mindfulness. *See* Buddhism
Ministry of Youth Affairs, 144
modeling, social learning theory, and media usage, 325–27
Monitoring the Future, 191, 266
moral authority, sources of, 127
moral-emotional responsiveness, 124–25
moral individuation, 131
moral judgments, 125
moral sense, 342–44
moral valuation, 125
moral volition, 125–26
morality
  and attachment, 19, 20–21, 42, 123–24
  and authority, 127
  and character development, 356
  and civil society, 342, 343
  and conscience, vii, viii, 19, 123–26, 127
  and developmental process, vii, viii, 10, 19–20, 42, 123–26, 342
  and emotions, 124–25
  and ideals/idealizations, 20–21
  and individuation, 131

and judgments, 125
and prosocial conduct, 20–21
recommendations, 40
and spirituality/religion, 30–31, 151–60,
  298, 371
and values, 125
and volition, 125–26
See also spirituality
Morris, Desmond, 286
mortality. *See* death and dying
mother world, 373
Motherhood Project, 374
Mothering magazine, 372
mothers and mothering, 369–74, xi
  activism for change, 373
  deprivation of, 104, 106–7, 108–9, 112
  emotional attitude toward children, 105
  mother-infant/child attachment, viii, 11, 73,
    89–90, 103–19, 155, 371
  separating from, 284–86, 290–93
  as valuable and foundational, 371
  See also attachment; maternal
    responsiveness; nurturing; parents and
    parenting
Mothers' Council, 370–74, xi; Task Force on
  the Needs of Children, 370, 374
Motz, Lottie, 299
Mr. Rogers' Neighborhood (television
  program), 323
multigenerational communities, 29, 30. *See also*
  intergenerational participation
Murdoch, George, 284–85
Murray, Charles, 15
music and music videos. *See* media and
  technology
mysticism, 167, 168, 169, 171–73
myth
  and culture, 289
  and spirituality, 173–74, 178–79, 181

National Center for Clinical Infant Programs,
  117–18
National Heart, Lung, and Blood Institute, 191
National Institute for Healthcare Research, 166
National Institute of Child Health and Human
  Development, 13–14
National Institute on Drug Abuse (NIDA),
  193, 266
National Institute on Media and the
  Family, 326
National Institutes of Health (NIH), 340–41
National Longitudinal Study of Adolescent
  Health (Add Health), 340–41
National Research Council (NRC), 3, 345–46

National Research Council and Institute of
  Medicine, 138–39, 142
National Survey of Families and Households
  (NSFH), 235–41
nature, vs. nurture, 13–15, 48n45, 99
near-death experiences, 167
neighborhoods, recommendations, 39. *See also*
  community; low-income neighborhoods
neurobiology, v, 12. *See also* biology;
  psychobiology
neuropeptides, in brain, 11, 256
neuropsychology, and spirituality/religion,
  viii–ix, 165–83. *See also* psychology
neuroscience, 16, 71, xiii–xiv
neuroticism, 4
neurotransmitters, in brain, 11
New Haven, Connecticut, public schools in,
  36–37, 310, 315–20
Newberg, Andrew B., viii–ix, xxiv, 25
Newberg, Stephanie K., viii–ix, xxv
Newton, Niles, 285
Nhat Hanh, Thich, 252, 253, 255
Nicholson, Barbara, 374
Nickelodeon (cable television channel), 329
NIDA. *See* National Institute on Drug Abuse
Nierman, Joe, 347
NIH. *See* National Institutes of Health
Noll, Richard, 153
nonattachment or equanimity, 251
non-self or egolessness, 252–53
novelty seeking. *See* risk taking and novelty
  seeking
NRC. *See* National Research Council
NSFH. *See* National Survey of Families and
  Households
numinosity, vs. mysticism, 168
nurturing, 87–102, viii
  effects on gene transcription and brain
    circuitry, 12–13
  and learning, 28
  vs. nature (debate/paradigm), 13–15,
    48n45, 99
  protective effect, 87–89, 98–99
  and resilience, 12
  and spirituality, 21–22
  See also attachment; mothers and mothering;
    parents and parenting

obesity, childhood, and media usage, 328
Oedipal theme, 156, 286–87
O'Mara, Peggy, 372
organic religion. *See* religion, organic
orthodoxy. *See* religion
OT. *See* oxytocin
other, wholly, 171. *See also* self/other

OTRs. *See* oxytocin receptors
Otto, R., 168, 171
oxytocin (OT), in brain
  and bonding, biochemistry of, 11, 73–74,
    78–79, 81, 371
  molecular structure, 73
oxytocin receptors (OTRs), in brain, 74–75

pair bonding tests, biochemical. *See* attachment
parasympathetic system, and myth, 174
parents and parenting
  and attachment, 11
  authoritative, vs. authoritarian, 27, 227–28,
    233–34, 238
  biochemistry of commitment, 77–83
  British style, 105
  character development, fostering, x, 356–57
  and connectedness, 372
  emulated by children, 362–63
  intergenerational closure, 231, 232, 240
  mindful, 248, 250, 255
  patriarchal style, 228, 238
  and religion, ix, 56n109, 188, 227–42
  religious discourse on, 232–35
  and rules/rulemaking, 240–41, 359–60
  social-structural dimensions, 231–32
  time spent with children, 231, 232
  values absorbed by children, 358–59
  and well-being, ix, 227–42
  See also families; fathers and fatherhood;
    mothers and mothering; nurturing; role
    models
Parker, Lysa, 374
partner preference tests. *See* attachment
paternal care, biochemistry of, 79–83. *See also*
  fathers and fatherhood
patience, 254
patriarchy
  and parenting, 228, 238
  and religious right, 227
  and sons, 281–93
  See also fathers and fatherhood
peers and friends, 129–31, 132
Peterson, B., 197
pharmacology, 6–7, 74
phenomenology, 169
pheromones, 13
Piaget, Jean, 21, 126, 178
Plato, 56–57n117
Pleasant-Jones, Loretta, 374
pleasure, 143
pluralism, and conscience, 30
Popenoe, David, 343
poverty, 364–65, 366
Power Hour, tutoring program, 348

prefrontal cortex (PFC), and brain
  development, 269
Prep for Prep, tutoring program, 315–16
primordial institutions (e.g., religious bodies,
  families), 23–24, 228–29. *See also* social
  institutions
problem solving, triage approach, 8
professionalism, 28–29
prolactin, in brain, 77–79
Prometheus, 283
prosocial development and conduct, vii, viii
  and morality, 20–21
  as protection and protective factors, 20–21
  religion, organic, impact of, ix, 187–89,
    195–97, 198
  and resilience, 137–50
protection and protective factors
  dual strategy, 137
  and morality, 20–21
  and nurturing, 87–89, 98–99
  and personal devotion, 24
  and positive psychology, 158
  and prosocial conduct, 20–21
  religion, organic, impact of, ix, 187–95, 198
  research, 139
  and resiliency, 137–42
  See also safety; security
Protestantism, 227–28, 242
psychoanalysis, 152, 153, 154
psychiatry, viii, 151–60. *See also* child
  psychiatry; psychology
psychobiology, of adolescence, ix, 263–75. *See
  also* biochemistry; biology; neurobiology;
  psychology
psychology, viii, 151–60
  developmental, 139–40, 166
  positive/negative, 158–59
  transpersonal, 157, 159
  See also neuropsychology; psychiatry;
    psychobiology
psychopathology, 133, 273–74
psychopharmacology, 6. *See also* pharmacology
psychotherapy, 153–54, 157
puberty
  and hormones, 266–67
  rites of passage for boys, 287–89, 291–92
  and social changes, 18, 90–91
  and spirituality, developmental, 180, 299
  See also adolescence; sexual development
Public/Private Ventures, 346
punishment, as negative, 105
purpose, sense of, and spirituality/religion,
  171–73, 195–96

purposive institutions (e.g., corporations, state welfare agencies), 23–24, 228, 229–30. *See also* social institutions
Putnam, Robert D., 27, 32–34, 41, 65n171, 343–44

Raising Children with Character (Berger), 368
reading, and child development, 312
reality therapy, 158
Recreational Software Advisory Council, 334
reculturation, 293
rejoicing and joy, 250–51
religion
    and coping mechanisms, 23
    and depression, 298, 299–300
    devotion (spiritual), personal, 24, 297, 299, 300
    encouraged, 30
    and family stability, 239–40
    fundamentalism of, 295–96
    gender differences in, 298–300
    and hardships suffered, 53n87
    health-related outcomes, impact on, 55n103, 187, 189–95, 198, 20218
    international, 189
    and moral sense, 342–43
    neuropsychological model for, viii–ix, 165–83
    organic, ix, 187–198
    organic, defined, 187, 189
    orthodoxy, ix, 228–32
    and parenting, ix, 56n109, 188, 227–42
    protective impact of, ix, 187–95, 198
    prosocial impact of, ix, 187–89, 195–97, 198
    and resilience, ix, 194, 295–300
    and social outcomes, 187–88
    theological conservatism, 236–38
    and values, 194
    and well-being, ix, 22–24, 55n103, 159, 195, 196, 197, 219–25, 227–42
    and youth, 188–89
    See also Buddhism; faith; spirituality; specific religions and beliefs
"Religion and Child Abuse: Perfect Together," 227
religious conversions, 167
religious institutions, in low-income neighborhoods, 37
resilience and resiliency
    and attachment, 112
    best practices, 141–42
    and biochemistry, 71–85, vii
    and nurturing, 12
    and prosocial development, 137–50, viii
    and protective factors, 137–42

research, 139
    and spirituality/religion, x, 194, 295–300
    and youth development, 142–45
resistance, 140, 141, 363
Resnick, Michael D., viii, xxv, 20–21, 39–40, 146
resources, private and public, recommendations, 40–41
respect, 31
responsibility, 31, 132, 143
reward deficiency, 16
rhesus monkeys (*Macaca mulatta*)
    aggression, individual differences in, 88, 90, 93–98
    early peer rearing, effects of, 90, 95–97, 98
    fear, individual differences in, 89–90, 91–93, 95–98
    gene-environment interactions, 97–98
    protective effect of good nurturing, 14, 87–99
    socioemotional regulation, normative development, 89–91
    socioemotional regulation, proficiency, 87–89
risk taking and novelty seeking
    during adolescence, 265, 266
    connected to brain structure and function, 15–17
    consequences, 16
    and resiliency, 138
    See also delinquency
rites of passage, and puberty, for boys, 51n70, 287–89, 291–92
rituals, 181, 284
Rivers, Eugene, 346–47
Robertson, James, 109
rodents, attachment studies, 71–83
Rogers, Carl, 157–58
role models, for boys/sons, ix–x, 281–93. *See also* parents and parenting; teachers
Rowan, J., 167
Rubinstein, Y. Y., 234
rules and rulemaking, by parents, 240–41, 359–60. *See also* expectations

sacred, and spirituality, 166
sacrifice, as necessary, 372, 373
sadness, and healing, 253–54
SafeSurf, 334
safety, 342, 345, 358, 359. *See also* protection and protective factors; security
satisfaction, 143
Sawhill, Isabel V., 41
SAY. *See* Survey of Adults and Youth
schizophrenia, 274
scholars, recommendations, 41–42

School Development Program (SDP), 310, 315–20

School Planning and Management Team (SPMT), 316–18

schools. *See* education and schooling; learning

Schore, Allan N., 10–11

science and scientific findings, and authoritative communities, 9–25

Scientific Advisory Committee on Television and Social Behavior (Surgeon General), 325

SDP. *See* School Development Program

Search Institute (Minneapolis), 27, 341, vi, xvii–xviii

security, 89–90, 95, 103, 110–11, 115, 143, 232. *See also* protection and protective factors; safety

security-empathy-oughtness representation, 19, 123–24, 126, 134

self
  defined, 252
  expanded power, 131
  fabricated, 252
  and spirituality, developmental, 176
  See also ego

self-actualization, 157–58, 167, 259

self-concept, 258–59

self-confidence, 140. *See also* confidence

self-control, 117

self-direction, 124

self-discovery, 127, 128

self-discipline, 358

self-esteem, 23, 127, 196, 286–87, 290, 357

self-expression, 144, 298

self-fulfillment, 159, 160

self-interest, 361

self-knowledge, 159

self/other dichotomy, 169. *See also* other

self-questioning, 127

self-realization, 153–54, 159

self-reflection, 144

self-reliance, 245

self-respect, 231, 232, 360

self-restraint, 31

self-sufficiency, 319

self-understanding, 159

Seligman, Martin, 27, 156, 158–59

serotonin, 94, 97

service delivery model, vs. social change model, xiv,

Sesame Street (television program), 323

sexual development, 299–300. *See also* puberty

sexual images, in media. *See* media and technology

sexuality
  and psychoanalysis, 152
  and spirituality/religion, 180, 192–93, 299

sexually transmitted diseases (STDs), prevalence, 5, 192–93

shame, 105

shared memory, 29

Siddhartha, 245–46

Simmons, Leo, 288

Skinner, B. F., 158

Smart, Ninian, 168, 171

Smith, John, 257

social attachments, biochemical processes for, 72–77

social capital, 64n168, 343–44

Social Capital Index, 34, 343–44

social change
  ecology, changes for, 372–73
  goals and recommendations for, 38, 39–42
  vs. service delivery, xiv

Social Commission of the United Nations, 107–9

social connectedness, 33

social contexts (environment), 13–17

social development. *See* prosocial development

social environment, and attachment, 115–19

social institutions
  and connectedness, 32–33
  decline in, 32–33
  as inclusive, 27–28
  See also primordial institutions; purposive institutions

social interest, 154

social network (SN), and child development, 314, 317

Social Skills Curriculum for Inner City Children (SSCICC), 318–19

Society for the Scientific Study of Religion, 227

socioemotional regulation
  early peer rearing, effects, 90, 95–97, 98
  gene-environment interactions, 97–98
  normative development, 89–91
  proficiency development, 87–89
  understanding, 98–99
  See also aggression; fear

soul, 282

spanking, 234, 236

Spear, Linda Patia, ix, xxv, 16

spirituality
  during adolescence-early adulthood, 180–81
  during adulthood, 181–83
  and attachment, 21–22
  during childhood, developmental, 177–79
  and depression, 299–300
  developmental, 165–83

encouraged, 30
gender differences in, 298–300
indiviudative-reflective stage, 181–82
during infancy, developmental, 175–77
intuitive-projective stage, 177–78
and morality, viii, 151–60
and mysticism, 167, 168, 169, 171–73
and myth, 173–74, 178–79, 181
mythic-literal stage, 178–79
neuropsychological model for, viii–ix,
    165–83
nonenvironmental contributions to, 296
and nurturing, 21–22
and phenomenology, 169
recommendations, 40
and resilience, in adolescent girls, x, 295–300
sacred, defined, 166
search, defined, 166
synthetic-conventional stage, 180–81
and unity, 171
and well-being, 22–24
and wholeness, 171–73
See also faith; morality; religion
Spitz, René, 107
SPMT. See School Planning and Management
    Team
sports, 23, 144, 239, 241, 331
SSCICC. See Social Skills Curriculum for Inner
    City Children
Stace, W. T., 168, 173
Stages of Faith (Fowler), 174–75
Stanczykiewicz, Bill, x, xxv, 9
Stand and Deliver (film), 344
State-Trait Anxiety Inventory, 257
STDs. See sexually transmitted diseases
Stenson, James, 233
stereotypes, portrayed in media and
    technology, 328–29
Stern, Daniel, 253
Stilwell, Barbara M., viii, xxv, 19, 20
Strange Situation research, 111–13
stress
    and poverty, 364–65
    responsiveness, 272–73
Strong-Willed Child, The (Dobson), 233
suicide, adolescent, 4, 5, 192
Suomi, Stephen J., viii, xxv–xxvi, 13–14
Surgeon General's Scientific Advisory
    Committee on Television and Social
    Behavior, 325
Survey of Adults and Youth (SAY), 235–41
Swedish study, 33

Tamminen, K., 174, 298
Taoism, 168, 177

TCI. See Temperament and Character
    Inventory
teachers
    and character development, 360–62
    and citizenship, promotion of, 360–62
    support for working with troubled
        children, 118
    See also education and schooling
technocratic efficiency, 28–29
technology and media. See media and
    technology
teenage pregnancy and births, 4–5, 45n17,
    192–93
teenagers. See adolescence
teleology, 152
television. See media and technology
testosterone, 11, 17, 51n68
Temperament and Character Inventory
    (TCI), 259
Ten Point Coalition (Dorchester, Mass.), 346
theology. See religion; spirituality
therapy, reality, 158
Thomas, Julie E., ix, xxvi, 56n109
Thompson, Ermil, 339–41
Thondup, Tulku, 253
Thornton, Arland, 63n161
Thurman, A. F., 252
Tocqueville, Alexis de, 59n141
tolerance, 357–58
Totem and Taboo (Freud), 53n83
transformation. See Buddhism
transitional object, 286
Traub, James, 344
triage approach, for problem-solving, 8
trust, 31, 285
Turner, Rebecca, 11
Two-Year-Old Goes to Hospital, A (film)

Unitary Consciousness, 168
United Nations Social Commission, 107–9
United Nations Universal Declaration of
    Human Rights (1948), 31
Urban Institute, 145

V-chip (violence chip), 324, 333, 334
valuational triangle, 125
values and value system
    absorbed by children, 358–59
    civic values, learned in school, 362
    and connectedness, 372–73
    moral, 125, 343
    and needs for human development, 144
    and religion, 194
    See also character; conscience; specific values

vasopressin, in brain
  and bonding, biochemistry of, 11, 73–74, 79
  molecular structure, 73
video games. *See* media and technology
violence, in media. *See* media and technology
virtue/virtues, 30, 156
Vitz, Paul C., viii, xxvi, 22
volunteerism, 41, 138, 140

Wallace, John, 191, 193
Warren, Mobi, 255
Weber, Max, 57n123
Weiss, Jay, 256
well-being
  at-risk youth, promoting, x, 305–21
  and gender, 17–18
  and parenting, 227–42, ix
  and religion, ix, 22–24, 195, 196, 197, 219–15,
    227–42
  and self-fulfillment, 160
  and spirituality, 22–24
  statistics, 4
  See also Buddhism
Welwood, J., 252
West Side Story, 131
Western Civilization in Biological Perspective:
  Patterns in Biohistory (Boyden), 143

Whiting, John, 288–89
WHO. *See* World Health Organization
Wilcox, W. Bradford, ix, xxvi, 24
Williams, Olgen, 347
Wilson, James Q., 342–44
Wilt, Chuck, 347
Winnicott, D. W., 154–55
work-family advocates, 39
workplaces, recommendations, 39
World Health Organization (WHO), 107–9,
  115, 138
Wuyek Lisa A., ix, xxvi

Yale Child Study Center, 316
Yale University, 27
YMCA, xvii, 27, 30, 315, 344
YWCA, 315
Young, Larry J., vii, xxvi, 12
youth and child development, 137–46, 310–15.
  See also adolescence
youth organizations and programs, 134, 144,
  344–46

Zen meditation, 257–58. *See also* meditations
Zero to Three report, 117–18

Printed in the United States
104202LV00002B/1-72/A